Patient-Centric 6G

The healthcare industry is poised for a transformative leap, driven by the convergence of next-generation wireless technologies and the growing demand for patient-centered care. In the 6G era, connectivity is no longer merely a supporting tool—it is the foundation upon which healthcare delivery is being built. *Patient-Centric 6G: A New Era in Smart Healthcare* is a guide to understanding and harnessing this revolution, where technology and compassion converge to redefine how care is provided and experienced.

This book explores the multifaceted impact of 6G on healthcare, merging a futuristic vision with practical insights. It starts with a foundational understanding of patient-centered care, explaining how 6G's technological advancements support this transition. By incorporating discussions on machine-type communication, extensive device connectivity, and ultra-reliable low-latency communication (URLLC), it underscores the crucial role these innovations play in creating a hyperconnected and responsive healthcare ecosystem.

By connecting abstract technological concepts to their real-world applications, this book offers practical examples, case studies, and comprehensive analysis to demonstrate how 6G is transforming the healthcare landscape. Examining the ethical challenges linked to patient-centric 6G, it explains creating systems that reflect moral values while preserving the trust of patients and stakeholders. A roadmap for continued research, innovation, and collaboration, this book encourages healthcare professionals, technologists, and researchers to work together to shape a healthcare system where connectivity fosters both precision and compassion.

Dr. Rajeev Kumar is currently serving as Professor in the Computer Science and Engineering Department, Moradabad Institute of Technology, Moradabad, Uttar Pradesh, India.

Dr. Ankush Joshi is an Associate Professor at COER University, India. Dr. Joshi specializes in the dynamic fields of artificial intelligence, machine learning, and data science. His extensive expertise and dedication make him a valuable asset in shaping the academic landscape at COER.

Dr. Preeti Bajaj is an electronics engineer and currently holds the position of Vice Chancellor of Lovely Professional University, India.

Dr. Danila Parygin is Head of the Department of Digital Technologies for Urban Studies, Architecture and Civil Engineering and Associate Professor of the Department of CAD (Computer-Aided Design), Volgograd State Technical University, Russia.

Advances in Computational Collective Intelligence
Series Editor
Dr. Subhendu Kumar Pani

Emotional Intelligence in the Digital Era: Concepts, Frameworks, and Applications
Edited by Pushan Kumar Dutta, Sachin Gupta, Shafali Kashyap, Anita Gehlot, Rita Karmakar, and Pronaya Bhattacharya

Deep Learning and Blockchain Technology for Smart and Sustainable Cities
Edited by Subramaniyaswamy V, G Revathy, Logesh Ravi, N. Thillaiarasu, and Naresh Kshetri

Computational Intelligence for Analysis of Trends in Industry 4.0 and 5.0
Edited by Joseph Bamidele Awotunde, Kamalakanta Muduli, and Biswajit Brahma

Metaverse and Blockchain Use Cases and Applications
Edited by Dileep Kumar Murala, Sandeep Kumar Panda, and Sujata Priyambada Dash

Leveraging Artificial Intelligence in Cloud, Edge, Fog and Mobile Computing
Edited by Shrikaant Kulkarni, P. William, Vijaya Prakash, and Jaiprakash Narain Dwivedi

Using AI to Develop Sustainability Strategies for a Changing Global Economy
Edited by A.V. Senthil Kumar, Ankita Chaturvedi, Atul Bansal, and Rohaya Latip

Artificial Intelligence, Geographic Information Systems, and Multi-Criteria Decision-Making for Improving Sustainable Development
Edited by Sujoy Kumar Jana, Kamalakanta Muduli, Indrajit Pal, and Purushottam Meena

Advanced AI and Data Science Applications
Edited by Dr. D. Sivabalaselvamani, Dr. G Revathy, and Dr. Ranjit Singh Sarban Singh

Intelligent Business Analytics
Edited by Nitendra Kumar, Lakhwinder Kaur Dhillon, Mridul Dharwal, Elena Korchagina, and Vishal Jain

Augmented Reality and Sustainability: Goals and Challenges
Edited by Sonal Trivedi, Vishal Jain, Balamurugan Balusamy, Subhendu Pani, and Danish Ather

Patient-Centric 6G: A New Era in Smart Healthcare
Edited by Rajeev Kumar, Ankush Joshi, Preeti Bajaj, and Danila Parygin

https://www.routledge.com/Advances-in-Computational-Collective-Intelligence/book-series/ACCICRC

Patient-Centric 6G
A New Era in Smart Healthcare

Edited by
Rajeev Kumar
Ankush Joshi
Preeti Bajaj
Danila Parygin

CRC Press
Taylor & Francis Group
Boca Raton London New York

CRC Press is an imprint of the
Taylor & Francis Group, an **informa** business
AN AUERBACH BOOK

Designed cover image: Shutterstock

First edition published 2026
2385 NW Executive Center Drive, Suite 320, Boca Raton FL 33431

and by CRC Press
4 Park Square, Milton Park, Abingdon, Oxon, OX14 4RN

CRC Press is an imprint of Taylor & Francis Group, LLC

ISBN: 978-1-032-82696-7 (hbk)
ISBN: 978-1-032-85109-9 (pbk)
ISBN: 978-1-003-51659-0 (ebk)

DOI: 10.1201/9781003516590

Typeset in Times
by SPi Technologies India Pvt Ltd (Straive)

Contents

Contributors

Joji Abey
Kingdom University
Riffa, Kingdom of Bahrain

Afreen N.
Anand College of Pharmacy
Agra, India

Shikha Agarwal
Department of Information
    Technology
Ajay Kumar Garg Engineering College
Ghaziabad, India

Wesam Ahmed
Department of Information
    Technology
Faculty of Computers and Artificial
    Intelligence
South Valley University
Hurghada, Egypt

Deep Chandra Andola
Amrapali University
Haldwani, India

Manisha Deep Andola
Surajmal University
Anjania, India

Tarun Bhardwaj
Department of Artificial Intelligence
G H Raisoni Institute of Engineering &
    Technology
Nagpur, India

Abhay Bhatia
Department of Computer Science and
    Engineering
Roorkee Institute of Technology
Roorkee, India

R. Bhuvaneswari
Dr. Mahalingam College of Engineering
    and Technology
Coimbatore, India

Vandana Bisht
Amrapali University
Haldwani, India

Vibha Bora
BETiC
G H Raisoni College of Engineering
Nagpur, India

Aarti Chaudhary
Department of Information Technology
Ajay Kumar Garg Engineering College
Ghaziabad, India

Anil Chauhan
Department of Information Technology
Ajay Kumar Garg Engineering College
Ghaziabad, India

Naman Chauhan
COER University
Roorkee, India

Sharda Chhabria
Department of Artificial Intelligence
G H Raisoni Institute of Engineering &
    Technology
Nagpur, India

Nita Dakhare
Department of Computer Science and
    Application
School of Allied Sciences
Faculty of Science and Technology
DMIHER (Deemed to be University)
Wardha, India

Sourav Deb
Department of Computer Science and
   Engineering
Roorkee Institute of Technology
Roorkee, India

Chitra Dhawale
Department of Computer Science and
   Application
School of Allied Sciences
Faculty of Science and Technology
DMIHER (Deemed to be University)
Wardha, India

K. Sankar Ganesh
Sharda University
Andijan, Uzbekistan

R. Sankar Ganesh
Vel Tech Rangarajan Dr Sagunthala
   R&D Institute of Science and
   Technology
Chennai, India

Ruhi Gedam
Department of Artificial Intelligence
G H Raisoni Institute of Engineering &
   Technology
Nagpur, India

Aishwarya Jain
STES
Sinhgad College of Pharmacy
Pune, India

Ankush Joshi
COER University
Roorkee, India

Anuj Kumar
COER University
Roorkee, India

Rachit Kumar
Anand Engineering College
Agra, India

Vikash Kumar
COER University
Roorkee, India

Khusboo Kumari
Department of Computer Science and
   Engineering
Roorkee Institute of Technology
Roorkee, India

Amena Mahmoud
Computer Science Department
Faculty of Computers and
   Information
Kafrelsheikh University
Kafr El Sheikh, Egypt

Sushil Mankar
N. K. P. Salve Institute of Medical
   Sciences & Research Centre and
   Lata Mangeshkar Hospital
Nagpur, India

Roohi Naaz
Department of Commerce
Graphic Era Deemed to be
   University
Dehradun, India

J. Nirubarani
Department of Management Studies
Dr. SNS Rajalakshmi College of Arts
   and Science
Coimbatore, India

S. Padmanabhan
ST. Francis College
Bengaluru, India

Awadesh Pandey
Anand Engineering College
Agra, India

Preeti Pandey
Amrapali University
Haldwani, India

Priya A.
Brindavan College
Bengaluru, India

P. Radha
School of Commerce
Jain (Deemed – to – be University)
Bengaluru, India

Birendra Kumar Ray
Government Polytechnic
    Aurangabad
Aurangabad, India

Nasreen Sayyed
School of Commerce
Jain (Deemed – to – be University)
Bengaluru, India

Riya Sharma
Department of Commerce
Graphic Era Deemed to be University
Dehradun, India

Kiran Deep Singh
Chitkara University Institute of
    Engineering and Technology
Chitkara University
Rajpura, India

Prabh Deep Singh
Department of Computer Science and
    Engineering
Graphic Era Deemed to be University
Dehradun, India

Yashvir Singh
COER University
Roorkee, India

Ananya Singhal
Department of Computer Science &
    Engineering
Ajay Kumar Garg Engineering College
Ghaziabad, India

Devansh Singhal
Department of Information
    Technology
Ajay Kumar Garg Engineering College
Ghaziabad, India

J. Sudarvel
Karpagam Academy of Higher Education
Coimbatore, India

M. Sudha
Department of Pharmacology
Saveetha College of Pharmacy
Saveetha Institute of Medical and
    Technical Sciences (Deemed to be
    University)
Chennai, India

Vijay Surve
Department of Orthopedics
N. K. P. Salve Institute of Medical
    Sciences & Research Centre and
    Lata Mangeshkar Hospital
Nagpur, India

Gesu Thakur
COER University
Roorkee, India

Ravi Thirumalaisamy
Modern College of Business and
    Science
Muscat, Sultanate of Oman

Sai Satya Navya Sri Vasamsetti
CSE Department
Pragati Engineering College
Surampalem, India

R. Velmurugan
Karpagam Academy of Higher
    Education
Coimbatore, India

Gisala Venkatesh
CSE Department
Pragati Engineering College
Surampalem, India

Manas Kumar Yogi
CSE Department
Pragati Engineering College
Surampalem, India

Preface

The healthcare industry is poised for a transformative leap, driven by the convergence of next-generation wireless technologies and the growing demand for patient-centered care. As we enter the 6G era, connectivity is no longer merely a supporting tool—it is the foundation upon which the future of healthcare delivery is being built. This book, *Patient-Centric 6G: A New Era in Smart Healthcare*, serves as a guide to understanding and harnessing this revolution, where technology and compassion converge to redefine how care is provided and experienced.

The goal of "patient-centric care" has long been a goal in healthcare, but with 6G, it becomes a fully achievable reality. Through unprecedented connectivity, ultra-low latency, and seamless communication, 6G empowers healthcare systems to deliver personalized and proactive care. It transforms the way patients interact with providers, offers unparalleled diagnostic accuracy, and equips healthcare professionals with the tools to make informed decisions in real time.

This book explores the multifaceted impact of 6G on healthcare, merging a futuristic vision with practical insights. It starts with a foundational understanding of patient-centered care, explaining how 6G's technological advancements support this transition. By incorporating discussions on machine-type communication, extensive device connectivity, and ultra-reliable low-latency communication (URLLC), the book underscores the crucial role these innovations play in creating a hyperconnected and responsive healthcare ecosystem.

Our journey doesn't end at technical marvels. We examine how 6G empowers patients, allowing them to actively engage in their health management through real-time data and insights. At the same time, healthcare providers acquire new capabilities to deliver care with precision and empathy. By connecting abstract technological concepts to their real-world applications, this book offers practical examples, case studies, and comprehensive analysis to demonstrate how 6G is transforming the healthcare landscape.

However, with great power comes great responsibility. As we embrace these technological advances, it is vital to consider the ethical implications that accompany them. This book devotes substantial attention to navigating the ethical challenges linked to patient-centric 6G, emphasizing data privacy, informed consent, and equitable access. It highlights the necessity of creating systems that reflect moral values while preserving the trust of patients and stakeholders.

The final section of this book looks ahead, offering a roadmap for continued research, innovation, and collaboration. By outlining future possibilities and challenges, we encourage healthcare professionals, technologists, and researchers to work together to shape a healthcare system where connectivity fosters both precision and compassion.

Patient-Centric 6G: A New Era in Smart Healthcare is not merely a book for technologists or healthcare providers—it is a manifesto for the future of healthcare. It encourages its audience to envision a world where technology empowers, connects, and humanizes care. Whether you are a healthcare educator, telehealth executive, researcher, digital health entrepreneur, or technology consultant, this book offers the insights and inspiration needed to spearhead the healthcare revolution that 6G connectivity will undoubtedly spark.

Let this book be your guide to understanding the profound impact of 6G technologies and your companion in shaping a healthcare system where connectivity and compassion work together to enhance lives. Welcome to the future of patient-centric healthcare—welcome to the 6G era!

1 Interdisciplinary Collaboration
Health IT Meets 6G

P. Radha, J. Nirubarani, Nasreen Sayyed,
S. Padmanabhan, and Priya A.

INTRODUCTION

The rapid advancement of wireless communication technologies has paved the way for significant innovations across various sectors, including healthcare. The imminent advent of 6G technology, characterized by its ultra-high speed, low latency, massive connectivity, and enhanced security features, presents a transformative opportunity for the healthcare industry. Concurrently, Health Information Technology (Health IT) has been at the forefront of modernizing healthcare delivery through electronic health records (EHRs), telemedicine, wearable health devices (Guo et al., 2016), and data analytics. Despite the progress, challenges such as data security, interoperability, real-time data processing (Evans, 2016), and efficient remote monitoring remain critical concerns in Health IT. The integration of 6G technology promises to address these challenges by providing a robust and efficient communication infrastructure. This interdisciplinary collaboration between Health IT and 6G aims to explore and harness these synergies to improve patient outcomes, enhance healthcare delivery, and streamline operations (Chaabane et al., 2020).

This study delves into the potential of 6G to revolutionize Health IT, examining how its capabilities can be leveraged to overcome current limitations and drive innovation. By bridging these two dynamic fields, we seek to create a comprehensive framework that guides future research, policy-making, and practical applications. The ultimate goal is to ensure that the healthcare sector can fully capitalize on the advancements in 6G technology, fostering a new era of connected, efficient, and patient-centric healthcare.

THEORETICAL FRAMEWORK OF THE STUDY

This study explores the theoretical framework for interdisciplinary collaboration between Health IT and 6G wireless technology. By integrating advanced Health IT systems with the high-speed, low-latency, and ubiquitous connectivity of 6G, we aim to enhance real-time health monitoring, telemedicine, and personalized healthcare. The framework is built on principles of cyber-physical systems, Internet of Things

(IoT), and artificial intelligence (AI), fostering seamless data exchange and robust security measures. This convergence promises to revolutionize healthcare delivery, improve patient outcomes, and drive innovation through collaborative research and development across these dynamic fields.

STATEMENT OF THE PROBLEM

The healthcare sector is undergoing a significant transformation driven by the integration of advanced digital technologies (Botta et al., 2016). Health IT has become crucial in managing patient data, facilitating telemedicine, and enhancing overall healthcare delivery. However, despite these advancements, several critical challenges persist, including data security, real-time data processing, interoperability, and accessibility, particularly in remote and underserved areas. With the advent of 6G wireless communication technology, which promises ultra-low latency, massive connectivity, high-speed data transfer, and enhanced security, there is a unique opportunity to address these challenges. However, the integration of 6G into Health IT is fraught with complexities and uncertainties. The healthcare sector must navigate technical, regulatory, and operational hurdles to effectively leverage 6G technology.

The problem at hand is to identify and evaluate the specific ways in which 6G can enhance Health IT, to overcome existing limitations, and to facilitate a seamless, secure, and efficient healthcare delivery system. This study aims to provide a comprehensive framework for understanding the potential impacts and practical applications of 6G in Health IT, guiding stakeholders in making informed decisions and fostering innovation in healthcare.

OBJECTIVES OF THE STUDY

- To improve the efficiency and accuracy of real-time health monitoring and diagnostics, ensuring timely interventions and better patient outcomes.
- To expand and improve telemedicine services, providing high-quality remote consultations and care regardless of geographical barriers.
- To support personalized treatment plans and precision medicine, tailored to individual patient needs and conditions.
- To develop robust frameworks for secure, seamless data exchange and storage, protecting patient privacy while enabling comprehensive data analytics and interoperability across healthcare systems.
- To promote collaborative research and development between Health IT and 6G technology fields, driving innovations that address current healthcare challenges and anticipate future needs.

SIGNIFICANCE OF THE RESEARCH

The significance of this study lies in its potential to transform healthcare through the integration of Health IT and 6G technology. By leveraging 6G's ultra-fast speeds, low latency, and massive connectivity, healthcare services can achieve unprecedented levels of efficiency and accuracy. This collaboration enables real-time remote monitoring, advanced telemedicine, and personalized treatment plans, enhancing patient care and outcomes. Furthermore, it drives innovation in medical research and health data analytics, paving the way for predictive and preventative healthcare. Ultimately, this interdisciplinary approach addresses critical challenges in healthcare delivery, making it more accessible, efficient, and responsive to patient needs.

REVIEW OF THE LITERATURE

Saad et al. (2020) outline the vision for 6G technology, highlighting its expected features such as terahertz frequency bands, AI-driven network management, and unprecedented data rates and connectivity. It emphasizes how these advancements will enable new applications in various sectors, including healthcare.

Evans (2016) discusses the current state and future trends in Health IT, covering key areas like EHRs, telemedicine, health data analytics, and wearable health technologies. It identifies existing challenges such as data interoperability, security, and real-time data processing.

Latif et al. (2017) examine the role of advanced wireless technologies, particularly 5G, in transforming healthcare services. It explores applications in telemedicine, remote surgery, and mobile health, and speculates on the future impact of 6G technology.

Radanliev et al. (2020) address the critical issue of data security and privacy in the healthcare sector. It reviews current security measures and highlights emerging threats and solutions, particularly focusing on how advancements like 6G could provide enhanced security features.

Ohannessian et al. (2020) explore the evolution of telemedicine, driven by advancements in communication technologies. It examines the impact of high-speed internet and mobile technologies on telemedicine practices and discusses how 6G could further revolutionize this field by providing real-time, reliable, and secure connections.

These articles collectively provide a comprehensive overview of the current state and future potential of integrating 6G technology with Health IT. They highlight the advancements, applications, challenges, and the transformative impact this interdisciplinary collaboration could have on healthcare delivery and patient outcomes.

RESEARCH GAP

Despite significant advancements in both Health IT and wireless technology, a research gap exists in comprehensively integrating 6G capabilities into healthcare systems. Current studies primarily focus on individual technologies, lacking a holistic approach to merging these fields. Challenges such as ensuring robust data security, managing vast amounts of health data efficiently, and addressing interoperability issues between diverse healthcare systems remain underexplored. Additionally, the ethical and regulatory implications of such integration need thorough investigation (Kumar et al., 2024). This study aims to bridge these gaps by developing a cohesive framework that leverages 6G's potential to enhance Health IT, ultimately transforming healthcare delivery and outcomes.

RESEARCH DESIGN

This study employs a mixed-methods research design, combining qualitative and quantitative approaches to comprehensively explore the integration of 6G technology into Health IT. Initially, a literature review will be conducted to identify existing challenges and potential synergies. Subsequently, expert interviews and focus groups with healthcare professionals and technology experts will provide qualitative insights. Quantitative data will be gathered through surveys assessing the current state of Health IT infrastructure and readiness for 6G adoption. Additionally, case studies of pilot projects utilizing 6G in healthcare settings will be analyzed to evaluate practical applications and outcomes, ensuring a holistic understanding of the subject.

ANALYSIS

The analysis phase of this interdisciplinary collaboration study involves several key steps to comprehensively evaluate the integration of 6G technology with Health IT:

- Technical Assessment: Conducting a technical evaluation of 6G features such as ultra-low latency, high-speed data transfer, and enhanced security to understand their potential impact on Health IT systems.
- Infrastructure Analysis: Assessing the existing Health IT infrastructure to identify compatibility and readiness for 6G adoption, including considerations for hardware, software, and network capabilities.
- Interoperability Testing: Examining the interoperability between 6G-enabled devices and existing Health IT systems to ensure seamless data exchange and communication.
- Performance Evaluation: Analyzing the performance metrics of 6G-enabled healthcare applications, including data transfer speeds, latency reduction, and reliability, compared to traditional technologies.
- Cost–Benefit Analysis: Conducting a cost–benefit analysis to determine the economic feasibility and potential return on investment of integrating 6G technology into Health IT systems.
- User Experience Assessment: Evaluating the user experience of healthcare professionals and patients when using 6G-enabled Health IT solutions, including ease of use, accessibility, and satisfaction.
- Security and Privacy Analysis: Assessing the security measures and privacy protections implemented in 6G-enabled healthcare systems to mitigate risks of data breaches and unauthorized access.
- Impact on Healthcare Delivery: Examining the broader impact of 6G integration on healthcare delivery, including improvements in patient outcomes, operational efficiency, and access to healthcare services.
- Regulatory Compliance: Ensuring compliance with relevant regulations and standards, such as HIPAA (Health Insurance portability and Accountability Act) for patient data privacy and security, and identifying any regulatory barriers to 6G adoption in healthcare.

Hypotheses based on Conceptual Model:

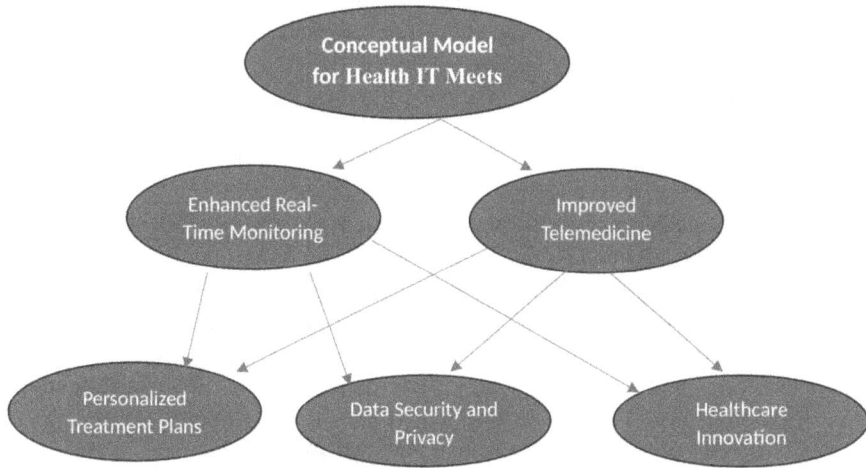

FIGURE 1.1 Conceptual model for health IT meets 6G.

- Ethical Considerations: Addressing ethical implications related to the use of 6G technology in healthcare, including equity of access, informed consent, and data stewardship.

By conducting a comprehensive analysis across these dimensions, this study aims to provide valuable insights into the potential benefits, challenges, and implications of interdisciplinary collaboration between Health IT and 6G technology, informing decision-making and guiding future research and implementation efforts (Figure 1.1).

FACTORS AFFECTING THE CONCEPTUAL MODEL

- Technological Infrastructure: The availability and development of 6G infrastructure are crucial for integrating Health IT systems. This includes network coverage, bandwidth, and the presence of advanced communication hardware.
- Data Security and Privacy: Ensuring robust cybersecurity measures is vital. Factors like encryption standards, data protection regulations, and secure communication protocols significantly impact the reliability and acceptance of the integrated system.
- Interoperability: The ability of different Health IT systems to work seamlessly with 6G technology affects the overall effectiveness. Standards for data exchange, compatibility of software and hardware, and integration protocols are key considerations.
- Regulatory Environment: Compliance with healthcare regulations and standards, such as HIPAA in the United States or GDPR (General Data Protection Regulation) in Europe, influences how Health IT and 6G technologies can be deployed. Regulatory support for innovation can accelerate adoption.

- User Acceptance and Training: The willingness of healthcare professionals and patients to adopt new technologies affects the implementation success. Adequate training, ease of use, and perceived benefits are critical for wide-spread acceptance.
- Cost and Economic Factors: The cost of deploying 6G infrastructure and integrating it with existing Health IT systems can be a significant barrier. Economic incentives, funding, and cost–benefit analyses influence the feasibility of large-scale adoption.
- Ethical Considerations: Ethical issues, such as patient consent, data ownership, and the potential for digital divide, must be addressed. Ensuring ethical standards are maintained is essential for the trust and legitimacy of the integrated system.
- Innovation and Research: Continuous research and development in both Health IT and 6G technologies drive improvements and innovations. Investment in R&D (Research and Development) and interdisciplinary collaboration fosters advancements and practical applications.
- Healthcare Policies and Support: Government policies and support for digital health initiatives and 6G deployment play a crucial role. Policy frameworks that encourage innovation and provide financial and logistical support are beneficial.
- Cultural and Societal Factors: Societal attitudes toward technology, cultural acceptance of telemedicine, and public awareness of the benefits of 6G-enabled Health IT systems can influence the adoption and effectiveness of these innovations.

HYPOTHESIS TESTING

Hypothesis 1:

Integrating 6G technology with Health IT will significantly improve the accuracy and responsiveness of real-time health monitoring systems.

Hypothesis 2:

The use of 6G networks will lead to a measurable improvement in the quality and reliability of telemedicine services.

Hypothesis 3:

Combining AI-driven Health IT with 6G connectivity will facilitate the development of highly personalized treatment plans, resulting in better patient outcomes and satisfaction.

Hypothesis 4:

Implementing advanced 6G security protocols within Health IT systems will enhance data security and privacy, reducing the risk of data breaches and ensuring compliance with healthcare regulations.

ABCD ANALYSIS

ABCD analysis is a strategic tool used to evaluate the Advantages, Benefits, Constraints, and Disadvantages of a project or initiative. Here, we apply it to the interdisciplinary collaboration between Health IT and 6G technology.

ADVANTAGES

- Ultra-Low Latency: 6G offers extremely low latency, which is crucial for real-time health applications like remote surgeries and instant patient monitoring.
- High-Speed Data Transfer: The high-speed capabilities of 6G facilitate the rapid transfer of large medical data sets, including high-resolution imaging and comprehensive patient records.
- Enhanced Connectivity: 6G supports massive connectivity, enabling seamless integration of numerous medical devices, sensors, and wearables, fostering an interconnected healthcare ecosystem.
- Improved Data Security: Advanced security features in 6G can enhance the protection of sensitive health data, mitigating risks of breaches and ensuring patient privacy.

BENEFITS

- Improved Patient Care: Enhanced communication and real-time data processing can lead to better diagnosis, timely interventions, and personalized treatment plans.
- Operational Efficiency: Streamlined data flows and automated processes can reduce administrative burdens, allowing healthcare professionals to focus more on patient care.
- Access to Remote Areas: 6G can expand the reach of telemedicine services, providing high-quality healthcare to remote and underserved regions.
- Innovative Healthcare Solutions: The integration of Health IT and 6G can drive innovation, leading to the development of new healthcare applications and services that improve overall health outcomes.

CONSTRAINTS

- Infrastructure Requirements: The deployment of 6G technology requires significant investment in infrastructure, including new antennas, base stations, and upgraded network equipment.
- Interoperability Issues: Ensuring seamless integration between existing Health IT systems and new 6G technologies can be complex and challenging.
- Regulatory Hurdles: Compliance with healthcare regulations and standards, such as HIPAA, can complicate the adoption of new technologies.
- Technical Challenges: Overcoming technical issues related to signal penetration, network coverage, and device compatibility is essential for successful implementation.

DISADVANTAGES

- High Costs: The initial costs of adopting 6G technology can be prohibitive for some healthcare providers, especially in resource-limited settings.
- Learning Curve: Healthcare professionals may require training to effectively use new 6G-enabled systems and tools, which can temporarily disrupt workflows.
- Data Privacy Concerns: Despite enhanced security features, the increased connectivity and data exchange inherent in 6G networks could raise additional privacy and cybersecurity concerns.
- Technology Dependence: An over-reliance on advanced technologies might reduce the emphasis on essential human elements of healthcare, such as patient-physician interactions and personalized care.

By conducting this ABCD analysis, we gain a comprehensive understanding of the potential and challenges associated with integrating 6G technology into Health IT, allowing stakeholders to make informed decisions and strategic plans for future development and implementation.

MAJOR FINDINGS

The interdisciplinary collaboration between Health IT and 6G technology yields significant findings that underscore its potential to revolutionize healthcare delivery.

- Enhanced Connectivity: The integration of 6G technology enables seamless connectivity between healthcare devices and systems, facilitating real-time data exchange and communication and leading to more efficient healthcare delivery and improved patient outcomes.
- Ultra-Low Latency: 6G's ultra-low latency capabilities support critical healthcare applications such as remote surgeries and telemedicine consultations, ensuring minimal delays and enhancing the quality of care, particularly in emergency situations.
- Improved Data Security: Advanced security features inherent in 6G networks bolster data protection in healthcare settings, mitigating risks of breaches and unauthorized access, thereby safeguarding patient privacy and confidentiality.
- Innovative Healthcare Solutions: The convergence of Health IT and 6G fosters innovation in healthcare, leading to the development of new applications and services that optimize clinical workflows, enable remote monitoring, and personalize patient care.
- Operational Efficiency: 6G-enabled Health IT systems streamline administrative tasks, reduce manual intervention, and optimize resource allocation, enhancing operational efficiency and allowing healthcare professionals to focus more on patient care.

These findings highlight the transformative potential of interdisciplinary collaboration between Health IT and 6G technology, offering promising avenues for improving healthcare delivery, advancing medical research, and enhancing patient experiences.

SCOPE OF THE STUDY

This study examines the intersection of Health IT and 6G wireless communication technology, focusing on the potential benefits, challenges, and applications arising from their integration. The scope includes the following key areas:

- Technological Advancements: Analyzing the specific features and advancements of 6G technology, such as ultra-low latency, enhanced data security, massive connectivity (Singh & Joshi, 2024), and its potential impact on Health IT.
- Healthcare Applications: Exploring how 6G can enhance various aspects of healthcare, including telemedicine, remote patient monitoring, EHRs, wearable health devices, and real-time data analytics.
- Data Security and Privacy: Investigating the implications of 6G on data security and privacy in healthcare, including the protection of sensitive patient information and compliance with regulatory standards.
- Interoperability and Integration: Assessing the challenges and solutions related to integrating 6G technology with existing Health IT systems, ensuring seamless interoperability and efficient communication across different platforms and devices.
- Patient Outcomes and Healthcare Delivery: Evaluating the potential improvements in patient outcomes and overall healthcare delivery efficiency that can be achieved through the adoption of 6G-enabled Health IT solutions.
- Policy and Regulation: Reviewing the policy and regulatory considerations necessary to support the successful implementation of 6G in healthcare, including standardization, infrastructure development, and ethical considerations.
- Future Research and Development: Identifying key areas for future research and development to fully realize the potential of 6G in Health IT, providing a roadmap for industry stakeholders, researchers, and policymakers.

By addressing these areas, the study aims to provide a comprehensive understanding of how the convergence of 6G and Health IT can revolutionize healthcare, offering actionable insights and recommendations for stakeholders involved in this interdisciplinary collaboration.

RECOMMENDATIONS

Based on the findings of this interdisciplinary collaboration between Health IT and 6G technology, the following recommendations are proposed:

- Investment in Infrastructure: Allocate resources for the development and deployment of 6G infrastructure to support seamless integration with Health IT systems.
- Interdisciplinary Research: Encourage collaborative research initiatives between healthcare professionals, technologists, and policymakers to explore innovative applications and solutions leveraging 6G technology.

- Training and Education: Provide training programs and educational resources to healthcare professionals on the use of 6G-enabled Health IT systems to ensure effective implementation and utilization.
- Regulatory Support: Establish clear regulatory frameworks and standards for 6G-enabled healthcare applications to ensure compliance with data security and privacy regulations.
- Continuous Evaluation: Regularly assess the performance, security, and usability of 6G-enabled Health IT solutions to identify areas for improvement and optimization.
- Implementing these recommendations will facilitate the successful integration of 6G technology into Health IT, maximizing its potential to enhance healthcare delivery, improve patient outcomes, and drive innovation in the healthcare sector.

CONCLUSION

The interdisciplinary collaboration between Health IT and 6G technology presents a transformative opportunity to revolutionize healthcare delivery. Through this partnership, we have explored the potential synergies, benefits, and challenges associated with integrating 6G into Health IT systems. Our analysis reveals that 6G technology offers unprecedented capabilities such as ultra-low latency, enhanced connectivity, and improved data security, which can significantly enhance healthcare services. From enabling real-time remote surgeries to optimizing patient monitoring and improving data exchange, the potential applications of 6G in healthcare are vast and promising. However, successful integration requires careful consideration of technical, regulatory, and operational factors. Investments in infrastructure, interdisciplinary research, training, and regulatory support are essential to realize the full potential of this collaboration.

In conclusion, the convergence of Health IT and 6G technology holds immense promise for improving healthcare delivery, advancing medical research, and ultimately, enhancing patient outcomes. By embracing this interdisciplinary approach and implementing our recommendations, we can usher in a new era of connected, efficient, and patient-centric healthcare. Together, let us embark on this journey to harness the power of Health IT meets 6G for the betterment of healthcare worldwide.

BIBLIOGRAPHY

Botta, A., De Donato, W., Persico, V., & Pescapé, A. (2016). Integration of cloud computing and internet of things: A survey. *Future Generation Computer Systems*, 56, 684–700.

Chaabane, S., Mani, F., Laurent, M., & Chelouah, R. (2020). The internet of things for healthcare: A comprehensive survey. *Journal of Network and Computer Applications*, 170, 102808.

Evans, R. S. (2016). Electronic health records: Then, now, and in the future. *Yearbook of Medical Informatics*, 25(S 01), S48–S61.

Guo, Y., Liu, Y., Oerlemans, A., Lao, S., Wu, S., & Lew, M. S. (2016). Deep learning for visual understanding: A review. *Neurocomputing*, 187, 27–48.

Jiang, F., Jiang, Y., Zhi, H., Dong, Y., Li, H., Ma, S., ... Wang, Y. (2020). Artificial intelligence in healthcare: past, present and future. *Stroke and Vascular Neurology*, 5(3), 230–243.

Kannan, V. R., & Parthiban, L. (2020). Leveraging artificial intelligence for healthcare delivery: A review. *Journal of King Saud University-Computer and Information Sciences*.

Kumar, R., Joshi, A., Sharan, H. O., Peng, S., & Dudhagara, C. R. (Eds.). (2024). *The Ethical Frontier of AI and Data Analysis*. IGI Global. doi:10.4018/979-8-3693-2964-1

Latif, S., Qadir, J., Farooq, S., & Imran, M. A. (2017). How 5G wireless (and concomitant technologies) will revolutionize healthcare. *Future Internet*, 9(4), 93.

Ohannessian, R., Duong, T. A., & Odone, A. (2020). Global telemedicine implementation and integration within health systems to fight the COVID-19 pandemic: A call to action. *JMIR Public Health and Surveillance*, 6(2), e18810.

Perumal, Radha and Aithal, P. S., Exploring (2023), The Nexus between human resource management (HRM) and enterprise resource planning (ERP) in manufacturing: A comprehensive examination of strategies, challenges, and integration dynamics. *International Journal of Applied Engineering and Management Letters (IJAEML)*, 7(4), 249–258. ISSN: 2581-7000.

Radanliev, P., De Roure, D., Nicolescu, R., Huth, M., & Cannady, S. (2020). Future developments in standardization of cyber risk in the Internet of Things (IoT). *SN Applied Sciences*, 2(2), 168.

Radha, P. & Aithal, P. S. (2024). The evolution of workplace diversity and its impact on organizational success: A comprehensive examination of diversity management strategies, *International Journal of Case Studies in Business, IT, and Education (IJCSBE)*, 8 (1), 221–239, DOI: 10.47992/IJCSBE.2581.6942.0342

Saad, W., Bennis, M., & Chen, M. (2020). A vision of 6G wireless systems: Applications, trends, technologies, and open research problems. *IEEE Network*, 34(3), 134–142.

Shamsi, J. A., & Sareen, S. (2020). Integrating internet of things and blockchain technology for enhanced security in smart healthcare ecosystems: A review, solutions, and future research directions. *Future Generation Computer Systems*, 111, 721–743.

Singh, B. P. & Joshi, A. (2024). Ethical considerations in AI development. In R. Kumar, A. Joshi, H. Sharan, S. Peng, & C. Dudhagara (Eds.), *The ethical frontier of AI and data analysis* (pp. 156–179). IGI Global Scientific Publishing. doi:10.4018/979-8-3693-2964-1.ch010

Taylor, N. K. (2019). Health information technology: Turning the corner in healthcare quality improvement. *Clinical Journal of Oncology Nursing*, 23(2), 127–129.

Wang, C., Dong, H., Dai, H., & Ma, X. (2020). Blockchain-enabled secure internet of things for industry 4.0: A comprehensive survey. *Journal of Industrial Information Integration*, 18, 100129.

Yang, Y., & Song, H. (2020). The emerging role of blockchain technology in science. *Science China Information Sciences*, 63(2), 120301.

Yang, Y., Zhang, Y., Ren, G., Li, C., Xue, R., & Wang, W. (2020). Research on the Internet of Things architecture, technology, and application prospects. *Sustainability*, 12(8), 3226.

2 6G Revolutionizing Healthcare

Speed, Connectivity, and Patient-Centered Care

Aishwarya Jain

INTRODUCTION TO 6G HEALTHCARE TRANSFORMATION

As fifth-generation (5G) and sixth-generation (6G) wireless technology merge, a new age of connectivity with unmatched speed, dependability, and creativity begins. More than its predecessors, 6G is expected to handle a large number of connected devices per square kilometre, ultra-low latency of less than 1 millisecond, and data throughput at the terabits per second (Tbps) level.

To attain unmatched performance, researchers at the Massachusetts Institute of Technology (MIT) have devised a vision for 6G networks that use cutting-edge technology, including integrated photonics, terahertz (THz) spectrum, and intelligent surfaces. 6G networks can transport data at speeds of more than 1 Tbps by utilizing THz frequencies. This allows for the use of applications like immersive virtual reality (VR) experiences and real-time holographic communication.

Furthermore, the integration of intelligent surfaces, consisting of reconfigurable meta-materials, can enhance signal strength and coverage, particularly in indoor environments where traditional wireless signals may be attenuated. Integrated photonics, which utilizes light instead of electrons to transmit data, offers the potential for ultra-high-speed communication with minimal energy consumption, making it ideal for future 6G networks (Tripathi et al., 2021).

IMPLICATIONS FOR HEALTHCARE

The introduction of 6G wireless technology has far-reaching consequences for the healthcare industry, providing significant prospects to improve patient care, streamline clinical operations, and enable novel healthcare applications. With ultra-high data rates and ultra-low latency, 6G networks can enable a wide range of healthcare applications, including real-time remote monitoring, telemedicine consultations, and surgical robotics. For example, researchers at the University of Tokyo established the viability of employing 6G-enabled wearable sensors to monitor patients' vital signs and physiological characteristics in real time. These sensors, which include advanced

DOI: 10.1201/9781003516590-2

biosensors and communication capabilities, can continuously communicate data to healthcare providers, allowing for early diagnosis of health conditions and timely interventions.

Furthermore, the combination of 6G technology with future trends like artificial intelligence (AI) and the Internet of Medical Things (IoMT) expands its potential impact on healthcare delivery. AI algorithms can analyse large amounts of healthcare data generated from 6G-enabled devices to deliver individualized insights and treatment recommendations. IoMT devices can promote seamless connections between medical devices and electronic health record (EHR) systems.

The 6G wireless technology launch marks a paradigm breakthrough in healthcare delivery, providing unprecedented speed, dependability, and connectivity. Healthcare providers can maximize the promise of 6G technology to improve patient outcomes and revolutionize the healthcare landscape by adopting patient-centric methods and incorporating sophisticated connectivity technologies (Gargrish et al., 2023).

INTEGRATION OF ADVANCED TECHNOLOGIES

EXPLORING AI, IoT, AND DATA ANALYTICS IN 6G-ENABLED HEALTHCARE ECOSYSTEMS

The integration of AI, the Internet of Things (IoT), and data analytics in healthcare ecosystems made possible by 6G technology represents a tremendous opportunity to transform healthcare services. When these technologies are seamlessly integrated, they can improve clinical operations and patient care and enable healthcare institutions to make data-driven decisions.

ARTIFICIAL INTELLIGENCE (AI)

AI, namely machine learning (ML) and deep learning algorithms, has emerged as an effective tool for evaluating healthcare data and extracting valuable insights (Joshi & Goyal, 2019) to enhance patient outcomes. In the context of 6G-enabled healthcare, AI can be used to analyse medical imaging scans, forecast illness development, and tailor treatment approaches to unique patient characteristics.

Stanford University researchers, for example, have developed AI algorithms capable of accurately detecting irregularities in medical imaging, allowing for the early diagnosis of illnesses such as cancer and cardiovascular disease. When deployed in conjunction with 6G networks, these AI-powered diagnostic technologies can give real-time findings to healthcare providers, accelerating treatment decisions and enhancing patient care (Hoeks et al., 2011).

INTERNET OF THINGS (IoT)

The network of linked objects that are integrated with sensors, actuators, and communication features that allow them to gather and share data is known as the IoT. IoT devices are essential in the healthcare industry for gathering patient-generated health data and enabling remote patient monitoring. Examples of these devices include wearable sensors, smart medical equipment, and remote monitoring systems.

Thanks to 6G networks' extremely high data rates and low latency, IoT devices may now communicate with each other and healthcare providers' systems more effectively. Continuous monitoring of patients' vital signs, early identification of health problems, and prompt action are made possible by this seamless connectivity, which improves healthcare outcomes and lowers healthcare costs (Johnson Healthcare Solutions, 2022).

DATA ANALYTICS

Data analytics encompasses the process of analysing large volumes of healthcare data to uncover patterns, trends, and insights that can inform clinical decision-making and improve patient care. In the context of 6G-enabled healthcare, data analytics techniques such as predictive analytics, prescriptive analytics, and real-time analytics play a vital role in extracting actionable insights from diverse sources of healthcare data.

For instance, researchers at Harvard Medical School have developed predictive analytics models that leverage EHRs, genetic data, and environmental factors to identify patients at risk of developing chronic diseases such as diabetes and hypertension. By deploying these analytics models on 6G-enabled platforms, healthcare providers can proactively intervene to prevent disease progression and improve population health outcomes (Rajkomar et al., 2019).

TECHNOLOGIES CONVERGE TO ENHANCE HEALTHCARE DELIVERY AND CONNECTIVITY

Incorporating AI, IoT, and data analytics into 6G-enabled healthcare ecosystems facilitates a more cooperative approach to connectivity and healthcare treatment. AI algorithms analyse data from IoT devices, like wearable sensors and smart medical devices, to generate useful insights that support clinical decision-making. 6G networks are then used to communicate this data in real-time to patients and healthcare practitioners, enabling prompt interventions and customized treatment plans.

The incorporation of AI, IoT, and data analytics into healthcare ecosystems provided by 6G signals a revolutionary shift in the way healthcare is delivered and connected. Healthcare professionals may be able to provide patients with more individualized, effective, and efficient care by utilizing the potential of these cutting-edge technologies, which will ultimately improve patient outcomes and advance healthcare (Beam & Kohane, 2018).

PATIENT-CENTRIC CARE PARADIGMS

The goal of patient-centric care, which aims to customize interventions and treatments to meet the requirements of each patient, has been a noticeable movement in healthcare in recent years. Technological developments, especially the introduction of 6G cellular technology, have further enabled this change. In this section, we'll look at how 6G technology makes individualized healthcare delivery possible and talk about how important it is to customize therapies for each patient (Chen & Zhao, 2020).

PERSONALIZED HEALTHCARE DELIVERY EMPOWERED BY 6G TECHNOLOGY

6G technology provides previously unheard-of levels of connectivity, data speed, and dependability, allowing medical professionals to give more individualized treatment than ever before. Healthcare workers can access real-time patient data, such as vital signs, medical histories, and treatment plans, from any location at any time with 6G-enabled devices and networks. As necessary, this seamless connectivity makes it possible to monitor patients' health continuously and to act quickly.

Wearable sensors with 6G connectivity, for instance, can track patients' physiological indicators in real-time, including blood pressure, glucose levels, and heart rate. Instantaneous transmission of this data to healthcare providers enables proactive management of chronic illnesses and early identification of health problems. Personalized care delivery is further enhanced by the incorporation of AI algorithms supported by 6G technology. These algorithms analyse patient data to find patterns and forecast health outcomes (Rappaport et al., 2019).

IMPORTANCE OF TAILORING TREATMENTS TO INDIVIDUAL PATIENT NEEDS

Improving health outcomes and raising patient satisfaction require individualized treatment plans and interventions. Each patient is distinct, having a varied genetic composition, way of life, and set of preferences that can affect how they react to treatment. Healthcare professionals can maximize treatment efficacy, reduce side effects, and enhance patient adherence to treatment regimens by customizing healthcare delivery.

Mayo Clinic research has shown how customized medicine can improve patient outcomes in several different medical specialties, such as cardiology, rheumatology, and oncology. Healthcare practitioners can choose the best courses of action for each patient by utilizing genetic data, biomarkers, and other patient-specific information. This improves clinical results and lowers healthcare expenditures (Kvedar et al., 2014).

REMOTE MONITORING AND TELEHEALTH

Essential elements of contemporary healthcare include telehealth and remote monitoring, which allow patients to receive care without physically visiting hospitals. These services are going to see major improvements because of the introduction of 6G technology, which will fundamentally alter how healthcare is provided and received.

ENHANCED CONNECTIVITY AND SPEED

The unprecedented speeds and connectivity offered by 6G technology are crucial for the real-time transfer of large datasets, movies, and high-resolution medical imaging. Thanks to this better connectivity, medical practitioners may now continuously and in real-time monitor patients' vital signs, health issues, and treatment outcomes.

Wearables with sensors, for instance, can quickly collect and transmit data, such as oxygen saturation, blood pressure, glucose levels, and heart rate, to medical doctors. The exceptionally low latency of 6G ensures that any anomalies or emergencies are detected and handled promptly, significantly reducing reaction time.

INTEGRATION OF AI AND MACHINE LEARNING

AI and ML combined with 6G technology could further revolutionize remote monitoring and healthcare. AI algorithms can analyse large patient data sets and identify patterns, predict potential health issues, and suggest preventive measures (Joshi, A., & Tiwari, H. 2023). AI, for example, may monitor patient information with a history of cardiac problems and predict the likelihood of a cardiac event, allowing for timely interventions. ML models can improve their accuracy and predictive potential by continuously learning from new data, progressively developing into more intelligent and trustworthy remote monitoring systems.

HIGH-QUALITY VIRTUAL CONSULTATIONS

Virtual consultations and telemedicine are two services that notably benefit from 6G's high-speed and low-latency capabilities. A near-in-person experience can be had through high-definition video conversations, which allow doctors to do comprehensive examinations and consultations from a distance. Patients who live in remote or underserved locations and may find it difficult to get to medical facilities may especially benefit from this. With 6G, medical photos, test results, and other diagnostic data may be shared in real-time during virtual consultations, enabling thorough medical assessments and precise diagnosis (Dorsey & Topol, 2016).

IMPROVING ACCESS TO HEALTHCARE

BRIDGING THE GEOGRAPHIC DIVIDE

The capacity to overcome geographical barriers is one of the most important benefits of 6G-powered telehealth and remote monitoring services. Due to the dearth of nearby medical facilities and specialists, patients residing in remote or rural locations frequently encounter difficulties in obtaining high-quality healthcare. Regardless of their location, 6G technology can link these patients with healthcare professionals, guaranteeing that they receive prompt and sufficient medical assistance. There may be fewer discrepancies in healthcare availability and quality as a result of this democratization of access to care.

CONTINUOUS AND PERSONALIZED CARE

Continuous and individualized care is made possible via remote monitoring, and this is especially crucial for the management of chronic illnesses. Individuals with respiratory disorders, diabetes, or hypertension can benefit from prompt treatment plan modifications based on real-time data and ongoing monitoring. AI-driven insights from the gathered data can be used to create personalized treatment plans, ensuring that every patient receives interventions that are specifically designed to meet their individual health needs (Topol, 2019).

FACILITATING PROACTIVE INTERVENTIONS

EARLY DETECTION AND PREVENTION

One of the biggest benefits of telehealth and remote monitoring services is that they are proactive. The early identification of any health problems before they develop into serious illnesses is made possible by ongoing monitoring. For instance, an abrupt rise in a patient's heart rate or a decrease in oxygen saturation levels might warn medical professionals right away, allowing for timely intervention and possibly even life-saving measures. To avoid problems, lower hospital admission rates, and save healthcare expenses, early detection is essential.

EMPOWERING PATIENTS

Patients can take an active role in managing their health with the use of telehealth services and remote monitoring. Patients can access their health information, better comprehend their medical conditions, and follow personalized recommendations to maintain or improve their health. This empowerment leads to improved patient participation, better overall health outcomes, and adherence to treatment plans. Telehealth platforms can integrate instructional materials and support networks to provide patients with the knowledge and abilities they need to take charge of their health.

REDUCING HEALTHCARE SYSTEM BURDENS

Telehealth and remote monitoring services can lighten the load on healthcare systems by enabling proactive actions. Disease progression can be stopped with early detection and ongoing monitoring, which lowers the need for emergency care and hospital stays. This enhances patient outcomes while simultaneously relieving the burden on healthcare resources, enabling medical professionals to concentrate on more urgent situations and boosting the system's overall effectiveness (Krittanawong et al., 2017).

PREDICTIVE ANALYTICS AND PRECISION MEDICINE

Utilizing statistical algorithms, ML methods, and historical data, predictive analytics determines the probability of future events based on historical trends. Predictive analytics can be used to create educated predictions about patient health in the context of 6G-enabled healthcare by utilizing the massive volumes of data gathered from numerous sources, including wearable technology, genetics, EHRs, and medical imaging.

DATA INTEGRATION AND REAL-TIME PROCESSING

With 6G technology, the integration and real-time processing of diverse and large datasets become feasible. The ultra-fast data transfer rates and low latency allow for seamless aggregation of patient data from multiple sources. For instance, continuous monitoring data from wearable devices, lifestyle information, genetic profiles, and historical medical records can be combined to create a comprehensive health profile for each patient. This holistic view enables more accurate and timely predictions about potential health risks.

EARLY DETECTION OF DISEASES

Early disease identification can be facilitated by 6G-powered predictive analytics. Predictive models can detect biomarkers and subtle indicators of the start of diseases, including diabetes, cancer, and cardiovascular disorders, by examining patterns and trends in patient data. To predict the chance of a patient getting a specific disease, for instance, a predictive model may examine alterations in the patient's vital signs, blood test results, and imaging investigations. This would enable early intervention and preventive measures.

PERSONALIZED RISK ASSESSMENTS

Tailored risk evaluations are another service that predictive analytics may offer. Predictive models assess an individual's chance of getting a particular ailment by taking into account characteristics including age, lifestyle choices, medical history, and genetic predispositions. By customizing preventative methods and interventions to each patient's specific risk profile, healthcare practitioners can increase the efficacy of preventive care (Floridi & Taddeo, 2016).

PRECISION MEDICINE IN 6G-ENABLED HEALTHCARE

Precision medicine, sometimes referred to as personalized medicine, is the practice of customizing medical care to each patient's unique needs. To provide more targeted and efficient treatments, this method takes into account lifestyle, environmental, and genetic factors that affect health and disease.

GENOMIC DATA INTEGRATION

Large-scale genomic data integration and analysis are supported by 6G technology. Complex genomic datasets can be handled effectively thanks to high-speed data transfer and processing capabilities. Precision medicine can find genetic variants and mutations that affect treatment response and illness risk by combining clinical and genetic data analysis on a patient. The targeted medicines that are most likely to work for each patient can be chosen with this information in mind.

TAILORED TREATMENT PLANS

Customized treatment regimens based on the distinct qualities of every patient are made possible by precision medicine. In oncology, for instance, genomic profiling of tumours might reveal certain genetic abnormalities promoting the development of cancer. Afterwards, targeted medicines that block these mutations can be chosen, resulting in less harmful and more effective treatments than conventional chemotherapy. Similar to this, pharmacogenomics aims to maximize drug selection and dosage, reduce side effects, and enhance therapeutic outcomes by comprehending how a patient's genetic composition influences how they respond to pharmaceuticals (Mittelstadt et al., 2016).

HOW THESE TECHNOLOGIES CONTRIBUTE TO MORE ACCURATE DIAGNOSES AND TARGETED TREATMENTS

IMPROVED DIAGNOSTIC ACCURACY

The combination of predictive analytics and precision medicine enhances diagnostic accuracy. Predictive models can analyse vast amounts of data to identify patterns and correlations that might be missed by traditional diagnostic methods. For instance, ML algorithms can analyse medical images, such as MRI or CT scans, to detect early signs of diseases with greater accuracy than human radiologists. Additionally, integrating genomic data with clinical information can reveal underlying genetic causes of diseases, leading to more precise diagnoses.

TARGETED THERAPIES

Precision medicine is characterized by targeted medicines, which aim to treat diseases at their molecular source. Precision medicine can pinpoint precise targets for treatment by comprehending the genetic and molecular causes of diseases. For instance, tailored medications in cancer treatment can selectively block proteins or metabolic processes linked to tumour growth, protecting healthy cells and minimizing adverse effects. This focused strategy improves patient outcomes and quality of life in addition to increasing therapeutic efficacy.

ENHANCED PREDICTIVE CAPABILITIES

The use of predictive analytics improves the capacity to anticipate and address possible health problems. Predictive models can estimate the probability of hospital readmissions for patients who have chronic diseases. This information enables healthcare practitioners to take preventive interventions aimed at preventing readmissions. Predictive analytics is useful in the management of diabetes because it can forecast blood glucose patterns and provide prompt interventions to avoid hypo- or hyperglycemia.

Personalized Preventive Measures

Personalized preventive measures are another significant benefit of predictive analytics and precision medicine. By identifying high-risk individuals and understanding their unique risk factors, healthcare providers can develop customized prevention strategies. For instance, patients with a genetic predisposition to certain cancers can undergo more frequent screenings and adopt lifestyle changes to reduce their risk. Personalized preventive care leads to early detection and intervention, ultimately improving health outcomes (Taleb et al., 2017).

Ethical and Regulatory Considerations

To ensure the proper use of these innovations, several ethical and regulatory challenges posed by the use of 6G technology in healthcare must be carefully considered. 6G technology raises concerns about privacy, security, equity, and accountability since it allows for hitherto unheard-of levels of data collecting, processing, and networking.

Privacy and Data Security

Highly sensitive personal health information is among the vast amounts of data that 6G-enabled healthcare systems produce and transmit Protected Health Information (PHI) (Kumar et al., 2024). It is crucial to protect the security and privacy of this data since security lapses can result in serious consequences like identity theft, discrimination, and diminished confidence in the healthcare system.

Consent and Data Ownership

Setting precise rules for consent and data ownership is essential, given the volume of data being gathered. Patients need to know exactly what information is being gathered, how it will be put to use, and who will be able to access it. Furthermore, individuals ought to be in charge of their data, with the option to revoke consent and ask that their information be deleted.

Equity and Accessibility

Ensuring fair access is crucial for the adoption of 6G technologies to prevent the escalation of current healthcare inequities. Due to limited infrastructure, getting 6G-enabled services may be difficult for underserved and rural regions. Furthermore, there is a chance that new medical technology will only help the wealthy, thereby creating a greater divide between various socioeconomic classes.

Algorithmic Bias and Fairness

Algorithmic bias and fairness are issues that arise with the application of AI and ML in 6G-enabled healthcare. Predictive models that are trained on biased data may provide algorithms that reinforce or even worsen already-existing disparities. To preserve confidence and equity in healthcare, AI systems must be clear, comprehensible, and equitable.

ACCOUNTABILITY AND LIABILITY

Determining accountability and liability in 6G-enabled healthcare systems is complex. With AI and automated decision-making systems playing a significant role, it becomes challenging to identify who is responsible when something goes wrong. Establishing clear guidelines and regulatory frameworks for accountability is essential to address these issues (Zhang et al., 2019).

IMPORTANCE OF ENSURING PATIENT PRIVACY AND DATA SECURITY

THE VALUE OF PRIVACY FOR PATIENTS

A basic right and a pillar of the patient-provider relationship is patient privacy. To keep people's faith in the healthcare system, personal health information must be protected. Patients must have faith that their privacy is protected and that their sensitive information is safe. In the absence of this trust, patients can be unwilling to divulge important information, which could impede a precise diagnosis and efficient care (Porter & Heppelmann, 2014).

LEGAL AND REGULATORY FRAMEWORKS

Strong legal and regulatory frameworks must be in place to protect patient privacy. Clear guidelines for data protection, such as those about data encryption, safe storage, and restricted access, should be outlined in these frameworks. While laws like the United States' Health Insurance Portability and Accountability Act (HIPAA) offer a starting point, they must change to meet the unique difficulties presented by 6G technologies.

DATA SECURITY MEASURES

Protecting patient data from cyber-attacks, breaches, and unwanted access requires the implementation of data security procedures. Robust security strategies must include mechanisms for secure authentication, sophisticated encryption techniques, and ongoing system vulnerability surveillance. To guarantee continuous adherence to security requirements, it is also necessary to do frequent security audits and compliance inspections.

ETHICAL USE OF DATA

The ethical use of patient data extends beyond privacy and security. It involves ensuring that data is used in ways that benefit patients and do not harm them. This includes using data to improve healthcare outcomes, advance medical research, and inform public health strategies while avoiding misuse for commercial gain or discriminatory purposes (Singh & Joshi, 2024).

TRANSPARENCY AND PATIENT EMPOWERMENT

Transparency in how patient data is collected, used, and shared is crucial. Patients should be informed about data practices in clear and understandable terms. Providing patients with control over their data, including options for consent and the ability to access and correct their information, empowers them and reinforces trust in the healthcare system (Chesbrough, 2006).

INFRASTRUCTURE AND CONNECTIVITY

A strong and sophisticated infrastructure is required for the deployment of 6G technologies in the healthcare industry to guarantee reliable connectivity and effective data transfer. The tremendous data capacity, high speed, and low latency that 6G promises must be supported by this infrastructure.

ADVANCED NETWORK ARCHITECTURE

Advanced architecture is needed for 6G networks to facilitate massive machine-type communications (mMTC) and ultra-reliable low-latency communications (URLLC). To achieve wide coverage and capacity, dense networks of small cells and large Multiple Input Multiple Output (MIMO) antennas are used. To move data processing closer to the source, lower latency, and speed up reaction times for crucial healthcare applications, the architecture must also allow edge computing.

HIGH-BANDWIDTH BACKHAUL NETWORKS

To support the high data rates of 6G, the backhaul network—connecting base stations to the core network—must provide high bandwidth and low latency. Fibre-optic cables are the preferred medium for backhaul networks due to their high capacity and reliability. However, innovative solutions such as millimetre-wave (mmWave) and THz wireless backhaul can also play a role in areas where laying fibre is impractical.

EDGE AND CLOUD COMPUTING INTEGRATION

For 6G healthcare networks, edge and cloud computing integration is crucial. Real-time data processing near the data source is made possible by edge computing, and this is essential for applications like remote surgery and real-time patient monitoring (Joshi et al., 2024). Cloud computing offers huge datasets, such as genetic data and medical records, scalable processing power, and storage. Healthcare applications are guaranteed to be able to make use of the advantages offered by both cloud and edge computing paradigms when they are integrated seamlessly.

IoT AND WEARABLE DEVICE INTEGRATION

The infrastructure needs to be integrated with a wide range of wearables and IoT devices that collect and transmit health data. This necessitates robust device management platforms, secure communication protocols, and standardized interfaces to ensure compatibility and reliability. Low-power wide-area networks (LPWANs) can also be utilized to ensure long battery life and wide coverage while giving wearable devices the connectivity they need.

NETWORK SLICING

A crucial component of 6G is network slicing, which enables the development of virtual networks customized for particular uses. Diverse network slices can be set aside for diverse uses in the healthcare industry, each with specific performance and security needs. Examples of these uses include emergency services, telemedicine, and remote monitoring. By doing this, it is ensured that vital healthcare applications have the resources they require and the quality of service (QoS) they require without being interfered with by other network traffic (Marmot et al., 2008).

INNOVATIONS IN NETWORK INFRASTRUCTURE TO SUPPORT HIGH-SPEED HEALTHCARE APPLICATIONS

Innovations in network infrastructure are crucial to realizing the full potential of 6G in healthcare. These innovations aim to enhance connectivity, reliability, and speed, enabling a wide range of high-speed healthcare applications.

TERAHERTZ (THz) COMMUNICATIONS

THz communications, operating in the frequency range of 0.1 to 10 THz, offer extremely high data rates and are a promising innovation for 6G. THz waves can support data transmission rates up to 100 Gbps and beyond, making them ideal for applications requiring large data transfers, such as high-resolution medical imaging and real-time telemedicine. However, THz waves have limited penetration and range, necessitating advancements in antenna design and signal propagation techniques.

INTELLIGENT REFLECTING SURFACES (IRS)

A developing technology that can improve signal transmission in 6G networks is called Intelligent Reflecting Surfaces (IRS). IRS can regulate electromagnetic wave reflection and refraction to increase signal strength and coverage, especially in difficult-to-reach places like cities and interior structures. The IRS can guarantee dependable connectivity for remote monitoring equipment and indoor medical facilities in the healthcare industry.

QUANTUM COMMUNICATION

Utilizing quantum mechanics, quantum communication offers extremely secure data transfer. By guaranteeing that encryption keys are transferred with complete confidentiality, quantum key distribution (QKD) keeps private medical information safe from prying eyes. Quantum communication can be extremely helpful in protecting patient privacy and data integrity as 6G networks handle ever-more-sensitive health information.

AI-DRIVEN NETWORK MANAGEMENT

AI can optimize network performance and reliability through intelligent network management. AI algorithms can predict traffic patterns, allocate resources dynamically, and identify potential faults before they impact service. In healthcare, AI-driven network management ensures that critical applications, such as remote surgery and emergency communications, maintain high performance and reliability.

ENHANCED MOBILITY SOLUTIONS

To provide seamless connectivity for mobile healthcare applications, increased mobility solutions will be supported by 6G networks. This includes sophisticated handover protocols that keep devices connected even when they switch between network cells. For situations like mobile health units or ambulance telemedicine, dependable connectivity is necessary for real-time data transfer and professional communication (Schwab, 2016).

GREEN AND SUSTAINABLE NETWORKS

Sustainability is a key consideration in the design of 6G infrastructure. Innovations in energy-efficient hardware, renewable energy integration, and intelligent energy management can reduce the environmental impact of 6G networks. For healthcare facilities, adopting green network technologies can lower operational costs and support environmental sustainability initiatives.

6G healthcare networks will require a significant and diverse infrastructure, including advanced network architecture, high-bandwidth backhaul, integration of edge and cloud computing, support for wearable devices and the IoT, and network slicing. For high-speed healthcare applications to be supported, innovations like THz communications, IRS, quantum communication, AI-driven network management, improved mobility solutions, and sustainable network designs are crucial. Stakeholders can guarantee that 6G technology delivers on its promise of transforming healthcare delivery, boosting patient outcomes, and improving the overall effectiveness of healthcare systems by funding and implementing these technologies (Bi et al., 2014).

HEALTHCARE INNOVATION ECOSYSTEM

The development and deployment of 6G technologies in healthcare necessitate a collaborative approach involving multiple stakeholders. These stakeholders include technology providers, healthcare institutions, government agencies, academic researchers, and patients. Collaboration and partnerships are vital in driving innovation, ensuring interoperability, and addressing the complex challenges associated with integrating 6G into healthcare systems.

TECHNOLOGY PROVIDERS AND HEALTHCARE INSTITUTIONS

Technology suppliers are essential in building the tools and infrastructure required for 6G healthcare applications. These providers include telecoms, device makers, and software developers. Working together with healthcare organizations guarantees that these solutions satisfy clinical standards and are customized to fit the unique requirements of patients and healthcare professionals.

ACADEMIC AND RESEARCH INSTITUTIONS

By performing fundamental research on 6G technologies and their applications in healthcare, academic and research organizations contribute to innovation in healthcare. These organizations can work with technology firms and healthcare providers to test and create novel solutions, confirm their efficacy, and make sure they are grounded in sound scientific principles.

GOVERNMENT AGENCIES AND REGULATORY BODIES

The establishment of regulations, provision of funds, and monitoring of adherence to laws are all made possible by government agencies and regulatory bodies. Partnerships between these organizations and other interested parties contribute to the development of a regulatory framework that encourages innovation while preserving patient security and privacy. Through grants, subsidies, and policy assistance, public-private partnerships can also quicken the development and uptake of 6G healthcare solutions.

PATIENTS AND PATIENT ADVOCACY GROUPS

A great source of information about end-user wants and preferences is patient advocacy groups and actual patients. Patients are better served by developing technologies that are easy to use, solve practical issues, and improve patient care when they are included in the innovation process. To increase acceptance and awareness of new technology, collaborations with patient advocacy groups can be helpful.

CROSS-INDUSTRY COLLABORATIONS

Healthcare innovation within the 6G ecosystem can benefit from cross-industry collaborations, such as partnerships with the pharmaceutical industry, insurance companies, and data analytics firms. These collaborations can lead to the development of comprehensive solutions that integrate medical treatments, insurance coverage, and advanced data analytics, providing holistic care for patients (Bauer et al., 2020).

IMPORTANCE OF FOSTERING AN ECOSYSTEM CONDUCIVE TO INNOVATION

Creating an ecosystem conducive to innovation is critical for the successful integration of 6G technologies in healthcare. This ecosystem should promote collaboration, provide the necessary infrastructure and resources, and support an environment where new ideas can be developed and tested rapidly.

COLLABORATIVE INNOVATION HUBS

Stakeholders can pool resources and ideas by establishing cooperative innovation hubs, such as research parks, innovation labs, and technological incubators. These hubs provide a physical or virtual space where academics, businesspeople, medical professionals, and tech developers may work together on joint projects, share expertise, and have access to cutting-edge resources.

OPEN STANDARDS AND INTEROPERABILITY

Open standards and interoperability must be encouraged to ensure that 6G healthcare technology can seamlessly interface with current systems and equipment. Healthcare providers can use the best options available when suppliers can collaborate more freely and there is less chance of vendor lock-in, thanks to open standards. Treatment continuity and coordination are improved when many systems share patient data thanks to interoperability.

FUNDING AND INVESTMENT

Adequate funding and investment are crucial for fostering innovation. Governments, venture capitalists, and private investors can support the development of 6G healthcare technologies by providing financial resources for research and development, pilot projects, and large-scale deployments. Funding mechanisms should also be in place to support startups and small businesses, which often drive disruptive innovations.

REGULATORY SUPPORT AND FLEXIBILITY

It takes a flexible and encouraging regulatory environment to promote innovation while maintaining patient safety. To comprehend the ramifications of emerging technology and create policies that safeguard patients without impeding innovation, regulatory agencies should collaborate closely with entrepreneurs. Regulatory sandboxes, which offer a controlled environment for testing new technologies, can aid in striking a compromise between these requirements.

EDUCATION AND WORKFORCE DEVELOPMENT

Creating a staff with the necessary skills is crucial to implementing 6G healthcare technologies successfully. Specialized training and programmes in fields like biomedical engineering, data science, telecommunications, and healthcare informatics should be provided by educational institutions. It's crucial for IT specialists and healthcare practitioners to have access to ongoing professional development opportunities to stay up to date with emerging technologies.

ETHICAL AND SOCIAL CONSIDERATIONS

To promote a responsible innovation environment, it is essential to address ethical and social factors. The ethical ramifications of emerging technology, including data privacy, equity, and patient permission, must be taken into account by stakeholders. To make sure that innovations are in line with social values, it might be helpful to detect and address potential ethical difficulties by interacting with ethicists, sociologists, and the larger community.

ACCELERATED TESTING AND DEPLOYMENT

Rapid testing and deployment of new technologies are crucial for bringing innovations to market quickly. This requires efficient clinical trial processes, fast-track regulatory approvals, and agile project management methodologies. Pilot projects and real-world testing environments, such as living labs, allow for the practical evaluation of new technologies and provide valuable feedback for further refinement.

It is impossible to overestimate the importance of partnerships and collaborations in fostering healthcare innovation inside 6G ecosystems. Developing and implementing successful 6G healthcare solutions requires a cooperative strategy combining technology providers, healthcare facilities, university researchers, governmental organizations, patients, and cross-industry partners. Establishing cooperative hubs, encouraging open standards and interoperability, providing sufficient funding, providing regulatory support, developing a skilled workforce, addressing ethical issues, and facilitating quick testing and deployment are all necessary to foster an ecosystem that is favourable to innovation. Stakeholders may fully utilize 6G technology to revolutionize healthcare delivery, enhance patient outcomes, and spur the next wave of innovation in the field by establishing such an ecosystem (Bashshur et al., 2015).

GLOBAL IMPACT AND EQUITY

The introduction of 6G technology into the healthcare industry has the potential to have a profound global impact, changing how medical services are delivered and made accessible to all people. But to reach its full potential, equitable access issues must be resolved, and the advantages of 6G healthcare must be distributed internationally.

ENHANCED GLOBAL CONNECTIVITY

Improved connectivity is expected to be available everywhere with 6G technology, including in isolated and underdeveloped places. 6G can close the digital gap by providing huge connections, low latency, and greater data transfer speeds, allowing even the most remote areas to access cutting-edge healthcare services. Improved healthcare results can be achieved in places with limited medical resources through the use of telemedicine, remote monitoring, and real-time health interventions made possible by this global connectedness.

CROSS-BORDER COLLABORATION

Cross-border partnerships between healthcare providers, researchers, and institutions can be facilitated via 6G healthcare. 6G can support global research collaborations, clinical trials, and collaborative care models by facilitating smooth data sharing and communication. This has the potential to hasten the creation and adoption of medical breakthroughs and best practices, which will benefit patients everywhere.

HEALTH DATA AND RESEARCH

The vast amounts of health data generated by 6G-enabled devices can provide valuable insights for global health research. By aggregating and analysing data from diverse populations, researchers can identify trends, track disease outbreaks, and develop more effective treatments. This global perspective can lead to advancements in public health, epidemiology, and personalized medicine.

DIGITAL HEALTH SERVICES

The broad use of digital health services, such as telemedicine, e-prescriptions, and virtual consultations, can be facilitated by 6G. These services can improve healthcare delivery efficiency, decrease the need for in-person visits, and cut expenses.

CONSIDERATIONS FOR EQUITABLE ACCESS

To ensure equitable access to 6G healthcare, several considerations must be addressed:

Infrastructure Development: It is essential to build the required infrastructure in underserved areas. This entails developing 6G networks, making sure power sources are dependable, and offering reasonably priced internet access. Infrastructure projects can be greatly aided by the funding and support of governments and international organizations.

Affordability: Making 6G healthcare services affordable for all populations is essential. This may involve subsidizing costs for low-income individuals, offering affordable healthcare plans, and leveraging economies of scale to reduce prices.

Digital Literacy: Enhancing digital literacy and providing education on using 6G healthcare technologies can empower individuals to take advantage of new services. Training programmes for both patients and healthcare providers are necessary to ensure widespread adoption and effective use of 6G tools.

Regulatory Frameworks: It is essential to establish national, international, and local regulatory frameworks that uphold patient rights and advance equity. Fair access to healthcare services, security, and data privacy should all be protected by regulations.

STRATEGIES TO ADDRESS HEALTHCARE DISPARITIES AND IMPROVE ACCESS TO ADVANCED SERVICES

Policy reforms, focused interventions, and creative solutions are all necessary components of a multimodal strategy to address healthcare inequities and increase access to advanced treatments.

POLICY AND ADVOCACY

Universal Healthcare Coverage: Enacting laws that guarantee everyone has access to necessary medical treatment is one way to guarantee that everyone has access to healthcare. This entails raising the scope of insurance plans and offering low-income people subsidies.

Incentives for Healthcare Providers: Encouraging medical professionals to work in underprivileged communities can contribute to a more equitable distribution of medical expertise. Financial incentives, loan forgiveness plans, and professional development opportunities are a few examples of this.

International Aid and Collaboration: High-income countries and international organizations can provide financial aid, technical support, and expertise to low-income countries to build healthcare infrastructure and implement 6G technologies.

TARGETED INTERVENTIONS

Targeted interventions can directly address specific healthcare disparities:

Mobile Health Units: Deploying mobile health units equipped with 6G connectivity can bring medical services to remote and underserved areas. These units can provide routine care, preventive services, and emergency care, reducing the burden on fixed healthcare facilities.

Telehealth Programmes: Enhancing access to specialized care and follow-up consultations can be achieved by extending telehealth services to underserved and rural communities. Mental health care and the management of chronic diseases can benefit greatly from telehealth.

Community Health Workers: Local healthcare delivery can be improved by providing 6G-enabled gadgets to community health workers and training them in their use. These professionals can do health screenings, provide knowledge, and help patients and healthcare providers communicate (Kruse et al., 2018).

INNOVATIVE SOLUTIONS

Innovation in healthcare technology and service delivery can address disparities:

- **Low-Cost Devices and Wearables**: A larger population will be able to access modern healthcare technology with the development of reasonably priced 6G-enabled gadgets and wearables. These gadgets offer real-time health data, facilitate telemedicine, and track health parameters.
- **Localized Health Platforms**: Creating localized health platforms that consider cultural, linguistic, and regional differences can enhance the relevance and effectiveness of healthcare services. These platforms can provide tailored health information, appointment scheduling, and remote consultations.
- **AI and Machine Learning**: By analysing health data with AI and ML, at-risk populations can be found and healthcare requirements can be anticipated. By directing early interventions and resource allocation, predictive analytics might enhance health outcomes in marginalized groups (Collins & Varmus, 2015).

6G healthcare will have a significant global influence and can change healthcare delivery and accessibility globally. To avoid escalating already-existing gaps, it is imperative to guarantee equitable access to these breakthroughs. Stakeholders may build an ecosystem for accessible healthcare by concentrating on infrastructure development, affordability, digital literacy, and strong regulatory frameworks. It is imperative to employ tactics like policy advocacy, focused interventions, and creative problem-solving to tackle healthcare inequities and enhance the availability of cutting-edge services. By working together, the advantages of 6G technology may be used to build a more just and effective global healthcare system, which will eventually improve people's health and well-being everywhere.

EMERGING TRENDS AND OPPORTUNITIES

With the introduction of several new trends and opportunities, the introduction of 6G technology has the potential to completely change the healthcare industry. These changes could improve patient outcomes, increase operational efficiency, and change how medical services are delivered.

ULTRA-RELIABLE LOW-LATENCY COMMUNICATION (URLLC)

Real-time applications are critical to the healthcare industry, and 6G's highly dependable low-latency communication capabilities make this possible. This includes remote procedures that enable doctors to do precise operations from a distance and real-time telemedicine consultations that provide patients with timely, effective care.

ENHANCED TELEMEDICINE AND TELEHEALTH

With the advent of 6G, telemedicine will advance and provide more engaging and interactive experiences via VR and augmented reality (AR). With the use of tactile feedback technology and high-definition video, doctors may do comprehensive examinations remotely, enhancing the standard of care offered by telehealth services.

AI AND MACHINE LEARNING INTEGRATION

Personalized treatment plans and improved diagnosis accuracy will result from the integration of AI and ML with 6G networks. Large-scale real-time data analysis is possible thanks to AI algorithms, which may also provide personalized treatment suggestions, risk assessment, and predictive analytics for early disease identification.

INTERNET OF MEDICAL THINGS (IoMT)

The potential of 6G to connect a large number of devices at the same time will help the IoMT spread rapidly. Wearable health monitors, smart implants, and connected medical devices all capture and send health data in real-time for monitoring and analysis.

ADVANCED REMOTE MONITORING

The possibilities of remote monitoring will be greatly enhanced by 6G technology, enabling low-latency and continuous observation of patients' health indices. This reduces hospital readmission rates and enhances the management of chronic illnesses by enabling prompt modifications to treatment plans and proactive interventions.

PRECISION MEDICINE

6G will help precision medicine by enabling the use of big data and sophisticated analytics to customize treatments for each patient according to their genetics, way of life, and surroundings. Massive genomic datasets may be processed and analysed quickly because of 6G's high-speed data transport.

SMART HOSPITALS

Smart hospitals equipped with 6G infrastructure can improve operations through automation and real-time data analytics. From sophisticated patient management systems to automated supply chain logistics, 6G enables hospitals to increase efficiency, lower costs, and provide better patient care.

VIRTUAL HEALTH ASSISTANTS

With the advent of 6G, AI-powered virtual health assistants will proliferate and offer patients round-the-clock access to prescription reminders, appointment scheduling, medical advice, and health education. These helpers can provide customized assistance by utilizing real-time data analysis (Raghupathi & Raghupathi, 2014).

POTENTIAL FOR FURTHER ADVANCEMENTS AND INNOVATIONS IN THE FIELD

The potential for further advancements and innovations in 6G-enabled healthcare is immense, promising to push the boundaries of what is currently possible and create new paradigms in healthcare delivery.

QUANTUM COMPUTING INTEGRATION

The integration of quantum computing with 6G networks has the potential to transform the healthcare industry by resolving intricate issues that are presently unsolvable by traditional computers. This includes treatment protocol optimization based on large-scale datasets and drug development, where quantum algorithms can model molecular interactions with unparalleled accuracy.

HOLOGRAPHIC COMMUNICATION

Holographic communication, enabled by 6G's high bandwidth and low latency, can transform telemedicine and medical training. Doctors can interact with 3D holograms of patients for remote diagnosis and treatment, and medical students can learn from holographic simulations of surgical procedures.

PERSONALIZED HEALTHCARE ECOSYSTEMS

The development of personalized healthcare ecosystems will be accelerated by 6G. These ecosystems integrate various digital health tools, including wearables, mobile apps, and EHRs, to provide holistic and personalized healthcare experiences tailored to individual needs.

DECENTRALIZED CLINICAL TRIALS

Decentralized clinical trials can benefit from 6G technology, which allows for remote monitoring, real-time data collection, and virtual consultations. This makes it easier to involve various people in trials, which improves the generalizability of research findings and speeds up the development of new medicines.

BIO-INTEGRATED WEARABLES AND IMPLANTS

6G connectivity will enable seamless integration with the biological systems of the body, enabling advancements in bio-integrated wearables and implants. These gadgets can instantly connect with healthcare professionals, deliver therapeutic actions, and continually monitor physiological data.

ADVANCED ROBOTICS AND AUTOMATION

6G will accelerate robotics and automation in healthcare, allowing for more precise and autonomous surgical robots, automated diagnostic systems, and intelligent care robots that help with patient care, rehabilitation, and geriatric care.

DIGITAL TWIN TECHNOLOGY

Digital twin technology, which generates virtual clones of physical entities, can be used to simulate patient-specific models for personalized treatment planning and medical equipment predictive maintenance. 6G allows for real-time synchronization between the digital twin and the actual entity, resulting in accurate and up-to-date simulations.

BLOCKCHAIN FOR HEALTH DATA SECURITY

Blockchain technology with 6G can improve the security and interoperability of health data. Blockchain ensures data security and permits safe information exchange between various healthcare systems by offering a decentralized, immutable ledger for medical records.

Healthcare is about to witness revolutionary developments and prospects with the advent of 6G technology. These include extremely dependable low-latency connections, improved telemedicine, AI integration, IoMT, sophisticated remote monitoring, precision medicine, smart hospitals, and virtual health assistants. Further developments and innovations have the potential to completely transform healthcare delivery and enhance patient outcomes. Examples of these include the integration of quantum computing, holographic communication, decentralized clinical trials, personalized healthcare ecosystems, bio-integrated wearables, advanced robotics, digital twin technology, and blockchain for health data security. As these technologies develop further, new avenues for medical innovation will open up, improving healthcare's effectiveness, individualization, and accessibility for people all over the world (Zhang et al., 2018).

CONCLUSION AND FUTURE SCOPE

The exploration of 6G technology's transformative potential in healthcare underscores its pivotal role in ushering in a new era of patient-centred smart healthcare. By leveraging its extraordinary speed, connectivity, and data management capabilities, 6G promises to revolutionize healthcare delivery, improve patient outcomes, and enhance overall healthcare efficiency. Technological advancements such as ultra-low latency, mMTC, and AI-driven data analytics enable real-time interactions critical for telemedicine, remote surgery, and emergency response systems. These capabilities also facilitate continuous patient monitoring and personalized medicine through advanced data processing capabilities. Applications span telemedicine, remote monitoring, personalized medicine, and emergency response systems, where real-time data from wearable devices can trigger immediate responses to patient emergencies, while AI algorithms analyse vast datasets to tailor treatment plans based on individual patient profiles. Deploying 6G in healthcare requires addressing critical challenges, including data privacy, cybersecurity, and equitable access. Robust data protection measures and regulatory compliance are essential to safeguard sensitive health information and bridge the digital divide for fair access to 6G technology. Future directions should focus on optimizing healthcare delivery systems, enhancing remote patient monitoring capabilities, and advancing personalized medicine through the integration of genetic, environmental, and lifestyle data. Collaboration among healthcare providers, technology developers, policymakers, and regulatory bodies is crucial to ensure global implementation success, prioritizing standards development, interoperability, and ethical guidelines. In conclusion, 6G technology represents a transformative shift in healthcare, promising a more responsive, efficient, and patient-centred healthcare environment with the potential to improve health outcomes and enhance patient satisfaction.

REFERENCES

Bashshur, R. L., Shannon, G. W., Smith, B. R., & Alverson, D. C. (2015). The empirical foundations of telemedicine interventions for chronic disease management. *Telemedicine and e-Health*, 20(9), pp. 769–800.

Bauer, H., Patel, M., & Veira, J. (2020). *The next generation of connectivity: The implications of 5G for business*. McKinsey & Company.

Beam, A. L., & Kohane, I. S. (2018). Big data and machine learning in health care. *JAMA*, 319(13), pp. 1317–1318. doi:10.1001/jama.2017.18391

Bi, Z., Da Xu, L., & Wang, C. (2014). Internet of things for enterprise systems of modern manufacturing. *IEEE Transactions on Industrial Informatics*, 10(2), pp. 1537–1546.

Chen, S., & Zhao, J. (2020). The requirements, challenges, and technologies for 6G of terahertz communication. *IEEE Communications Magazine*, 58(3), pp. 36–42.

Chesbrough, H. W. (2006). *Open innovation: The new imperative for creating and profiting from technology*. Harvard Business School Press.

Collins, F. S., & Varmus, H. (2015). A new initiative on precision medicine. *New England Journal of Medicine*, 372(9), pp. 793–795.

Dorsey, E. R., & Topol, E. J. (2016). State of Telehealth. *The New England Journal of Medicine*, 375, pp. 154–161.

Floridi, L., & Taddeo, M. (2016). What is data ethics? *Philosophical Transactions of the Royal Society A: Mathematical, Physical and Engineering Sciences*, 374(2083), p. 20160360.

Gargrish, S., Chauhan, S., Gupta, M., & Obaid, A. J. (2023). 6G-enabled IoT wearable devices for elderly healthcare. In *6G-enabled IoT and AI for smart healthcare* (pp. 157–169). CRC Press. doi:10.1201/9781003321668-8

Hoeks, L. B. E. A., Greven, W. L., & De Valk, H. W. (2011). Real-time continuous glucose monitoring system for treatment of diabetes: a systematic review. *Diabetic Medicine*, 28(4), 386–394. doi:10.1111/j.1464-5491.2010.03177.x

Johnson Healthcare Solutions. (2022). Transforming Healthcare with 6G-Powered Telemedicine Platforms.

Joshi, A., & Goyal, S. B. (2019). Comparison of various round robin scheduling algorithms. *2019 8th International Conference System Modeling and Advancement in Research Trends (SMART)*. Moradabad, India, pp. 18–21, doi: 10.1109/SMART46866.2019.9117345

Joshi, A., Kumar, V., Thakur, G., Pant, H. V., & Singh, B. P. (2024). The impact of cloud computing on data science and engineering: Opportunities and challenges. *2024 International Conference on Electrical Electronics and Computing Technologies (ICEECT)*, 1–4. https://doi.org/10.1109/ICEECT61758.2024.10739285

Joshi, A., & Tiwari, H. (2023). An Overview of Python Libraries for Data Science. *Journal of Engineering Technology and Applied Physics*, 5(2), 85–90. https://doi.org/10.33093/jetap

Krittanawong, C., Johnson, K. W., Rosenson, R. S., De Fer, T., & Henry, T. D. (2017). Deep learning for cardiovascular medicine: a practical primer. *European Heart Journal*, 40(25), pp. 2058–2073.

Kruse, C. S., Karem, P., Shifflett, K., Vegi, L., Ravi, K., & Brooks, M. (2018). Evaluating barriers to adopting telemedicine worldwide: a systematic review. *Journal of Telemedicine and Telecare*, 24(1), pp. 4–12.

Kumar, R., Joshi, A., Sharan, H. O., Peng, S. L., & Dudhagara, C. R. (Eds.). (2024). *The Ethical Frontier of AI and Data Analysis*. IGI Global.

Kvedar, J., Coye, M. J., & Everett, W. (2014). Connected health: a review of technologies and strategies to improve patient care with telemedicine and telehealth. *Health Affairs*, 33(2), pp. 194–199.

Marmot, M., Friel, S., Bell, R., Houweling, T. A., & Taylor, S. (2008). Closing the gap in a generation: Health equity through action on the social determinants of health. *The Lancet*, 372(9650), pp. 1661–1669.

Mittelstadt, B. D., Allo, P., Taddeo, M., Wachter, S., & Floridi, L. (2016). The ethics of algorithms: mapping the debate. *Big Data & Society*, 3(2), p. 2053951716679679.

Porter, M. E., & Heppelmann, J. E. (2014). How smart, connected products are transforming competition. *Harvard Business Review*, 92(11), pp. 64–88.

Raghupathi, W., & Raghupathi, V. (2014). Big data analytics in healthcare: Promise and potential. *Health Information Science and Systems*, 2(1), p. 3.

Rajkomar, A., Oren, E., Chen, K., Dai, A. M., Hajaj, N., Hardt, M., & Zhang, M. W. (2019). Scalable and accurate deep learning with electronic health records. *npj Digital Medicine*, 2(1), pp. 1–10. doi:10.1038/s41746-018-0029-1

Rappaport, T. S., Xing, Y., MacCartney, G. R., Molisch, A. F., Mellios, E., & Zhang, J. (2019). Overview of millimeter wave communications for fifth-generation (5G) wireless networks—With a focus on propagation models. *IEEE Transactions on Antennas and Propagation*, 65(12), pp. 6213–6230.

Schwab, K. (2016). *The fourth industrial revolution*. World Economic Forum.

Singh, B. P., & Joshi, A. (2024). Ethical considerations in AI development. In R. Kumar, A. Joshi, & H. O. Sharan (Eds.), *The ethical frontier of AI and data analysis* (pp. 156–179). IGI Global. doi:10.4018/979-8-3693-2964-1.ch010

Taleb, T., Samdanis, K., Mada, B., Flinck, H., Dutta, S., & Sabella, D. (2017). On multi-access edge computing: A survey of the emerging 5G network edge architecture & orchestration. *IEEE Communications Surveys & Tutorials*, 19(3), pp. 1657–1681.

Topol, E. (2019). High-performance medicine: The convergence of human and artificial intelligence. *Nature Medicine*, 25, pp. 44–56.

Tripathi, S., Sabu, N. V., Gupta, A. K., & Dhillon, H. S. (2021). Millimeter-wave and terahertz spectrum for 6G wireless. In *6G mobile wireless networks* (pp. 83–121). Springer International Publishing. doi:10.1007/978-3-030-72777-2_6

Zhang, Q., Yang, L. T., Chen, Z., & Li, P. (2018). A survey on deep learning for big data. *Information Fusion*, 42, pp. 146–157.

Zhang, Z., Xiao, Y., Ma, Z., Xiao, M., Ding, Z., Lei, X., Karagiannidis, G. K., & Fan, P. (2019). 6G wireless networks: Vision, requirements, architecture, and key technologies. *IEEE Vehicular Technology Magazine*, 14(3), pp. 28–41.

3 Towards a Connected Healthcare Future
Global Insights on 6G Adoption

Wesam Ahmed and Amena Mahmoud

INTRODUCTION

Dealing with disasters, such as the COVID-19 epidemic, remains challenging, despite innovations in technology. Hospitals struggled to manage patient traffic due to a lack of preparation. After the pandemic announcement, many people globally did not have access to necessary medical care. COVID-19 collapsed the healthcare system due to increased patient numbers, lack of medical services, failure to prevent infection, and delayed reaction. Healthcare systems in developed nations struggled to offer quick and secure medical facilities for personnel and patients, limiting the damage. The application of current digital health systems and the adoption of the ever-growing 5th Generation (5G) of wireless communication technology in healthcare have paved the way for achieving the provision of the Internet of Medical Things (IoMT). Despite the promises of 5G, the healthcare IoT ecosystem is still in its adolescence and needs further improvement in search of reliable, low-latency, ultra-reliable communication, and minimal sluggish behaviour. Inquisitiveness and research work for the development of the immensely talented and dynamically blazing frontiers of the Sixth-Generation (6G) of wireless technology in 2026 are already on the right track (Nayak & Patgiri, 2021).

In low- and middle-income countries, the most promising use-cases addressed by rural extended reality (XR) aimed solutions are planned on-demand services for providing remote onsite technical assistance to users of automated diagnostic equipment at selected self-care community health units. Only one rural ambulance would be enough for the transportation of patients to medical centres staffed with emergency health care professionals if needed. This tele-health solution can provide a globalized answer to alleviate the rapid population aging of rural areas in developed countries with a declining birth rate in the long-term scenario. Reciprocally, the third technological mode, massive broadband conjoined communication (MBCC), which may help the long-term scenarios, depends on the resolution of technological bottlenecks, such as the development of 6G technology, which could guide future research (Akhtar et al., 2020).

DOI: 10.1201/9781003516590-3

The use of ultra-reliable low-latency communication (URLLC) information and communication technology (ICT) to improve healthcare is referred to in evidence-based approaches as e-health. Until today, 5G and its revised standard, Release 16, is still being deployed all over the world, with its aims of improving remote patient monitoring, providing tele-health services extended to underserved regions and populations (such as both urban and rural network not-spots and third-world populations), and advancing technical aids like massive machine-type communication (MTC), which aim to enable switched-off sensors enabling predictive tailored travel network solutions. These could help patients who receive notifications to be redirected to adapted, neighbouring medical care facilities just in time when risks of hospital-acquired infections (HAIs) occur. While some opportunities and challenges related to 6G networks have been envisioned recently, evidence for what a trusted base 6G infrastructure is required for governance of the distributed healthcare ecosystem from a global perspective is lacking. Through understanding and addressing these requirements, 6G will contribute to sustainable United Nations (UN) development goals as a key driver for inclusive and resilient societies (Mucchi et al., 2020).

The main contributions of the chapter lie in the following: (1) it reviews and determines the most likely proposals for 6G's healthcare adoption from a global perspective, providing the prospects for future 6G research. (2) It describes a scoping review search and a 6G vision survey to generate and rank 6G multidisciplinary, covering multiple user segments and society-building relevant healthcare, employing representatives from multiple geographic areas and user domain expertise using statistical methods to refine the results. (3) It devises a 6G Tran's disciplinary framework, the authors aim to model and expand through future collaborative work, providing the global user with valued initial feedback to the relevant standardization activities.

UNDERSTANDING 6G TECHNOLOGY

Well-designed measurement and data-gathering processes are essential for the evolution of—what is likely to be—6G wireless. Such processes could lead to collaborative public-private programmes and centres that serve as shared resources, dig into geographically distributed databases, and carry out data analytics, steering computation off of healthcare centres and lab sites, that, given multiple, complex alternatives, lead to overall, distributed measurement algorithms for metrics that are fit-for-purpose across use-cases that span the entire scope of medical needs.

From a technological perspective, it is vital to understand that the health sector must deal with a broad range of actors—both human and technical—whose behaviour is influenced by a similarly wide variety of incentives and motivations. Part of the success of 5G in markets where the major, early income earners, such as entertainment and gaming, remain is that the actors in these markets can often be assumed to interact together. However, both 5G and 6G market success in the healthcare domain will be premised on understanding a wider system where significant uncertainties and medical risks are important, the data and rules surrounding that data often need special handling, and multiple data stewards have legitimate concerns (Janjua et al., 2020).

DEFINITION AND KEY FEATURES

Recognized as a significant benefit for healthcare management (Enterprise Resource Planning (ERP)) applications, 6G technologies can be used similarly in the future. These use cases typically deal with big data and analytics issues, reflecting these characteristics. To effectively make this manipulation of data, however, previous studies have suggested that data lakes, artificial intelligence (AI), the Internet of Things (IoT), edge and fog computing, blockchain, and intelligent process automation (IPA) might be employed wisely. Healthcare will be disrupted by 6G technologies and new business models more than the internet, AI, or 5G networks did domestically and globally. Mega-trends such as demographic change (rising life expectancy, increasing childlessness, and aging societies), globalization, and increasing regulation are putting more and more pressure on healthcare systems around the world. Among other things, higher costs and the need to manage staff and resources more effectively are at the forefront of healthcare challenges. The search for practices, methodologies, and tools that deliver the best possible results at the lowest cost levels and that internalize sustainable development goals has come a long way and is expected to continue in the coming years. 6G networks are expected to provide considerable improvements over current 5G technology. Figure 3.1 summarizes the features and advantages of 6G networks. Here are some of the important features and probable advances related to 6G (Javaid et al., 2023):

- **High Data Transmission Rates**: 6G networks are predicted to significantly improve data transfer speeds, perhaps reaching up to 10 Tbps. This marks a huge increase above the current limit for 5G networks, which is 10 Gbps.
- **Low Latency**: 6G networks are projected to provide ultra-low latency, potentially as low as 0.1 ms, greatly improving the latency requirement of 5G networks, which is 1 ms.

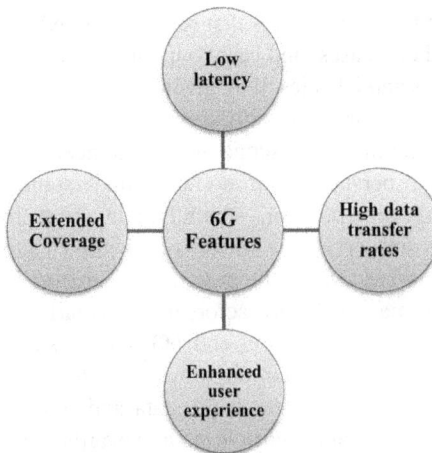

FIGURE 3.1   Characteristics of 6G networks.

- **Wider Coverage Range**: 6G networks could reach space, the deep sea, and underground locations. Space travel, deep-sea sightseeing, and industrial internet will all be enabled by this technology.
- **Enhanced User Experience**: The enhancement of user experience is expected to be caused by the enhancement of capabilities such as XR, augmented reality (AR), virtual reality (VR), and AI.
- **Increased Spectral Efficiency**: Spectral and network efficiency are projected to be ten times greater in 6G networks than in 5G networks.

HEALTHCARE INDUSTRY OVERVIEW

The inefficient systems present in healthcare come with real costs, not only to individuals but also to society and its members. There are numerous estimates of the size of this waste, all of which are significant. Certainly, some portions of healthcare waste are the result of conditions that are difficult to diagnose and treat. However, areas exist where a multitude of inefficient and suboptimal systems prevent efficient, effective care. These inefficiencies provided the impetus for the early adoption of the biggest and most ambitious healthcare revolution, before the emergence of 6G, the 6G of cellular and wireless connectivity. As we move into the 6G era, we consider what technologies will emerge and the role they may take in impacting the healthcare industry and its systems. We provide a high-level perspective of the types of healthcare impact that 6G advances could drive in the industry sector. The healthcare discussion is divided into two perspectives: the provider domain for those involved in directly delivering healthcare services and the consumer domain for general citizens who will take advantage of the services in the market (Rahman et al., 2022).

The healthcare industry has changed dramatically over the past decade, due mainly to forces outside of healthcare—mainly digital technologies, various industries' forays into healthcare, consumer demand for more affordable and more accessible care, and government efforts to accelerate transformation. This evolution has so far focused primarily on individual components of the industry without addressing the need for a broader system-level perspective for consideration of what is necessary to achieve better health outcomes. Healthcare overall is encumbered by an apparent paradox. Despite substantial improvements in medical knowledge, diagnostics, and therapeutics, healthcare delivery performance has lagged other industries in several important areas. Healthcare often fails to consistently deliver even basic, simple health advice and knowledge that is known to be impactful. Furthermore, healthcare costs have limited the ability of many to benefit from the developments in the field.

CURRENT TRENDS AND CHALLENGES

On the other hand, the digitalization of health records (such as diagnostic results, treatment practices, and billing details) and the inclusion of smart healthcare technologies have raised significant concerns about the privacy and security of patient data. The major challenge of healthcare is ensuring the confidentiality, privacy, and security of clinical data, personal records, and healthcare data. While in this paper, we talk about the importance of connecting health data, a further issue to convey is that although patient data have benefited from shared access, it is also associated with significant privacy, confidentiality, and security risks (e.g., unauthorized access, data leakage, misuse, and tampering). In the future, addressing cybersecurity, human rights, and ethical challenges in health very slightly and, apart from the lack of the digitalization effect, care should be taken for the security of data that is collected from different resources. Furthermore, data flows not only through IoT devices but also through the communication between these devices. Providing flexible, intelligent, trustworthy, and self-organized network management to 6G healthcare applications in support of Quality of Service (QoS) provisioning to the data flow in the access layer of the healthcare sensor networks while offering energy efficiency to the sensor devices (Wang et al., 2020).

Today, the number of elderly people has risen to 12% of the global population. As elderly people prefer living in the comfort of their own homes, increasing demand for remote healthcare will only continue. In other words, as well as providing medical services using advanced digital and technical means, these services are required for patients not needing to leave their location. Concerning the increasing share of the global population being elderly, the importance of 6G technologies and future networks in the healthcare system is also presented in various studies. Technologies to be developed during the 6G term, AI-IoT-based healthcare devices, and future communication technologies all have the potential to make significant contributions to the healthcare system, such as reducing the workloads of health professionals who care for elderly patients (Jiang et al., 2021).

POTENTIAL BENEFITS OF 6G IN HEALTHCARE

A brain-computer interface (BCI) is a communication pathway between a brain or nervous system and an external device, such as a computer. This operates on the principle of deciphering the user's mental activities. The applications of BCI include, among others, communication help for patients, monitoring brain states, and detecting brain function-related activities. AI, AR, and VR technologies can be used in BCI, and their effectiveness is enhanced in terms of treatment duration, effectiveness, and patient satisfaction. BCI applications can thus provide remote diagnosis and real-time support for patients in need of healthcare without a hospital visit, using 6G technology. The coronavirus pandemic has only increased the need for technologies that can help medical professionals remotely monitor and support patients without direct contact, particularly in cases where a patient needs continuous monitoring but does not require hospitalization (Padhi and Charrua-Santos, 2021).

AR and VR technologies, enhanced by 6G and its high-end technologies, can be used in different fields. AR/VR technology can help doctors create three-dimensional reconstructions of an image during an operation. Additionally, VR and AR technologies improve the rehabilitation of handicapped people. The speed of uploading data and images in 6G is expected to be very fast, and the image in 6G healthcare will be close to real-time. Therefore, doctors in one hospital can diagnose patients in another hospital. Utilizing AR/VR technology, telemedicine is enhanced, and it will be used for remote consultations between doctors or between a doctor and a patient, where the patient can consult to obtain a needed healthcare service (Jain et al., 2022).

IMPROVED TELEMEDICINE SERVICES

In the United States, where relative telemedicine vendor priorities in the telemedicine marketplace can be studied, the increasing emphasis on telemedicine by medical software developers should complement their introduction of truly free global mobile wireless and ecosystem platforms. During the COVID-19 pandemic, with consequent numerous healthcare data leaks, the United States' rational security for telemedicine wetware and infrastructure should be supported correspondingly. At present, remote telemedicine military healthcare is well-advanced, network-oriented, with global UAV (Unmanned Aerial Vehicle)/USV (Unmanned Surface Vehicle)/ UUV (Unmanned Underwater Vehicle) roaming networks synchronized to establish a methodology for coverage from coastlines inward to provide near-instantaneous data delivery to the most isolated of population dwellings. C-OT (Clinical Outreach Team)-enabled global healthcare provider access to primary digital diagnostic and healthcare services has enabled the military to execute more focused healthcare support in its battle to enhance military readiness and optimization using new 6G-powered technology demonstrators. The United States should capitalize on the telemedicine cost savings achieved to further incentivize the development of medical devices for the domestic global telemedicine network (Ishibashi et al., 2022).

In the United States alone, the 41% access to telemedicine services by the entire population represents a significant common denominator on the demand side compared to the anticipated global population of 7.83 billion to meet healthcare needs in 2025. Economies that disruptively integrate 6G for the provision of next-generation telemedicine services are thus expected to generate fast-growing healthcare solutions and to become market leaders in a sector focused on the 6Gs, incorporating supply chain sorting, customized onshore healthcare, personalized AI patient treatment suggestions, advanced instant surgical data processing, and real-time remote emergency support for ambulance and air ambulance providers above urban centres. In turn, this will lead large corporations in strategic locations to pay significant premiums for improved executive and employee healthcare for their avoidance of compromised system vulnerabilities and the potentially catastrophic impacts of cryptic bio agents, enhancing some smaller, isolated economies to monetize 6G as a primary sources of telemedicine for secure international remote patient access (Tataria et al., 2021).

A HEALTHCARE MONITORING SYSTEM

AI and the 6G revolution will revolutionize health monitoring by allowing for real-time data processing, remote monitoring, personalized care, predictive analytics, healthcare automation, and improved diagnosis and treatment. The low latency and high data transfer speeds of 6G networks make it possible to seamlessly transmit and analyse health data, resulting in prompt interventions and personalized healthcare recommendations based on individual data insights by systems that can analyse large databases to detect patterns, anticipate health trends, and automate healthcare operations. Combining AI and 6G technologies can improve patient care by making it more efficient, proactive, and personalized (Giordani et al., 2020).

BARRIERS TO ADOPTION

As in digital technology, all sectors—policy, business, and society—will have to adapt to 6G. Actors and regulators on both national and international scales should also take on these challenges. Furthermore, 6G seems to provide the functional transformation of capacity, speed, and latency. It would be wise for each sector to define its security objectives and the methods to achieve them. Once again, regulators must work with standardization organizations to incorporate safety into the design of future technological developments and remain at the heart of R&D (Research and Development) in press relations. This vision is key to defining a use case for the 6G generation of technology, which is geared towards a reassuring future for society. Successful adoption and integration of 6G wireless technology depend on its complex IT (Information Technology) infrastructure. Suppose it satisfies regulatory requirements for a global, potentially intergenerational patient pool. In contrast to 2G to 5G mobile services that have emerged from developed regions. In that case, 6G is harnessing global inclusivity and human needs as its primary design objective. Secondly, this technology raises the critical question of the available bandwidth on Earth due to spatial and frequency limits. However, emphasis on digital data encouraged investment in cable infrastructure, associated with cooperation among telecommunication companies. The capacity to deliver 10G, which will be deployed on fibre, involves a significant increase in infrastructure. The integration of 6G communication technology has its challenges. First and foremost is the uncertainty of penetration and equity of access to 6G connectivity in geographical areas worldwide. Subsequently, the need for development and investment, maintenance and rebooting, avoiding obsolescence, and cybersecurity defence has potential implications for increased operating costs and staff skills to meet the IT specialist requirements. This is a clear long-term cost. All these costs and vulnerabilities must be considered, as this is a highly sensitive area since personal and private data are at the heart of healthcare (Liu et al., 2020).

Legal and regulatory challenges are critical for 6G healthcare adoption. Interest in legal and regulatory concerns in healthcare technology innovation has increased in the last few years. A scoping review on legal frameworks for AI found that the application of AI in medicine and healthcare inherently deals with human lives, and therefore, legal and ethical issues surrounding AI in this domain are distinct and more extensive than in other industries, such as logistics or transport. Healthcare regulatory authorities usually function passively, waiting for stakeholders to realize and address the implications of a new technology. Once launched in the market, regulators are supposed to guarantee the safety, privacy, and effectiveness of the technology and its specific applications. Additionally, several studies described general barriers that legal issues can pose to healthcare technology, pointing out that the lack of understanding and awareness of IT legal issues can prevent organizations and companies from achieving their full potential (Murdoch, 2021).

CASE STUDIES OF 6G HEALTHCARE IMPLEMENTATION

Disasters cause 200,000 deaths globally and impair survivors' physical and mental health, worsen living conditions (potable water/food shortage), and lead to social disruptions and mental health problems, leading to around 250,000 deaths annually in the future. To provide immediate medical care and support the rescue work after a disaster occurs in a local area, in this study, we propose a 6G vital signals delivery system with intelligent networks capturing human life information. In our research, the ReRNN (Recalling-Enhanced Recurrent Neural Network) T&D (Transmission and Distribution) model is designed to transfer 12-lead ECG (Electrocardiogram) vital signal data across different satellite links with 28 GHz 6G frequency, and the intelligent signal movement co-generating scheme-enabled UAM (Urban Air Mobility) Drone/UGV (Unmanned Ground Vehicle) Robot to make intelligent transmission decisions. The designed system is used in a three-dimensional urban area scenario processed by 6G 3D intelligent networks. The proposed system is validated and simulated, and the practical test results demonstrate that it significantly enhances the disaster area's connectivity and healthcare resource flexibility and space-time-area metrics rapid diagnosis potential (Patgiri et al., 2021).

6G VITAL SIGNALS DELIVERY WITH DRONES FOR DISASTER REGION HEALTHCARE

There are a few factors that hamper the adoption of modern healthcare technologies in lower-income countries. While the low production costs tend to bring the prices down, procurement volume, such as limited state budgets and low device utilization rates, tends to make the production of custom devices and high-risk investments less attractive. Generally, patients and health professionals in developing countries are willing to participate in studies to develop high-tech applications since they view technology as a panacea for their local plight. This has led to an exponential increase in the number of studies in e-health, telemedicine, m-health, and Information and Communication Technologies for Development (ICT4D). We aim to develop new systems that can bridge the physical limitations and moral hazards encountered by private actors when investing in low-income telemedicine and m-health services. As we have some evidence that patients in developing countries are willing to contribute to e-health solutions and can get impressive results within a few days of operation, we decided to invest in systems with very low entry barriers, albeit with slight performance trade-offs (Mucchi et al., 2020).

DIGESTIBLE MEDICAL DEVICES AND HEALTHCARE DELIVERY SYSTEMS FOR LOWER-COST COUNTRIES

Stepping towards Affordable Healthcare Solutions. In today's world, revolutionary advancements continually shape the medical industry, particularly digestible medical devices and healthcare delivery systems. These groundbreaking technologies are poised to revolutionize healthcare accessibility, particularly in lower-cost countries. These devices offer promising solutions to bridge the gap between limited resources and ever-growing healthcare needs by combining innovation, portability, and cost-effectiveness. Digestible medical devices entail developing innovative technologies that patients can safely ingest, providing real-time data and insights about their health conditions. Such devices, often in the form of swallowable capsules or smart pills, enable healthcare providers to monitor a patient's vitals, deliver targeted treatments, and diagnose diseases more efficiently. These breakthrough devices are non-invasive and minimize the need for invasive surgical procedures, allowing for a more patient-friendly and cost-effective approach to healthcare. In conjunction with digestible medical devices, healthcare delivery systems tailored for lower-cost countries are becoming increasingly prominent. These systems focus on addressing the unique challenges faced by healthcare providers in resource-constrained regions (Javaid et al., 2023). They aim to provide comprehensive care and promote early intervention while considering the limited infrastructure, financial constraints, and shortage of skilled medical professionals. By leveraging technology and incorporating tele-health capabilities, these systems empower patients to access healthcare services remotely, reducing the burden on already overcrowded healthcare facilities.

The integration of digestible medical devices with tailored healthcare delivery systems has the potential to bring affordable and quality healthcare to millions of individuals in lower-cost countries. By utilizing these cutting-edge technologies, healthcare providers can monitor patient health, promptly identify potential health risks, and intervene proactively, ultimately preventing the progression of diseases. Additionally, these advancements enable remote patient monitoring, ensuring that individuals residing in rural or poor areas can access timely and specialized medical attention without the need for complicated travel arrangements. As digestible medical devices and tailored healthcare delivery systems continue to mature, their benefits are already being realized in lowering healthcare costs and improving patient outcomes. Their potential extends beyond traditional medical practices, reaching into various sectors such as clinical trials, drug administration, and preventive healthcare. The affordability and versatility of these solutions allow healthcare providers and policymakers to allocate resources more effectively, ensuring that every individual can receive the care they deserve.

In conclusion, digestible medical devices and healthcare delivery systems tailored for lower-cost countries mark a significant step towards achieving affordable and accessible healthcare worldwide. With their ability to monitor and treat patients remotely, bridge geographical barriers, and optimize healthcare delivery, these innovations hold immense promise in addressing the healthcare disparities prevalent in lower-cost regions. By prioritizing these technological advancements, a brighter and healthier future can be realized for individuals, regardless of their socioeconomic status or geographic location (Xiang et al., 2024).

REMOTE SURGERY

Tele-surgery, made possible by robotic technology and wireless networking, has transformed surgical practices by connecting patients and surgeons across distances. This novel strategy combines sophisticated communications and robots, leveraging the projected 6G network revolution and AI technologies. The 6G network's fast data transfer speeds and low latency allow for seamless communication between robotic surgical systems and doctors, bypassing geographical obstacles and providing high-quality care in remote places. AI-powered robotic equipment has precise and dexterous motions, helped by AI algorithms that continuously learn and adapt to improve surgical outcomes. AI systems evaluate and analyse data in real-time, allowing remote surgeons to make more educated decisions during tele-surgery procedures, ultimately enhancing patient safety and surgical precision (Nasralla et al., 2023).

SUCCESS STORIES AND LESSONS LEARNED

During this process, all participants sought appropriate solutions to optimize the advantages offered by the new communication capabilities of wireless systems in a continuous pursuit of excellence. In this programme, all the researchers worked exceptionally well with people who could demonstrate the real needs and deliverables that were identified as major demands by both the public and clinicians. Major achievements took place, but a significant number of pieces of research failed to answer the raised needs, as technological transfer to daily practice usually takes time and a complex chain of events tailored by dozens of successive professional entities. This is especially true with medicine, as we professionally serve a highly competent board where new ideas must be tested and established before transferring into daily or critical applications (Lu and Zheng, 2020).

Since the 1970s, Japanese scientists have been continually predicting the development capabilities of wireless generations over the coming decades. The prevailing opinion is that a new generation appears every 10 years. This prediction method has produced sumptuous results in recent years and, in 2013, the Japanese Ministry of Internal Affairs and Communications launched a programme entitled "Beyond 5G," to lead researchers from the Ministry of Health, Labour and Welfare to plan what possibly lies beyond 5G. This programme was initially organized by physicians, a funded robotics team, professors, and directly funded groups of medical experts. As real stakeholders at the national level, it was supported by government representatives seeking to improve and evolve the medical healthcare system, as well as the underlying architecture, at the local and regional levels.

ETHICAL CONSIDERATIONS

The application of AI and ML (Machine Learning) algorithms to analyse medical data has significantly improved clinical outcome measures. The widespread use of technology and advanced analytics carries risks, including exposure of research subjects to loss of privacy, loss of public trust in data-driven medical imaging and Omic'ss research, including future research that falls outside the realm of clinical use of the images, techniques, and approaches already developed, and loss of public trust resulting in delays and denials in access to research images and data. Indeed, research findings about what can be inferred from medical images have significant implications for individual medical privacy. Monitoring data collected when individuals are outside traditional hospital settings may even generate more privacy concerns due to the lack of strong security mechanisms and residential custodial care (Imoize et al., 2021).

There are numerous challenges involved in deploying 6G technology. Figure 3.2 illustrates some of them. We anticipate that ethical and privacy concerns will have a

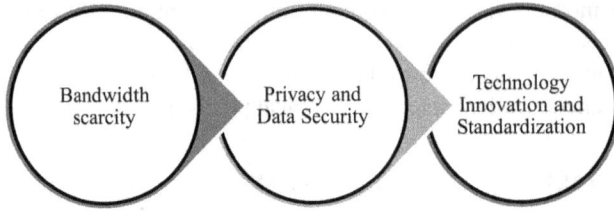

FIGURE 3.2   Some 6G deployment challenges.

significant impact on the deployment and adoption of 6G-connected health. Technological advances have supported an increasing shift of care technologies from conventional hospital/clinic settings to homes and communities. In doing so, reliance on IoT and social media, as well as sensor signals and algorithms, is increasing for remote daily monitoring, well-being assessment, chronic disease management, patient care, and even physical/mental intervention. With healthcare data collection becoming less dependent on medical facilities, this new paradigm has come under scrutiny for interoperability, interconnection, security, privacy, and confidentiality. For example, both the HeartToGo case, in which data was accessed at a remote site while being transferred from the device to the home base, and Medtronic's CareLink 2090 design flaw highlighted the importance of safety and security in the unintended event of medical device data being intercepted during transmission (Shafeeq et al., 2023).

PRIVACY AND DATA SECURITY

Data security is an issue for all technologies comprising next-generation wireless and 6G. The security measures can vary between the different technologies, requiring special attention from manufacturers, service providers, and the entities that decide the measures to be taken to protect health data. A general concern with all IT applications in healthcare, some of which frequently involve communications with individuals in person-responsibility arrangements, is the potential for unauthorized use and disclosure of sensitive personal health data. Moreover, customers of IT services in the healthcare sector increasingly want portable, interoperable, and transparent healthcare-related gadgets and applications that foster their personal health and wellness goals (Geetha and Lakshmi, 2021).

Privacy and data protection are salient in discussing technology seeking widespread healthcare adoption. In the emerging age, questions related to the technical ability to secure data and the resources required are additional dimensions of setting the story of privacy and data protection challenges. Major healthcare systems worldwide have been the victims of serious cyber-attacks, demonstrating that securing and protecting health data is not straightforward. Digital health, a growing healthcare sector, most of the time a domain whose service providers operate independently of heritage health systems, may have even fewer resources to apply against the risk of unauthorized disclosure of sensitive personal health data (Ahmad et al., 2022).

TECHNOLOGY INNOVATION AND STANDARDIZATION

Technical challenges exist in implementing new enabling technologies such as millimetre-wave and terahertz-wave communication, massive and ultra-massive MIMO (Multiple Input Multiple Output), AI, machine learning, quantum communication, and URLLC (Mohammed-Roberts et al., 2020).

BANDWIDTH SCARCITY

Finding and allocating enough bandwidth in the Terahertz (THz) frequency range for 6G is a major difficulty. THz frequencies have the potential for enormous data speeds, but they pose propagation issues and necessitate new regulatory frameworks (Fadda, 2020).

INTEROPERABILITY WITH EXISTING NETWORKS

Ensuring interoperability among diverse technologies across industries and use cases is a difficult task because many other networks utilize different standards and protocols.

GLOBAL PERSPECTIVES ON 6G HEALTHCARE ADOPTION

The recent rollouts of 5G networks and a major global pandemic have rapidly transformed the adoption of remote healthcare solutions. Such transformations are indicative of both early 6G healthcare characteristics and adoption, which should be addressed with sufficient capacity and affordability to provide quality care for everyone. This poses a question: whether an original dynamic and synergistic interaction among 6G cells, wearables, and IoTs can lower the socio-economic disparities, enable active living, and improve the quality of life via digital inclusion. To begin asking that question, this chapter presents a discussion on the evolution of wireless generations, the new actors in the healthcare market in the 6G era, along with technological enablers and health policies to foster the 6G healthcare adoption. The discussion distils three cornerstones from the current literature about global perspectives on 6G healthcare adoption, including opportunities for digital inclusion (Abdel Hakeem et al., 2022).

This chapter discusses the evolution of wireless generations, the new actors in the healthcare market in the 6G era, and the technological enablers and health policies to foster the 6G healthcare adoption. The chapter distils key elements from the current literature about global perspectives on 6G healthcare adoption and poses areas for future exploration. Preliminary findings of the linkages among Philadelphia's Digital Inclusion Roadmap, Microsoft Cities Digital Initiative, and three 6G technological enablers may provide opportunities and challenges to work for digital inclusion in 6G Philadelphia and other smart cities.

REGIONAL VARIANCES AND CULTURAL FACTORS

In contrast to the current STC (Standard Test Conditions) model for the deployment of healthcare devices and networks, where healthcare service providers are the primary clients, the future 6G model puts the individual user at the centre of the ecosystem of hierarchical communication and network systems that support the health and well-being of the user. The balance of power between healthcare consumers and healthcare service providers will change. Individual user choice will become the driving force for healthcare innovation because good ideas could spread rapidly over cluster markets, representing millions of potential users for the new healthcare service, instead of the years-long iterative clinical prospective animal and human trials. The time and financial costs for the development of new healthcare technologies are expected to drop, and the pool of capital available for venture investment in healthcare technology would rise. The healthcare ecosystem may thus quickly evolve around the preferences of users who choose what they want to adopt with significantly less formal intermediation. The market dominance of larger healthcare providers will necessarily tend to fall (Abedi, 2024).

This section explores the major global and regional variances and cultural factors that could significantly influence healthcare technology adoption, transforming healthcare globally. From devices connected to patients or worn on the body, to connected healthcare rooms and the use of various wireless communication networks for healthcare, to the establishment of IoT-integrated smart healthcare buildings and digital hospitals, and to the widespread use of tele-health and telemedicine that leverage the penetration of communication technology. The use of wireless networks, wearables, WPT (Wireless Power Transfer), and other technologies to enhance the health and well-being of people seems likely to continue evolving and extending further. The single-use 6G AIoT (Artificial Intelligence of Things) device that works with the 6G cellular network could transform the computer of users from a communication device to the omnipotent centre of users' lives.

FUTURE DIRECTIONS AND RESEARCH OPPORTUNITIES

Since there is currently a scarcity of research specifically in medical technologies, it would be particularly helpful if future researchers and policymakers from different disciplines interested in various forms of 6G technology in healthcare could address the issues discussed in this paper and, as a result, provide suggestions for further research on special research concerns. Finally, we suggest potential applications and implications, paving the way for future relevant research. The application of 6G technology in healthcare has significant implications and infinite possibilities. In the context of 6G technology innovations, the public will have opportunities to achieve life bacteriostasis, human ubiquity, and AI, unlimited medical quality, scope, and customization, and a far greater proportion of healthy and disabled lifespan than at any time in the last millennium. However, given the scarcity of research into healthcare provided using various forms of 6G technology, it is necessary to consider not just the benefits of differing 6G but also the potential social, ethical, privacy, and security issues in 6G (Banafaa et al., 2023).

EMERGING TECHNOLOGIES AND INNOVATIONS

These include fitness tracking, digital help, AR rehab systems, and MR (Mixed Reality). Speech recognition is another widespread application, providing the fastest interface for EHRs (Electronic Health Record). Finally, the consumer and commercial applications that support clinical telecommunication, such as schedule synchronization with patient ambition to adhere to instructions, remote interaction at visits and outpatient appointments, or medicines for suspected diseases, benefit from natural language, deep learning intellect, and DSS (Decision Support System). Typing is an alternative to speech recognition, but this alternative requires the review of important health advantages and disadvantages to ensure ease of use among all societies using a variety of procedures. (Chataut et al., 2024).

The transformative potential of 6G healthcare is beyond 5G healthcare settings, overlooking the current revolution, and can only if properly utilized in healthcare settings. What is currently possible is a result of the integration of various AI-supported technologies in clinical environments. Innovations in sensory systems involving non-invasive movements, natural interactions in mixed realities, and voice recognition encourage consumers and health services to interact with remote services and assistive robotics. Overlapping is another trend in the app market, driven by AI algorithms, such as apps detecting and regulating mood and behaviour, health applications in workers' workplace areas, and mindfulness and insomnia hours rest and raise attention. EHRs are related to the emergence of close-globe technology. These concentrate on real-time information about healthcare occasions near individuals, particularly through temporal, spatial, and context details (Xue et al., 2024).

DEVELOPING QUANTUM KEY DISTRIBUTION SCHEMES

Research should develop realistic, scalable quantum key distribution techniques that meet the high-speed and bandwidth requirements of 6G networks. More research on entanglement is needed for 6G networks to be secure and efficient. Researchers should investigate producing, distributing, and utilizing entangled quantum states to improve communication security and create new protocols with better performance (Zawish et al., 2024).

CASE STUDY: EXPLORING AND ANALYSING THE ROLE OF HYBRID SPECTRUM SENSING METHODS IN 6G-BASED SMART HEALTHCARE APPLICATIONS

Researchers are prioritizing the development of fast and real-time healthcare and monitoring systems due to the rapid technological advancements in the modern world. A highly effective choice is smart healthcare, which utilizes a range of sensors and devices worn on and off the body to continuously track patients' well-being and seamlessly share information with medical facilities and healthcare experts. Cognitive radio (CR) can be advantageous for efficient and intelligent healthcare systems to transmit and receive patient health data by utilizing the primary user (PU) spectrum. This study introduces a technique that integrates energy detection (ED) and cyclostationary (CS) spectrum sensing (SS) algorithms. This method was employed to evaluate the SS capabilities in CR-based smart healthcare systems. The suggested Enhanced Detection and Cooperative Sensing (ED-CS) technique enhances the accuracy of SS in CR systems. Due to its simple implementation, ED is primarily utilized for detecting unused frequency bands. If the electronic device is unable to locate the unused frequency range, the signals are detected using CS-SS, a technique that utilizes the cyclic statistical characteristics of the signals to distinguish the PUs from the interfering signals.

The simulation employed 20,000 samples, utilized 64-QAM (Quadrature Amplitude Modulation) modulation, employed a 64-point Fast Fourier Transform (FFT), had an overlapping factor of 4, and employed NOMA (Non-Orthogonal Multiple Access) waveform in the presence of a Rician channel. The simulation findings provide useful insights for examining concepts by creating a controlled environment to investigate hypothetical scenarios. Figure 3.3 presents an analysis of the detection performance of both the ED-CS and traditional approaches. The suggested ED-CS achieves the highest detection at a signal-to-noise ratio (SNR) of −2 dB, followed by CS at 2.1 dB, MF (Matched Filter) at 4.2 dB, and ED at 6.2 dB. Therefore, it may be inferred that the ED-CS performs better than the CS, MF, and ED by achieving a gain of 4.1 dB, 6 dB, and 7.9 dB, respectively.

It is observed that the maximum value of probability of detection (Pd) occurs at the false alarm probabilities of 0.1, 0.3, 0.55, and 0.62 for the methods ED-CS, CS, MF, and ED, respectively. Thus, it can be inferred that the suggested ED-CS demonstrates effective performance in scenarios with significant false alarm rates when compared to traditional methods (Figure 3.4).

In summary, the proposed hybrid ED-CS method improves and optimizes the spectral performance of the 6G NOMA waveform. The ED-CS approach is compared to the standard CS, ED, and MF methods under a Rician channel. The superiority of the ED-CS method over standard SS methods is evident in its performance in terms of Pd, false alarm probability (Pfa), BER (Bit Error Rate), and PSD (Power Spectral Density). The ED-CS demonstrated effective signal detection at low SNR and successfully mitigated the impact of Pfa.

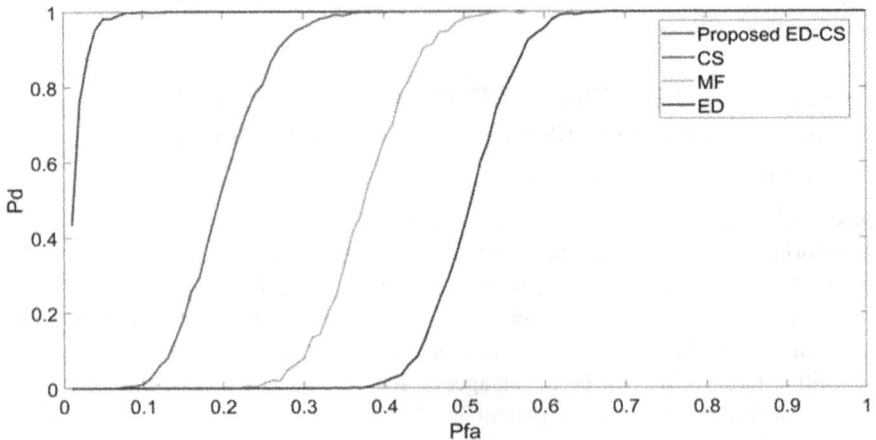

FIGURE 3.3 Comparison of signal-to-noise ratio (SNR) and probability of detection (Pd) in a Rician Channel.

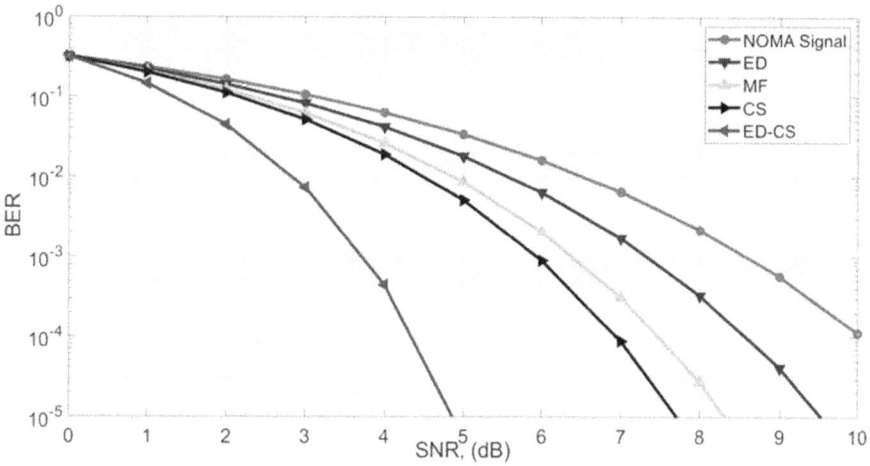

FIGURE 3.4 The relationship between the probability of a false alarm (Pfa) and the probability of detection (Pd) in a Rician Channel.

CONCLUSION AND FUTURE SCOPE

The sectors where the development of 6G will be the most effective are manufacturing, transport and logistics, resources, food, housing and construction, healthcare, tourism, recreation, entertainment, retail trade, public administration, and defence. Among all these industries, the healthcare sector stands out with technological development. The 6G technology will provide a technological leap to overcome the limitations of the 5G technology and make the currently commercialized digital systems by realizing them more functional and effective. This study shows the global trend of 6G technology through publication analysis. It can be considered a guide for useful insights regarding countries' global positioning and for managing world-leading research institutions in a particular research area that utilizes 6G technology. In this article, we have reviewed existing literature, summarized various forms of 6G technology in healthcare, and analysed the techno-behavioural enablers influencing healthcare stakeholders, particularly consumers, medical providers, and institutions, in their 6G adoption decision-making. In addition to contributing to the existing theoretical base, practical field experts and future researchers will also benefit from this article's discussions by proposing research and practical implications, addressing the application and problems of underused and invariant technologies in healthcare. Concise guidance and decision support can also be helpful for healthcare providers and institutions intending to enhance healthcare service accessibility, cost-effectiveness, and safety. In the future, we can further optimize the use of 6G networks in healthcare apps to boost the quality of experience for m-health services.

REFERENCES

Abdel Hakeem, S. A., Hussein, H. H., & Kim, H. (2022). Security requirements and chal-
    lenges of 6G technologies and applications. *Sensors*, 22(5), 1969.
Abedi, M. (2024). *Planning of wireless networks for 5G/6G applications* (Doctoral disserta-
    tion). Aalto University. ISBN 978-952-64-1669-4.
Ahmad, J., Ahmad, M. M., Su, Z., Rana, I. A., Rehman, A., & Sadia, H. (2022). A systematic
    analysis of worldwide disasters, epidemics and pandemics associated mortality of 210
    countries for 15 years (2001–2015). *International Journal of Disaster Risk Reduction*,
    76, 103001.
Akhtar, M. W., Hassan, S. A., Ghaffar, R., Jung, H., Garg, S., & Hossain, M. S. (2020). The
    shift to 6G communications: Vision and requirements. *Human-Centric Computing and
    Information Sciences*, 10(1), 53. https://doi.org/10.1186/s13673-020-00258-2
Banafaa, M., Shayea, I., Din, J., Azmi, M. H., Alashbi, A., Daradkeh, Y. I., & Alhammadi,
    A. (2023). 6G mobile communication technology: Requirements, targets, applica-
    tions, challenges, advantages, and opportunities. *Alexandria Engineering Journal*, 64,
    245–274.
Chataut, R., Nankya, M., & Akl, R. (2024). 6G networks and the AI revolution—Exploring
    technologies, applications, and emerging challenges. *Sensors*, 24(6), 1888.
Fadda, J. (2020). Climate change: an overview of potential health impacts associated with
    climate change environmental driving forces. In *Renewable Energy and Sustainable
    Buildings: Selected Papers from the World Renewable Energy Congress WREC 2018*
    (pp. 77–119). Springer International Publishing.
Geetha, R., & Lakshmi, T. (2021). Disaster Management-An Comprehensive Review.
    International Journal of Pharmaceutical Research (09752366), 13(1).
Giordani, M., Polese, M., Mezzavilla, M., Rangan, S., & Zorzi, M. (2020). Toward 6G net-
    works: Use cases and technologies. *IEEE Communications Magazine*, 58(3), 55–61.
Imoize, A. L., Adedeji, O., Tandiya, N., & Shetty, S. (2021). 6G enabled smart infrastruc-
    ture for sustainable society: Opportunities, challenges, and research roadmap. *Sensors*,
    21(5), 1709.
Ishibashi, K., Hara, T., Uchimura, S., Iye, T., Fujii, Y., Murakami, T., & Shinbo, H. (2022).
    User-centric design of millimeter wave communications for beyond 5G and 6G. *IEICE
    Transactions on Communications*, 105(10), 1117–1129.
Jain, P., Gupta, A., & Kumar, N. (2022). A vision towards integrated 6G communication net-
    works: Promising technologies, architecture, and use-cases. *Physical Communication*,
    55, 101917.
Janjua, M. B., Duranay, A. E., & Arslan, H. (2020). Role of wireless communication in health-
    care system to cater disaster situations under 6G vision. *Frontiers in Communications
    and Networks*, 1, 610879.
Javaid, M., Haleem, A., Singh, R. P., & Suman, R. (2023). 5G technology for healthcare:
    Features, serviceable pillars, and applications. *Intelligent Pharmacy*, 1(1), 2–10. https://
    doi.org/10.1016/j.ipha.2023.04.001
Jiang, W., Han, B., Habibi, M. A., & Schotten, H. D. (2021). The road towards 6G: A compre-
    hensive survey. *IEEE Open Journal of the Communications Society*, 2, 334–366.
Liu, G., Huang, Y., Li, N., Dong, J., Jin, J., Wang, Q., & Li, N. (2020). Vision, requirements
    and network architecture of 6G mobile network beyond 2030. *China Communications*,
    17(9), 92–104
Lu, Y., & Zheng, X. (2020). 6G: A survey on technologies, scenarios, challenges, and the
    related issues. *Journal of Industrial Information Integration*, 19, 100158.
Mohammed-Roberts, R., Ajumobi, O. B., & Guzman, A. (2020). *Learning from Disaster
    Response and Public Health Emergencies: The Cases of Bangladesh*, Bhutan, Nepal,
    and Pakistan.

Mucchi, L., Jayousi, S., Caputo, S., Paoletti, E., Zoppi, P., Geli, S., & Dioniso, P. (2020). How 6G technology can change the future wireless healthcare. In *2020 2nd 6G wireless summit (6G SUMMIT)*. Levi, Finland, 1–6.

Murdoch, B. (2021). Privacy and artificial intelligence: Challenges for protecting health information in a new era. *BMC Medical Ethics*, 22, 1–5.

Nasralla, M. M., Khattak, S. B. A., Ur Rehman, I., & Iqbal, M. (2023). Exploring the role of 6G technology in enhancing quality of experience for m-Health multimedia applications: A comprehensive survey. *Sensors*, 23(13), 5882.

Nayak, S., & Patgiri, R. (2021). 6G communication technology: A vision on intelligent healthcare. *Health Informatics: A Computational Perspective in Healthcare*, 1–18.

Padhi, P. K., & Charrua-Santos, F. (2021). 6G enabled tactile internet and cognitive internet of healthcare everything: Towards a theoretical framework. *Applied System Innovation*, 4(3), 66.

Patgiri, R., Biswas, A., & Roy, P. (Eds.). (2021). *Health informatics: a computational perspective in healthcare*. Singapore: Springer.

Rahman, M. M., Khatun, F., Sami, S. I., & Uzzaman, A. (2022). The evolving roles and impacts of 5G enabled technologies in healthcare: The world epidemic COVID-19 issues. *Array*, 14, 100178.

Shafeeq, K. Y., Manikappa, S. K., Raju, S. P., Doddamani, A. H., Tansa, K. A., Sadh, K., & Kasi, S. (2023, April). Integration of disaster management with public health: A capacity-building approach. In *Fifth World Congress on Disaster Management: Volume V* (pp. 363–368). Routledge.

Tataria, H., Shafi, M., Molisch, A. F., Dohler, M., Sjöland, H., & Tufvesson, F. (2021). 6G wireless systems: Vision, requirements, challenges, insights, and opportunities. *Proceedings of the IEEE*, 109(7), 1166–1199.

Wang, M., Zhu, T., Zhang, T., Zhang, J., Yu, S., & Zhou, W. (2020). Security and privacy in 6G networks: New areas and new challenges. *Digital Communications and Networks*, 6(3), 281–291.

Xiang, P., Wei, M., Liu, H., Wu, L., & Qi, J. (2024). How does technological value drive 6G development? Explanation from a systematic framework. *Telecommunications Policy*, 48, Article 102790. https://doi.org/10.1016/j.telpol.2024.102790

Xue, Q., Ji, C., Ma, S., Guo, J., Xu, Y., Chen, Q., & Zhang, W. (2024). A survey of beam management for mmWave and THz communications towards 6G. *IEEE Communications Surveys & Tutorials*, 26(3), 1520–1559. https://doi.org/10.1109/COMST.2024.3361991

Zawish, M., Dharejo, F. A., Khowaja, S. A., Raza, S., Davy, S., Dev, K., & Bellavista, P. (2024). AI and 6G into the metaverse: Fundamentals, challenges and future research trends. *IEEE Open Journal of the Communications Society*, 5, 730–778.

4 Future Proofing Healthcare
A Roadmap with 6G

Vikash Kumar, Ankush Joshi, Naman Chauhan, and Birendra Kumar Ray

INTRODUCTION

The arrival of 6G technology holds the potential to transform the healthcare sector in ways that were previously unthinkable (Abdel Hakeem et al., 2022). In an era where pandemics and aging populations pose tremendous difficulties to healthcare systems worldwide, it is more important than ever to integrate cutting-edge communication tools. Sixth-generation (6G) wireless technology is expected to serve as the foundation for a healthcare system that is more individualized, effective, and responsive. This chapter presents a thorough plan for utilizing 6G to future-proof the healthcare industry, outlining its advantages, possible uses, and implementation requirements (Porambage *et al.*, 2021).

UNDERSTANDING 6G TECHNOLOGY

The velocity, connectivity, and applicability of wireless technology have advanced exponentially from the first generation (1G) to the upcoming 6G. The healthcare industry has been significantly touched by the enormous changes that each generation has brought forth, shaping a variety of industries (Porambage *et al.*, 2021). It is anticipated that 6G will push the envelope even farther, providing previously unheard-of capabilities that will revolutionize patient outcomes and healthcare delivery. This section analyzes the main elements of 6G, defines its scope, and digs into the history of wireless technologies.

OVERVIEW OF THE DEVELOPMENT OF WIRELESS TECHNOLOGIES FROM 1G TO 6G

- **1G**: The first wireless technology generation, introduced in the 1980s, allowed for analog voice transmission. Although it was a big improvement over cable communication, its capacity and security were constrained (Solyman and Yahya, 2022).

DOI: 10.1201/9781003516590-4

- **2G**: Introduced in the 1990s, 2G allowed for text messaging, improved quality digital audio transmission, and encryption for security.
- **3G**: 3G was introduced in the early 2000s and offered quicker data transmission, making multimedia messaging, video calls, and mobile internet access possible (Thakur et al., 2022).
- **4G**: Developed in the latter part of the 2000s, 4G provided even faster speeds and more capacity, enabling mobile gaming, streaming HD videos, and more advanced internet apps.
- **5G**: Introduced in the latter part of the 2010s, the current standard offers extremely low latency and fast (Solyman and Yahya, 2022).

DESCRIBE 6G

It is projected that 6G will expand upon 5G's architecture and push the boundaries of technology even farther. It is anticipated to provide:

- **Terahertz Frequency Bands**: Possibly reaching 1 Tbps, these bands are used to deliver extremely fast data transfer speeds.
- **Latency in Microseconds**: Cutting latency down to the microsecond level will enable almost instantaneous communication.
- **Massive Device Connectivity**: Increasing the number of connected devices by an exponential amount and improving the Internet of Medical Things (IoMT) (Razdan and Sharma, 2022).
- **Intelligent Network Management**: Intelligent network management is the process of managing and optimizing networks dynamically by utilizing artificial intelligence (AI) (Thakur, 2012).

KEY FEATURES OF 6G

Ultra-connectivity

To create an IoMT that connects everything from wearable health monitoring to hospital equipment and patient records, 6G intends to connect a wide range of devices (Razdan and Sharma, 2022; Thakur et al., 2022). High levels of connectivity will make it possible to share and analyze data in real time, which will improve the coordination and effectiveness of healthcare services (Rahman et al., 2023; Solyman and Yahya, 2022).

Integration of Edge Computing and AI

With 6G, edge computing will move data processing closer to the location where the data is generated (Singh and Joshi, 2024). This lessens dependency on centralized data centers in the healthcare industry by enabling quicker data analysis and decision-making at the point of care. Predictive analytics, individualized treatment plans, and diagnostic accuracy will all improve with AI and edge computing integration (De Alwis et al., *2021*; Porambage et al., 2021).

Improved Privacy and Security

As the number of connected devices and data traffic rises, it is critical to protect patient privacy and data security. Sensitive health data will be protected with 6G's superior security standards and encryption methods. AI will also be involved in the real-time detection and mitigation of security issues (Singh and Joshi, 2024).

Innovative Uses of 6G in Healthcare

The potential of 6G technology to completely transform healthcare is becoming more and more apparent. 6G's ultra-fast speeds, low latency, and widespread device connection can support a wide range of creative applications in healthcare, greatly enhancing patient outcomes and revolutionizing the provision of healthcare services. The most cutting-edge and potential applications of 6G in healthcare are examined in this section, ranging from smart hospitals and precision medicine to telemedicine and remote monitoring (De Alwis et al., *2021*; Porambage et al., 2021).

Telemedicine and Remote Monitoring

Featuring 6G, telemedicine will be able to conduct real-time, high-definition consultations with extremely low latency, going beyond basic video conversations. To provide precise and prompt care, doctors will be able to remotely control medical equipment and use AI-driven diagnostic tools. With the use of high-resolution imaging, doctors will be able to remotely examine detailed scans and make more accurate diagnoses. Furthermore, virtual reality (VR) consultations will improve communication and patient involvement by enabling doctors and patients to engage in immersive virtual environments.

Wearable Medical Equipment

The IoMT will benefit from 6G since it will make it possible for sophisticated wearable technology to monitor health in real time. Early disease detection and proactive management will be made possible by the continuous collection and transmission of health data by these wearables. Continuous glucose monitors, for instance, will provide diabetic patients access to their blood sugar levels in real time, increasing the precision of their therapy. In a similar vein, wearable ECG (Electrocardiogram) monitors will identify abnormal cardiac rhythms and notify medical professionals right away, guaranteeing prompt treatment.

PERSONALIZED TREATMENT PLANS IN PRECISION MEDICINE

In enabling medical practitioners to create highly customized treatment plans based on a patient's genetic makeup, lifestyle, and medical history, 6G technology will be essential to the advancement of precision medicine. Doctors can improve treatment outcomes and reduce side effects by using AI-powered large-scale data analysis to forecast how patients will react to various medications. Pharmacogenomics is one important use, in which drugs are customized based on a patient's genetic profile to guarantee optimal efficacy while minimizing adverse effects. Furthermore, by integrating data from wearable technologies, genetics, and electronic health records, lifestyle integration will enable medical professionals to develop all-encompassing treatment plans, guaranteeing a patient-centered approach.

In addition to providing individualized care, 6G will transform genomics-based predictive analytics by greatly speeding up the processing and analysis of genetic data. This will result in advances in our knowledge of the genetic origins of illnesses and the creation of focused therapies. For example, research on genetic changes in malignant cells in the field of cancer genomics will aid in the development of highly customized cancer treatments, increasing patient survival rates. Furthermore, in order to identify illness risks and development and enable early treatments and preventative care, predictive health analytics will use AI to examine genetic data and other health indicators. Healthcare will change to a more proactive, accurate, and individualized approach using 6G's enhanced data processing and real-time analytics, which will eventually improve patient care and treatment effectiveness.

HOSPITALS USING SMART AUTONOMOUS SYSTEMS

6G will be used by smart hospitals to deploy autonomous systems for a range of activities, including patient care, logistics, and surgery. Healthcare delivery may be made more accurate and efficient with the use of robotics and AI-driven solutions (Tavakoli et al., 2020).

- **Robotic Surgery**: By minimizing invasiveness and performing intricate procedures with high precision, high-precision robotic devices can shorten recovery times and enhance results.
- **Automated Logistics**: Supply chain management can be done by AI-driven logistics systems, guaranteeing that prescription drugs and medical supplies are always available when needed.

ADVANCED MEDICAL DIAGNOSIS AND CARE

With facilitating lightning-fast data transfer and AI-powered analysis, 6G technology will greatly improve real-time diagnostics and enable prompt medical decision-making and treatment. By integrating AI, advanced imaging technology can identify abnormalities that the human eye might overlook, increasing the precision of diagnosis. Furthermore, quick and advanced medical tests at the patient's bedside will be made possible by mobile point-of-care testing devices, which will deliver immediate results for speedier actions. 6G will transform diagnosis with these developments, improving the effectiveness, accuracy, and responsiveness of healthcare.

6G'S ADVANTAGES FOR HEALTHCARE

6G networks will significantly increase access to healthcare by bringing strong connectivity to underserved and rural locations. Healthcare services like telemedicine, remote consultations, and emergency response systems can reach even the most remote regions thanks to lightning-fast networks and smooth data transmission, guaranteeing that no patient is left behind. Furthermore, by facilitating quick data exchange, real-time disease outbreak monitoring, and effective coordination during medical emergencies, 6G will boost global health initiatives and ultimately strengthen healthcare systems around the world.

Besides accessibility, 6G's automation, predictive analytics, and real-time monitoring will increase cost effectiveness and enhance medical results. Operational costs will be drastically decreased while preserving high-quality patient care by optimizing hospital operations with AI-powered automation and remote healthcare technologies. Hospital operations will be ensured by optimizing resource allocation through advanced data analytics. Additionally, real-time decision-making will be much improved, giving medical personnel instant access to accurate patient data, which will speed up diagnosis and treatment. Early disease detection, preemptive intervention, and improved overall patient outcomes will be made possible by continuous health monitoring via wearable technology and AI-driven analytics, ushering in a new era of accuracy and efficiency in healthcare.

FEDERATED LEARNING AND ITS TRAINING PROCESS

In addition to offering previously unheard-of connectivity and data transfer rates, 6G technology also creates new opportunities for sophisticated machine learning methods in the medical field (Zhang et al., *2021*). Federated Learning (FL) is one such method that preserves data privacy while enabling decentralized model training across numerous devices or organizations. The notion of FL, its significance in the context of 6G healthcare, and the comprehensive procedure for training machine learning models with this method are all covered in this part. FL is a decentralized machine learning technique in which models are cooperatively trained without the need to share raw data between many devices or organizations (Porambage et al., 2021). Rather, the model is trained locally on each participant's input, and only model changes (like gradients or parameters) are shared with the central server (Rahman et al., 2023). These updates are combined by the server to produce a global model, which is then redistributed to every participant for additional training.

RELEVANCE TO MEDICAL CARE

- **Data Privacy**: By keeping patient data localized and eliminating the need to move sensitive information across networks, FL improves data privacy.
- **Cooperation**: It allows for cooperative learning across various medical professionals, academic institutions, and even nations, promoting creativity while honoring privacy restrictions.

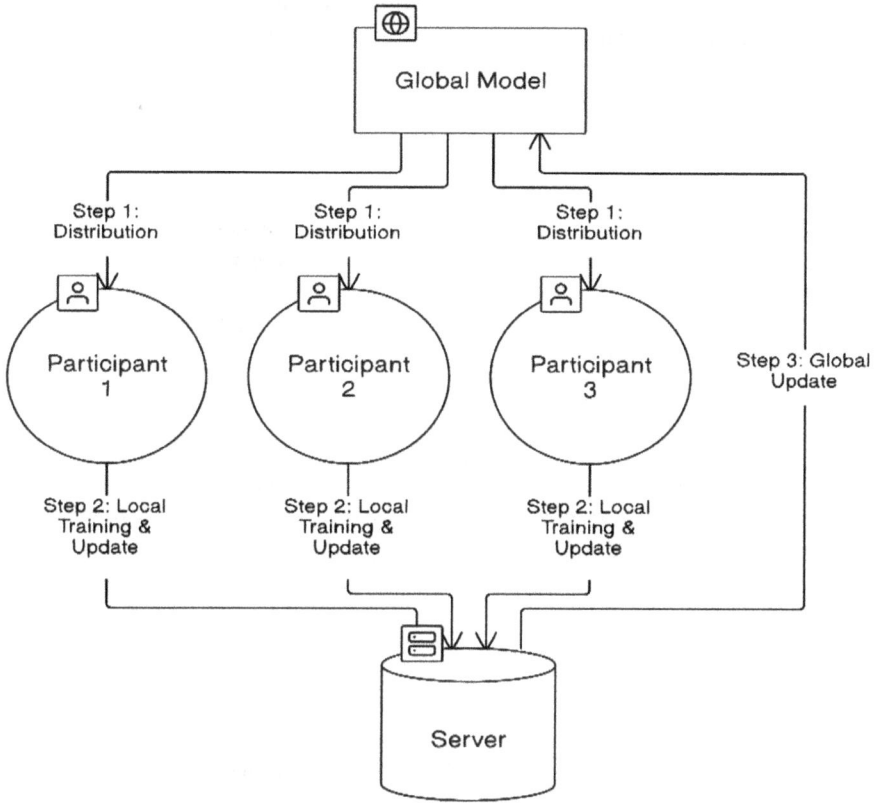

FIGURE 4.1 Federated learning and its training process.

- **Scalability**: FL is appropriate for the heterogeneous and pervasive nature of healthcare data since it can manage massive amounts of data dispersed across multiple sources (Figure 4.1).

THE STEP-BY-STEP TRAINING PROCESS FOR FEDERATED LEARNING

COMMENCEMENT

Global model initialization, which can be done with randomly supplied parameters or as a pretrained model, is the first step in the FL process. Sensitive data is kept safe and decentralized by distributing this global model to all participating devices or institutions, guaranteeing that every client has a copy to start local training.

REGIONAL INSTRUCTION

During a predetermined number of epochs or until a predetermined convergence condition is satisfied, each participating client trains the global model using its local dataset. To ensure that the model improves without sharing raw data, the client creates model updates—such as modified weights or gradients—after local training is finished. These updates reflect patterns learned from the local data.

Aggregation Model

Users submit their model updates to the central server after local training is finished, guaranteeing that raw data is kept private and that only model modifications—like updated weights or gradients—are shared. After that, the central server aggregates the data, usually by weighted average, considering how many training data points each client consumed. The global model is improved overall in terms of accuracy and efficacy by this aggregated update (Nguyen et al., 2022).

Update of the Global Model

The global model is improved and refined by the central server using the aggregated information, making it more precise and effective with each repetition. All participating clients receive the redistributed model after it has been changed, and they utilize it as the new baseline for their subsequent local training session. Until the model performs at its best, this iterative process continues.

Convergence and Iteration

Once the global model reaches an optimal state, the iterative training process is performed several times, including local training, model updates, aggregation, and redistribution. Following convergence, the model is tested and assessed on a different validation dataset to guarantee its efficacy, precision, and applicability in a range of real-world situations.

APPLICATIONS OF FEDERATED LEARNING IN HEALTHCARE

Disease Prediction and Diagnosis

- **Collaborative Diagnostics**: Hospitals can work together to train diagnostic models on a variety of patient data sets without disclosing private information, which produces diagnostic tools that are more precise and applicable to a wider range of patients (Zhang et al., 2021).
- **Predictive analytics**: By using FL to create patient outcome prediction models, proactive and individualized care can be provided.

Genomics and Drug Discovery

- **Genomic Research**: By working together to analyze genomic data, researchers can make faster discoveries while protecting the privacy of genetic information (Rahman et al., 2023).

- **Drug Efficacy Studies**: By working together to evaluate clinical trial data, pharmaceutical companies can evaluate the safety and efficacy of their drugs, accelerating the development of novel therapies (Zhang et al., *2021*).

FEDERATED LEARNING'S (FL) CHALLENGES WITHIN THE HEALTHCARE INDUSTRY

Greater Safety and Privacy: FL makes sure that private patient information stays on local devices, lowering the possibility of data breaches and adhering to laws like GDPR (General Data Protection Regulation) and HIPAA (Health Insurance Portability and Accountability Act). FL maintains strong security measures (Kumar et al., 2024) while reducing the attack surface for cyber threats by decentralizing data storage.

Scalable and Innovation: FL fosters different datasets for more accurate AI models by facilitating smooth collaboration between healthcare organizations without requiring the sharing of raw data (Joshi and Tiwari, 2023). This method guarantees scalable solutions that can be tailored to different healthcare applications while protecting patient privacy, expediting medical research, and enabling individualized treatment programs (Zhang et al., 2021).

ROADMAP TO IMPLEMENTATION

INTRODUCTION TO INFRASTRUCTURE DEVELOPMENT

To use 6G technology in the healthcare industry, a strong and well-thought-out infrastructure is needed. In addition to installing the digital and physical components required for 6G, building this network also entails making sure it interfaces seamlessly with the healthcare IT (Information Technology) systems that are currently in place (Akhtar et al., 2020). The procedures for building the infrastructure needed for the implementation of 6G in the healthcare industry are described in this part, along with methods for making sure the new system works well with the old one (Nayak and Patgiri, 2021).

BUILDING THE NETWORK STRUCTURE

Spectrum Distribution and Control

Authorities and regulatory bodies must set aside certain frequency bands to supply enough bandwidth for smooth medical applications, allowing for ultra-fast, low-latency communication, in order to guarantee the effective integration of 6G in healthcare. Furthermore, strict regulatory compliance mechanisms need to be put in place to guarantee that 6G networks follow safety, security, and privacy regulations, especially when handling sensitive medical data. These rules will guarantee that healthcare systems function safely and effectively within the 6G framework, protect patient information, and preserve data integrity (Joshi et al., 2025).

Material Infrastructure

A strong infrastructure is necessary for the effective deployment of 6G in healthcare, beginning with the installation of extensive fiber optic networks to guarantee ultra-low latency and high-speed data transfer. Furthermore, the deployment of 6G base stations and small cells will offer extensive and dense network coverage, especially in distant and medical environments where connectivity is essential. Data centers and edge computing nodes must be set up in order to effectively handle the enormous amounts of data produced by 6G-enabled medical devices. This will allow for the processing, storing, and analysis of medical data in real time, improving healthcare delivery.

Architecture of Networks

- **Infrastructure and Security Improvements**: In order to increase speed and dependability, the healthcare industry will need to implement 6G. Additionally, network slicing will be necessary to establish specialized virtual networks for various medical applications. Advanced encryption methods and AI-driven security measures will shield patient data from online attacks in order to guarantee data protection. To guarantee smooth interoperability between healthcare systems and devices, standardization initiatives will also be required, along with stringent testing and certification.
- **Integration, Difficulties, and Cooperation**: Assessing present infrastructure, identifying gaps, and putting open APIs (Application Programming Interface) and data standardization in place for seamless data sharing are all necessary for the successful integration of 6G with current healthcare IT systems. Prior to full deployment, 6G applications will be improved through a staged integration strategy that includes pilot projects and small enhancements. To effectively adapt, healthcare workers will need training courses and change management techniques. Large-scale 6G projects will require cooperation from public-private partnerships, healthcare providers, and industry leaders in order to be funded and carried out. To make 6G-powered healthcare solutions broadly available, major obstacles include managing infrastructure costs, addressing ethical AI concerns, protecting data privacy, and guaranteeing network stability (Abdel Hakeem et al., 2022).
- **6G Healthcare Integration**: To ensure smooth compatibility and interoperability, integrating 6G technology with current healthcare IT systems calls for a methodical approach. To examine the healthcare infrastructure's present capabilities and limits, a thorough inventory assessment must be carried out. A gap analysis must then be performed to determine what needs to be upgraded or replaced. Open APIs and data standardization must be put in place to promote interoperability and guarantee seamless communication between new 6G technologies and legacy systems. Prioritizing crucial areas like remote monitoring and emergency services, a staged integration plan that begins with pilot projects and small updates can assist in identifying potential issues prior to full-scale deployment. Healthcare workers should also be introduced to 6G apps through training programs, and change

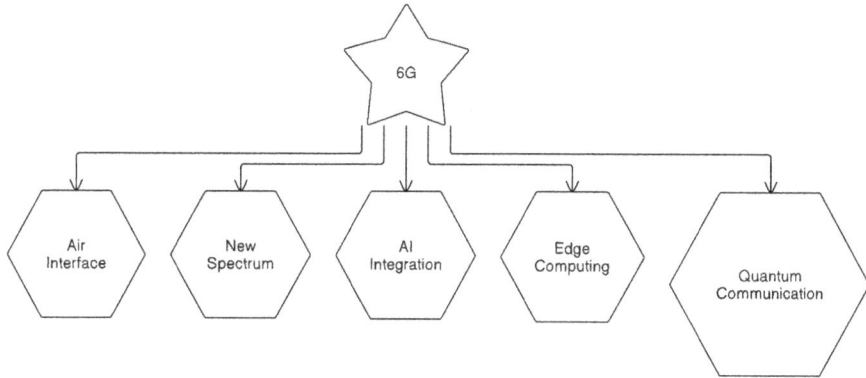

FIGURE 4.2 6G wireless network elements.

management techniques will help to avoid interruptions and guarantee seamless transitions. To pool resources, share expertise, and secure finance for large-scale 6G infrastructure projects—and eventually create a healthcare ecosystem that is more efficient and prepared for the future (Bhat and Alqahtani, 2021)—strong industry collaboration and public-private partnerships will be crucial (Figure 4.2).

CHALLENGES AND THINGS TO THINK ABOUT

Technical Difficulties

- **Network Stability**: Guaranteeing the stability and dependability of 6G networks, particularly in vital medical situations.
- **Interoperability**: Ensuring smooth communication between diverse medical equipment and systems.

Privacy and Ethical Issues

- **Data privacy**: Safeguarding private patient information in a networked world.
- **Ethical AI Use**: Ensuring that AI-driven healthcare decisions are impartial, open, and morally sound is known as ethical AI use (Abdel Hakeem et al., 2022).

Financial Consequences

- **Infrastructure Costs**: The substantial expenses related to creating and implementing 6G infrastructure.
- **Affordability**: Ensuring that all societal sectors can afford and utilize 6G healthcare solutions.

CONCLUSION

In conclusion, the introduction of 6G technology into healthcare systems has the potential to completely transform the sector by bringing previously unheard-of improvements in speed, connectivity, and intelligence. By tackling the present issues with telemedicine, remote patient monitoring, and health data management, these advancements will promote a more patient-centric, effective, and integrated healthcare environment (Smith and Doe, 2024). Real-time health interventions, personalized medicine, and predictive analytics will be made possible by the implementation of critical enablers such as edge computing, enhanced AI, and the IoMT (Razdan and Sharma, 2022). To protect patient rights and legal compliance, it is also critical to address the security, privacy, and ethical issues related to the deployment of 6G (Razdan and Sharma, 2022). The detailed roadmap intends to assist all relevant parties—from tech developers to legislators and healthcare providers—in utilizing 6G to build a future-proof healthcare ecosystem that is durable, flexible, and able to satisfy the changing demands of society.

REFERENCES

Abdel Hakeem, S. A., Hussein, H. H., & Kim, H. W. (2022). "Security requirements and challenges of 6G technologies and applications." *Sensors*, 22(5), 1969.

Akhtar, M. W., Hassan, S. A., Ghaffar, R., Jung, H., Garg, S., & Hossain, M. S. (2020). The shift to 6G communications: Vision and requirements. *Human-centric Computing and Information Sciences*, 10, 1–27.

Bhat, Jagadeesha R., and Alqahtani, S. A. (2021). "6G ecosystem: Current status and future perspective." *IEEE Access*, 9, 43134–43167.

De Alwis, C., Kalla, A., Pham, Q. V., Kumar, P., Dev, K., Hwang, W. J., & Liyanage, M. (2021). Survey on 6G frontiers: Trends, applications, requirements, technologies and future research. *IEEE Open Journal of the Communications Society*, 2, 836–886.

Joshi, A., Thakur, G., Kumar, V., Singh, Y., Joshi, D. (2025). Harnessing Big Data Visualization in Bioinformatics: From Data to Discovery. In: A. Choudhury, K. Kaushik, V. Kumar, B.K. Singh (Eds.) *Cyber-Physical Systems Security. Studies in Big Data*, vol 154. Springer, Singapore. https://doi.org/10.1007/978-981-97-5734-3_12

Joshi, A., & Tiwari, H. (2023). An overview of Python libraries for data science. *Journal of Engineering Technology and Applied Physics*, 5(2), 85–90. https://doi.org/10.33093/jetap.2023.5.2.10

Kumar, R., Joshi, A., Sharan, H. O., Peng, S., & Dudhagara, C. R. (Eds.). (2024). *The Ethical Frontier of AI and Data Analysis*. IGI Global. https://doi.org/10.4018/979-8-3693-2964-1

Nayak, S., and Patgiri, R. (2021). "6G communication technology: A vision on intelligent healthcare." *Health Informatics: A Computational Perspective in Healthcare*: 1–18.

Nguyen, D. C., Pham, Q. V., Pathirana, P. N., Ding, M., Seneviratne, A., Lin, Z., ... Hwang, W. J. (2022). Federated learning for smart healthcare: A survey. *ACM Computing Surveys (Csur)*, 55(3), 1–37.

Porambage, P., Gür, G., Osorio, D. P. M., Liyanage, M., Gurtov, A., & Ylianttila, M. (2021). The roadmap to 6G security and privacy. *IEEE Open Journal of the Communications Society*, 2, 1094–1122.

Rahman, A., Hossain, M. S., Muhammad, G., Kundu, D., Debnath, T., Rahman, M., ... Band, S. S. (2023). Federated learning-based AI approaches in smart healthcare: concepts, taxonomies, challenges and open issues. *Cluster Computing*, 26(4), 2271–2311.

Razdan, S., & Sharma, S. (2022). "Internet of medical things (IoMT): Overview, emerging technologies, and case studies." *IETE Technical Review*, 39(4), 775–788.

Singh, B. P. & Joshi, A. (2024). Ethical considerations in AI development. In R. Kumar, A. Joshi, H. Sharan, S. Peng, & C. Dudhagara (Eds.), *The Ethical Frontier of AI and Data Analysis* (pp. 156–179). IGI Global. https://doi.org/10.4018/979-8-3693-2964-1.ch010

Smith, J., & Doe, A. (2024). Future proofing healthcare: A roadmap with 6G. In R. Brown (Ed.), *Advancements in Healthcare Technology* (pp. 123–145). HealthTech Publishing.

Solyman, A. A. A., & Yahya, K. (2022). "Evolution of wireless communication networks: from 1G to 6G and future perspective." *International Journal of Electrical and Computer Engineering*, 12(4), 3943.

Tavakoli, M., Carriere, J., & Torabi, A. (2020). "Robotics, smart wearable technologies, and autonomous intelligent systems for healthcare during the COVID-19 pandemic: An analysis of the state of the art and future vision." *Advanced Intelligent Systems*, 2(7), 2000071.

Thakur, G. (2012). "Analysis of Different Congestion Control Formats for TCP/IP Networks."

Thakur, G., Kumar, Y., & Bhatnagar, G. (2022). "Challenges and opportunities presented by the Internet of Things (IoTs) in the hospitality industry." *Mathematical Statistician and Engineering Applications*, 71(4), 2582–2597.

Zhang, C., et al. (2021). "A survey on federated learning." *Knowledge-Based Systems*, 216: 106775.

5 Innovations in Healthcare Communication with 6G

Afreen N., Rachit Kumar, and Awadesh Pandey

INTRODUCTION

Researchers are increasingly drawn to 6G communication technology due to its advanced capabilities and promising potential. This next-generation technology is poised to revolutionize various industries, with the transformative impacts expected to become evident from 2030 onward. Extensive discussions on the features of 6G have taken place in leading forums, continuously shaping the requirements for its development.

Nayak and Patgiri have highlighted significant issues and challenges associated with 6G communication technology. Several countries have already embarked on 6G projects to ensure timely disposition. Finland originated its 6G project in 2018, followed by the United States, South Korea, and China in 2019. Japan also joined the forefront of 6G research with its own project starting in 2020. Numerous algorithms have been developed to support (Joshi & Goyal, 2019) the advancement of 6G.

It is crucial for countries to initiate 6G projects to remain competitive internationally. In contrast, while 5G communication technology is still in the process of being fully deployed worldwide, and beyond 5G (B5G) technologies are yet to be developed, they may have limitations in fully revolutionizing modern lifestyles, societies, and businesses (Awais et al., 2023).

The extensive accumulation of comprehensive healthcare (HC) data is accompanied by the trend of gathering various items, leading to advancements in medical procedures. These diverse methodologies serve as a roadmap for progress in the realm of clinical diagnosis.

Henceforth, both industry and academia have initiated the development of the upcoming 6G network, surpassing the capabilities of 5G. Notably, proponents of 6G network design advocate the integration of artificial intelligence (AI) into its foundational protocols and operations to achieve optimal performance and energy efficiency.

HC, once centered on hospitals and specialists, is rapidly transitioning toward dispersed, patient-centered care. The transition is driven by a multitude of technological progressions, where communication technology stands out for its pivotal role in facilitating personalized and remote HC services (Padhi & Charrua-Santos, 2021). Currently, the HC sector heavily relies on the 4G network and other communication technologies to support sophisticated applications, with continuous expansions underway to meet upcoming requirements. However, as the smart HC industry continues to grow, an increasing number of applications will generate diverse types of

DOI: 10.1201/9781003516590-5

data. Existing communication technologies are insufficient to handle the complex and dynamic requirements posed by these varied smart HC applications. Consequently, the 5G and forthcoming 6G networks are anticipated to facilitate smart HC applications that meet the majority of necessary provisions, including ultra-low latency.

These advancements aim to enhance network coverage, performance, and address security concerns. The global deployment of 5G innovation has been expedited, with its components proving ideal for driving significant advancements in HC applications. These include in-building information management, streamlined handling of large imaging datasets, remote patient monitoring, and virtualization capabilities. The HC landscape is on the brink of transformation with the emergence of 6G communication technology. Expected to revolutionize various sectors, including HC, 6G will usher in an era of AI-driven HC, fundamentally altering our lifestyle. Time and location barriers in HC delivery will be overcome by 6G, paving the way for enhanced accessibility and efficiency (Figure 5.1).

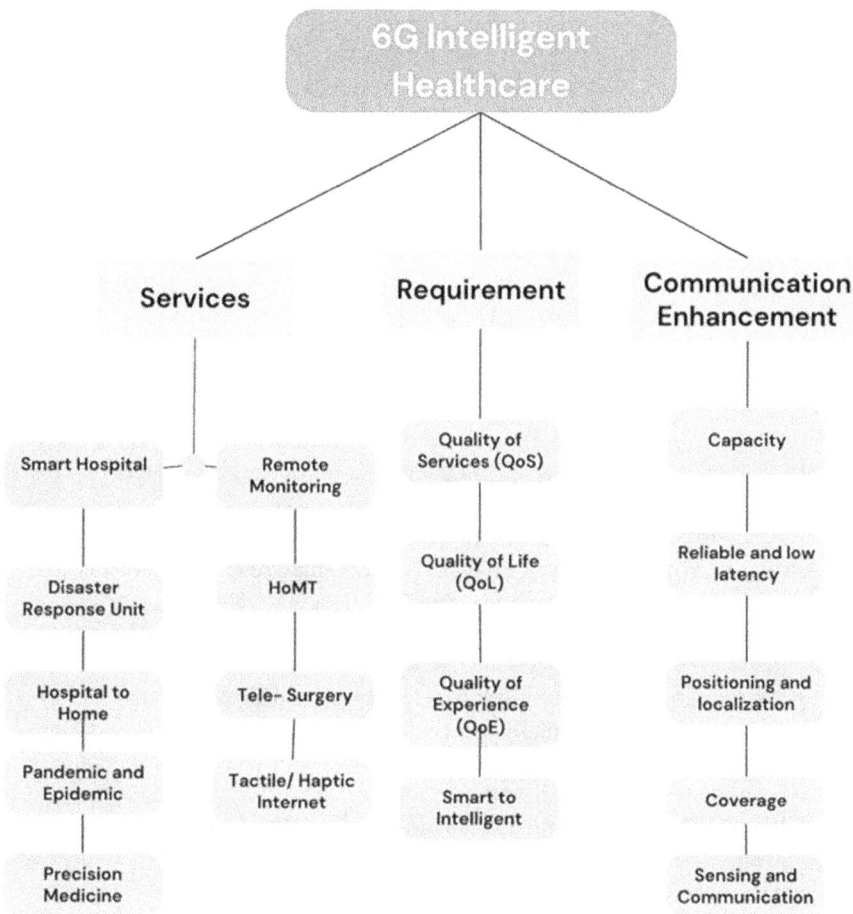

FIGURE 5.1   Taxonomy of 6G intelligent healthcare.

FEATURES OF 6G TECHNOLOGY

- **Enhanced Data Speeds and Bandwidth**: 6G is projected to achieve significantly higher data transmission speeds compared to 5G, possibly reaching terabits per second (Tbps) levels. This immense speed boost will facilitate seamless streaming of high-definition content, rapid data transfers, and instantaneous downloads and uploads. (Abdel Hakeem et al., 2022; Gerke et al., 2020)
- **Reduced Latency and Improved Reliability**: One of the defining characteristics of 6G will be its ultra-low latency, measured in microseconds or even nanoseconds. This minimal delay is critical for applications demanding real-time responsiveness, such as autonomous vehicles, telemedicine, and industrial automation. Additionally, 6G aims to enhance reliability through ultra-reliable communication (URC) features, ensuring consistent and dependable network connections. (Akhtar et al., 2020; Dangi et al., 2023)
- **Utilization of Advanced Frequency Bands**: 6G is expected to leverage a broader spectrum of frequencies, including millimeter wave (mmWave), terahertz (THz), and sub-terahertz bands. These higher frequency ranges offer increased bandwidth and data capacity, albeit with challenges related to signal propagation and coverage. (Banafaa et al., 2023; Qureshi et al., 2023)
- **Massive Connectivity for IoT**: Building upon the foundation of 5G's massive machine-type communication (mMTC), 6G will further support a vast network of interconnected Internet of Things (IoT) devices. This encompasses sensors, wearables, smart infrastructure, industrial equipment, and other IoT endpoints, fostering the growth of the Internet of Everything (IoE) ecosystem.
- **Integration of Artificial Intelligence (AI)**: AI will play a pivotal role in optimizing 6G networks, enabling intelligent resource allocation, predictive analytics, and automated network management. Edge computing capabilities will also be enhanced, allowing AI-powered applications to process data locally, reducing latency and enhancing overall efficiency.
- **Emphasis on Security and Privacy**: 6G will place a higher priority on strong security and privacy safeguards due to the growing complexity and size of connected devices. To protect user data and network integrity, this includes sophisticated encryption techniques, safe authentication procedures, and privacy-enhancing technology.
- **Environmental Sustainability**: 6G technology will aim to be more energy-efficient and environmentally sustainable. Innovations in hardware design, network architecture, and power management will contribute to reducing the carbon footprint of wireless networks. (Chen & Kang, 2023)
- **Global Collaboration and Standards Development**: Collaboration among industry stakeholders, standardization bodies, and regulatory authorities will be pivotal for the development and adoption of 6G technology. This includes defining technical standards, spectrum allocation, and interoperability frameworks to ensure seamless connectivity on a global scale. (Akhtar et al., 2020)

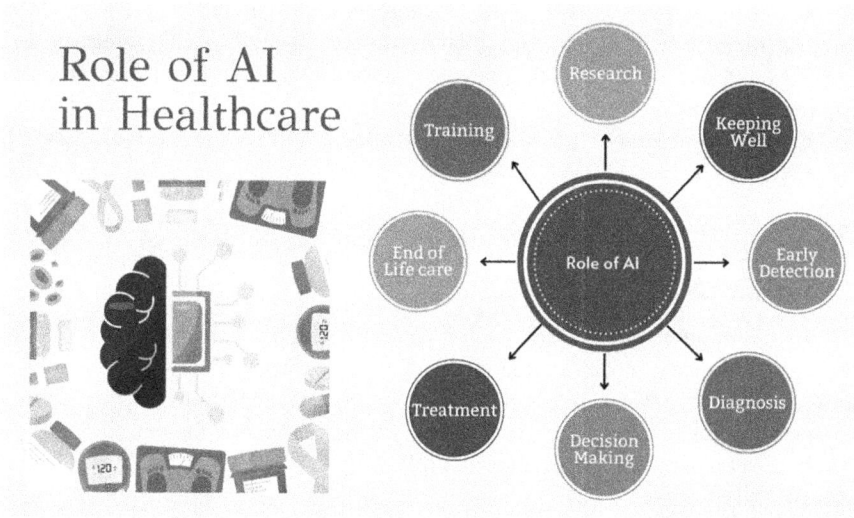

FIGURE 5.2   Role of artificial intelligence in healthcare.

The evolution toward 6G technology promises to unlock unprecedented possibilities in wireless communication, paving the way for transformative applications and driving innovation across industries. However, it's crucial to note that 6G is still in the early stages of research and development, with commercial deployment expected in the coming decade (Figure 5.2).

THE NEED FOR ADVANCED COMMUNICATION IN HEALTHCARE

In today's HC environment, the complexity of patient needs and the rapid pace of medical advancements necessitate more sophisticated communication systems. Traditional methods like face-to-face consultations and basic telephone interactions are often insufficient for modern HC's demands. This section delves into why advanced communication technologies are critical and how they can revolutionize HC delivery.

CURRENT CHALLENGES IN HEALTHCARE COMMUNICATION

One major challenge in HC communication is the fragmentation of information across different systems and providers. Often, patient data is stored in separate, incompatible databases, leading to significant difficulties in sharing information across various HC providers. This lack of integration can result in miscommunications, delayed diagnoses, and even medical errors.

Furthermore, existing telemedicine platforms often struggle with technical limitations such as low bandwidth, poor video quality, and high latency. These issues can compromise the quality of remote consultations, making it harder for HC providers to deliver effective care, especially in rural or underserved areas where connectivity may be poor.

Another pressing issue is the lack of interoperability among different HC technologies. Many systems are not designed to work together seamlessly, creating inefficiencies and barriers to adopting new technologies that could improve care. This disjointedness can slow down the integration of innovations like electronic health records (EHRs), wearable health devices, and telehealth services into existing HC frameworks (Kim et al., 2023).

THE ROLE OF COMMUNICATION IN PATIENT CARE AND MANAGEMENT

Effective communication is crucial for patient care and management, impacting everything from diagnosis to treatment adherence. Clear, timely communication between HC providers and patients can significantly enhance health outcomes. When patients fully understand their diagnoses and treatment plans, they are more likely to adhere to recommended therapies and follow-up appointments, which can lead to better overall health.

Advanced communication technologies enable continuous monitoring and proactive management of chronic conditions. For example, real-time data sharing allows HC providers to monitor patients' health metrics continuously, identify potential issues early, and adjust treatment plans promptly. This proactive approach can reduce hospital readmissions and improve patient quality of life.

Moreover, these technologies facilitate better collaboration among HC teams. Multidisciplinary teams can communicate more effectively, share insights, and make coordinated decisions, leading to comprehensive and integrated patient care. For instance, a cardiologist, primary care physician, and dietician can all access the same patient records and collaborate on a cohesive care plan, ensuring that all aspects of the patient's health are addressed.

Enhanced communication technologies also play a critical role in patient engagement and empowerment. Tools like mobile health applications and patient portals give patients easy access to their health information, allowing them to take an active role in managing their health. Patients are able to arrange appointments, ask for prescription refills, and communicate directly with their HC providers, which encourages a patient-centric approach to care.

In summary, the need for advanced communication in HC is evident. Addressing current challenges and leveraging modern communication technologies can improve efficiency, enhance patient outcomes, and ensure more equitable access to care. Integrating advanced communication solutions is essential for meeting the contemporary HC system's demands and providing high-quality care to all patients.

APPLICATIONS OF 6G TECHNOLOGY IN HEALTHCARE

Dynamic Remote Patient Monitoring

Utilizing 6G's ultra-responsive network capabilities, HC providers can implement dynamic remote patient monitoring solutions. These systems leverage wearable devices and medical sensors to continuously collect patient data, such as vital signs and activity levels, in real-time. This data is securely transmitted over the 6G network to HC professionals for immediate analysis. Any anomalies or concerning trends can prompt timely interventions, potentially preventing medical complications and reducing hospital readmissions. (Tijus et al., 2024; Suraci et al., 2023)

IMMERSIVE TELEMEDICINE EXPERIENCES

With the advent of 6G, telemedicine experiences will become more immersive and interactive. Through high-definition video streaming and augmented reality (AR) technologies, patients can engage in virtual consultations with HC providers as if they were in the same room. Specialists can remotely guide patients through self-examinations or demonstrate medical procedures with enhanced clarity and precision. This level of immersive telemedicine can foster stronger patient-provider relationships and improve health literacy among patients.(Daher et al., 2022; Jacobs et al., 2022; Kim et al., 2023)

PRECISION REMOTE SURGERY

6G's ultra-low latency and reliability open up possibilities for precision remote surgery. Surgeons equipped with haptic feedback devices and robotic surgical systems can perform intricate procedures from distant locations with minimal delay. The seamless transmission of high-resolution video feeds and real-time sensory feedback ensures that surgical interventions are conducted with utmost accuracy and safety. This capability is particularly beneficial for providing expert surgical care to patients in remote or underserved areas. (Ahmed Solyman & Yahya, 2022; Kharche & Kharche, 2023; Nasralla et al., 2023)

The term "telesurgery" refers to the practice of physicians performing surgery from a distance. Robots, nurses, and intermediaries between doctors who are remote are all necessary in this cutting-edge medical practice. Telesurgery requires very high data rates and ultra-reliable low-latency communication (URLLC) for effective communication, which current 5G and B5G technologies cannot completely enable. Thus, for telesurgery to be successful, 6G technology must be implemented. (Choi et al., 2018)

In telesurgery, communication in real time is essential. Physicians can give advice orally, via teleconferencing, or by teleassistance. More interactive verbal advice during surgery can be made possible via holographic communication with 6G technology. This enables doctors to virtually accompany patients throughout surgery and modify their vision to improve visibility of the operative area. Telestration is the practice of doing surgery remotely, frequently with the use of video. AR and virtual reality (VR) technology have the potential to improve communication in intelligent HC (Taghian et al. 2023). Furthermore, physicians can support the surgery through the use of tactile/haptic technology, which enables distant physical involvement. (Nasralla et al., 2023)

The requirements for effective telesurgery can be met by 6G communication technology, demonstrating that surgery can be performed beyond physical boundaries.

AI-DRIVEN HEALTHCARE INSIGHTS

Large-scale medical data can be transformed into useful insights by AI-driven HC analytics platforms, which are made possible by 6G's high-speed data transmission capabilities. AI systems are able to recognize trends, forecast the course of diseases, and suggest individualized treatment strategies through the analysis of patient records, diagnostic imaging, genomic data, and real-time monitoring data. In the end, this data-driven strategy improves patient outcomes and lowers HC costs by enabling HC practitioners to provide more accurate and efficient care. (Alowais et al., 2023; Secinaro et al., 2021; Sun & Zhou, 2023)

INTELLIGENT WEARABLE DEVICES (IWD)

Intelligent Wearable Devices (IWD) are internet-connected gadgets designed to transmit both psychological and physical data to testing and monitoring centers. These devices monitor various health indicators such as body weight, blood pressure, pulse rate, blood tests, and nutritional status. The results from these tests are quickly available. Additionally, IWDs learn from an individual's health history to provide personalized advice, such as recommending physical activities like walking or running (Nahavandi et al., 2022).

IWDs maintain a detailed personal history of health, nutrition, and habits, which allows them to offer dietary recommendations in case of deficiencies. By detecting minor health issues early, such as nutrient deficiencies, IWDs can reduce the frequency of hospital visits, thereby lowering medical expenses and allowing hospitals to focus on more complex cases. Furthermore, IWDs can analyze blood samples and transmit the data for pathological results, potentially enabling early detection of conditions like cancer. Consequently, IWDs can significantly improve overall health and longevity (Wu et al., 2023).

These devices are particularly crucial for elderly care, which demands intensive monitoring. Future iterations of IWDs will integrate multiple features into a single device, streamlining their functionality. While the initial versions of these comprehensive devices may be expensive, their cost is expected to decrease over time, making them affordable for the general population (Liu et al., 2021).

VIRTUAL REALITY MEDICAL TRAINING

VR technology with 6G support transforms medical education and training by offering immersive learning environments. In a virtual setting, medical professionals and students can practice operating on patients, dissecting anatomy, and interacting with them. These realistic simulations enhance learning retention, decision-making skills, and procedural proficiency without the need for physical cadavers or live patient encounters. As a result, HC professionals can continuously refine their skills and stay updated on the latest medical advancements. (Javaid & Haleem, 2020; Tene et al., 2024)

SECURE HEALTHCARE DATA MANAGEMENT WITH BLOCKCHAIN

Leveraging the security features of blockchain technology, 6G networks ensure the integrity and privacy of HC data. Blockchain-based systems enable tamper-proof storage and seamless sharing of EHRs across HC providers, insurers, and patients. Each transaction is cryptographically secured and transparently recorded on the distributed ledger, mitigating the risk of illegal access and data breaches. This secure data management framework promotes interoperability, patient-centric care, and trust within the HC ecosystem. (Anjelin & Kumar, 2023; Saeed et al., 2022)

COMMUNICATIONS IN-BODY, ON-BODY, AND OFF-BODY

By utilizing information and communication technology (ICT) capabilities, the concept of in-body, on-body, and off-body communications seeks to provide remote health monitoring. These many communication modalities are included in the Body-Layer idea. Data can be transmitted in real time to cloud and edge devices with off-body communications. The nanostructures or molecules that function as biological communication networks throughout the body are the sensors. (Ardiani et al., 2022; Ben Arbia et al., 2017; Salleh & Sam, 2016)

INTELLIGENT NANOSCALE INNER BODY COMMUNICATIONS

A new chapter in HC history is being ushered in by the development of intelligent Nanoscale inner body communications. Biological cells are laying the groundwork for the Internet of Bio-Nano Things (IoBNT) in the human body, making it possible to observe and manipulate internal organs. Medical data can now be more easily gathered and remotely shared with HC providers thanks to technology. Medical staff can take appropriate action after receiving this data. It is impossible to overestimate the importance of 6G technology in this context since it will make it possible for IoBNT and the Internet of Nano Things (IoNT) to be seamlessly integrated, revolutionizing HC monitoring and treatment. (Kuscu & Unluturk, 2021; Atta-Ur-Rahman & Alhiyafi, 2018)

HUMAN BOND COMMUNICATIONS

Using all five senses of the human body, Human Bond Communications is a cutting-edge method for data detection and transmission. The idea of sharing someone's ideas or experiences with another person may not be too far off. This progress is expected to be greatly aided by 6G technology, which will act as a material technology that interprets data from emotion sensors to improve the user experience. This invention creates opportunities for improved services like patient tracking, diagnosis, help, and therapy. (Atta-ur-Rahman et al., 2019)

These innovative applications demonstrate how 6G technology can revolutionize HC communication, delivery, and patient outcomes by enabling real-time monitoring, immersive telemedicine experiences, precision surgical interventions, AI-driven analytics, virtual medical training, and secure data management.

CHALLENGES OF 6G IN HEALTHCARE COMMUNICATION

Addressing the challenges of implementing 6G in HC communication requires a nuanced understanding of both technological limitations and the complexities of HC delivery. Here are some key challenges:

Infrastructure Deployment: Deploying 6G infrastructure, such as high-frequency small cell networks and massive Multiple Input, Multiple Output (MIMO) antennas, is a significant challenge. HC facilities, especially those in rural or underserved areas, may lack the necessary infrastructure to support 6G connectivity. Ensuring equitable access to 6G-enabled HC services requires extensive investment in infrastructure development and network expansion. (Ahad et al., 2024; Nasralla et al., 2023)

Security of Data and Privacy: The transmission of sensitive medical data over 6G networks raises concerns about data security and privacy. HC businesses need to have robust encryption technologies and data management policies to safeguard patient data from cyber threats and illegal access. Following regulations such as the Health Care Portability and Accountability Act is essential to preserving consumer confidence and regulatory compliance. (Ahad et al., 2024; Nasralla et al., 2023)

Interoperability and Standardization: Achieving seamless interoperability between disparate HC systems and devices remains a significant challenge in HC communication. 6G networks must support standardized protocols and data formats to facilitate the exchange of EHRs, medical imaging files, and real-time monitoring data across different platforms and devices. Collaborative efforts between HC stakeholders and technology providers are necessary to establish interoperability standards and ensure compatibility between 6G-enabled solutions. (Chataut et al., 2024; Porambage et al., 2021)

Digital Divide and Accessibility: The digital divide exacerbates disparities in access to HC services, particularly among marginalized and underserved populations. While 6G technology promises high-speed connectivity and advanced telemedicine capabilities, not all communities have equal access to these resources. Addressing the digital divide requires targeted interventions, such as subsidizing internet access, deploying mobile HC units, and providing digital literacy training to vulnerable populations. (Heeks, 2022; Pettersson et al., 2023)

Integration with Existing Healthcare Systems: Integrating 6G-enabled solutions into existing HC workflows and systems poses challenges in terms of compatibility, scalability, and usability. HC providers may face resistance to change from clinicians accustomed to traditional modes of care delivery. Seamless integration with EHR systems, clinical decision support tools, and billing systems is essential to maximize the benefits of 6G technology without disrupting existing workflows. (Chataut et al., 2024; Kongsen et al., 2024)

Ethical and Legal Considerations: Ethical dilemmas surrounding the use of emerging technologies in HC, such as AI-driven diagnostics and remote surgery, require careful consideration. HC providers must adhere to ethical guidelines and regulatory frameworks to ensure patient safety, autonomy, and informed consent (Kumar et al. 2024). Additionally, legal issues related to liability, malpractice, and licensure may arise in the context of remote HC delivery and cross-border telemedicine consultations. (Elendu et al., 2023; Gerke et al., 2020; Guni et al., 2024)

Addressing these challenges requires collaboration between technology providers, HC organizations, policymakers, and regulatory agencies to develop comprehensive strategies for deploying 6G technology responsibly and equitably in HC communication. By addressing infrastructure gaps, enhancing data security and privacy, promoting interoperability, bridging the digital divide, integrating with existing HC systems, and upholding ethical and legal standards, 6G has the potential to revolutionize HC delivery and improve patient outcomes.

FUTURE DIRECTIONS OF 6G IN HEALTH CARE

Plans are already in place for the construction of 6G networks, even though the implementation of 5G mobile communication networks is still in its early phases. The rise of technologies like blockchain, edge-cloud computing, federated and distributed learning, big data analytics, AI, and the IoT is the driving force behind this. These developments have made it easier for a wide range of sophisticated and dispersed smart city applications to proliferate. But as traffic demands continue to rise, current 5G networks might not be able to keep up with the many and demanding needs of these apps in terms of dependability, efficiency, and real-time operation.

Advanced technologies like holography may need data rates as high as 4.3 Tbps, and 5G networks might not be able to provide the ultra-low latencies and large data rates required for such applications. As a result, 6G networks are anticipated to outperform earlier network generations in meeting the needs of several intelligent and connected applications that have high demands for energy efficiency, wide frequency bands, ultra-low latency, and high data throughput. It is expected that AI would be crucial in facilitating these networks at different layers, such as the application, middleware, and network infrastructure layers.

6G networks stand to benefit greatly from AI's self-learning capabilities, which will make them more intelligent, nimble, flexible, and adaptive. Channel estimation purposes, modulation identification, network traffic categorization and forecasting, intelligent navigation, radio resource administration, error management, network power optimization, and the identification of intrusions, botnets, and anomalous traffic are just a few of the tasks that these advancements will make easier. Furthermore, AI will facilitate smart city application scheduling requests, effectively handle computing resources, maximize energy consumption for communication and computation, improve application performance, apply context-aware data caching, guarantee fault tolerance, and preserve data availability at the middleware layer.

AI will play a key role in enabling the development of applications across new technical paradigms in the field of smart city applications, including block chain technology, cloud computing, edge-cloud computing, healthcare (HC), Internet of Vehicles (IoV), Internet of Medical Things (IoMT), Internet of Drones (IoD), Internet of Robots (IoRT), and Industrial Internet of Things (IIoT).

CONCLUSION

The advent of 6G technology heralds a transformative era in HC communication, promising to address long-standing challenges and introduce unprecedented advancements. As we have explored, the limitations of current communication systems—such as fragmented information, technical inefficiencies, and lack of interoperability—significantly hinder the efficacy of HC delivery. However, 6G's potential to revolutionize these systems offers a glimpse into a future where these issues are mitigated.

With 6G, HC can benefit from ultra-reliable, low-latency communication networks that enhance remote patient monitoring, telemedicine, and real-time data sharing. These capabilities are particularly crucial in rural and underserved areas, where access to quality HC has been historically limited. By enabling high-quality video consultations and seamless data transmission, 6G can bridge the gap between patients and providers, ensuring equitable HC access.

Furthermore, the integration of 6G with advanced technologies such as AI, IoT, and AR/VR can facilitate smarter, more responsive HC environments. Smart hospitals equipped with interconnected devices can provide real-time insights, predictive analytics, and automated responses to patient needs, enhancing both the efficiency and quality of care. The role of augmented and VR, powered by 6G, in medical training, surgical procedures, and patient rehabilitation also points to a future where medical professionals can perform their duties with greater precision and patients can experience more engaging and effective treatment methods.

In addition to technological advancements, 6G's role in enhancing patient-provider communication and patient engagement cannot be overstated. With the ability to support extensive mobile health applications and patient portals, 6G empowers patients to take an active role in their HC journey. This heightened interaction results in stronger commitment to treatment regimens and enhanced health results.

6G has enormous potential for HC communication, but there are drawbacks as well. To fully reap the benefits of 6G, issues including data security, concerns regarding privacy, and the requirement for a strong infrastructure must be resolved. It is imperative that lawmakers, health care professionals, and technology developers work together to establish guidelines and structures that guarantee the secure and efficient deployment of 6G technologies.

In conclusion, 6G represents a significant leap forward in HC communication, offering solutions to existing problems and paving the way for innovative practices. By embracing these advancements, the HC industry can improve patient outcomes, enhance operational efficiencies, and provide more inclusive and accessible care. The future of HC, empowered by 6G, holds the promise of a more connected, responsive, and effective HC system.

REFERENCES

Abdel Hakeem, S. A., Hussein, H. H., & Kim, H. W. (2022). Vision and Research Directions of 6G Technologies and Applications. *Journal of King Saud University - Computer and Information Sciences*, 34(6), 2419–2442. https://doi.org/10.1016/J.JKSUCI.2022.03.019

Ahad, A., Jiangbina, Z., Tahir, M., Shayea, I., Sheikh, M. A., & Rasheed, F. (2024). 6G and Intelligent Healthcare: Taxonomy, Technologies, Open Issues and Future Research Directions. *Internet of Things*, 25, 101068. https://doi.org/10.1016/J.IOT.2024.101068

Ahmed Solyman, A. A., & Yahya, K. (2022). Evolution of Wireless Communication Networks: From 1G to 6G and Future Perspective. *International Journal of Electrical and Computer Engineering*, 12(4), 3943–3950. https://doi.org/10.11591/IJECE.V12I4.PP3943-3950

Akhtar, M. W., Hassan, S. A., Ghaffar, R., Jung, H., Garg, S., & Hossain, M. S. (2020). The Shift to 6G Communications: Vision and Requirements. *Human-Centric Computing and Information Sciences*, 10(1), 1–27. https://doi.org/10.1186/s13673-020-00258-2

Alowais, S. A., Alghamdi, S. S., Alsuhebany, N., Alqahtani, T., Alshaya, A. I., Almohareb, S. N., Aldairem, A., Alrashed, M., Bin Saleh, K., Badreldin, H. A., Al Yami, M. S., Al Harbi, S., & Albekairy, A. M. (2023). Revolutionizing Healthcare: The Role of Artificial Intelligence in Clinical Practice. *BMC Medical Education*, 23(1), 1–15. https://doi.org/10.1186/S12909-023-04698-Z

Anjelin, D. P., & Kumar, S. G. (2023). Blockchain Technology to Improve Security in Healthcare Data Breaches. *International Journal of Intelligent Systems and Applications in Engineering*, 11(7s), 332–339. https://ijisae.org/index.php/IJISAE/article/view/2958

Ardiani, G. A., Octaviani, S., & Iskandar, I. (2022). Simulation and Measurement of on-body and off-body Communication Propagation Channels by Using dual-band Magnetic Simulation and Measurement of on-body and off-body Communication Propagation Channels by using dual-band Magnetic Antenna Textile. *Saudi Journal of Engineering and Technology*, 7(7), 358–372. https://doi.org/10.36348/sjet.2022.v07i07.003

Atta-Ur-Rahman, & Alhiyafi, J. (2018). Health Level Seven Generic Web Interface. *Journal of Computational and Theoretical Nanoscience*, 15(4), 1261–1274. https://doi.org/10.1166/JCTN.2018.7302

Atta-ur-Rahman, Dash, S., Luhach, A. K., Chilamkurti, N., Baek, S., & Nam, Y. (2019). A Neuro-fuzzy Approach for User Behaviour Classification and Prediction. *Journal of Cloud Computing*, 8(1), 1–15. https://doi.org/10.1186/s13677-019-0144-9

Awais, M., Ullah Khan, F., Zafar, M., Mudassar, M., Zaigham Zaheer, M., Mehmood Cheema, K., Kamran, M., & Jung, W. S. (2023). Towards Enabling Haptic Communications over 6G: Issues and Challenges. *Electronics*, 12(13), 2955. https://doi.org/10.3390/ELECTRONICS12132955

Banafaa, M., Shayea, I., Din, J., Hadri Azmi, M., Alashbi, A., Ibrahim Daradkeh, Y., & Alhammadi, A. (2023). 6G Mobile Communication Technology: Requirements, Targets, Applications, Challenges, Advantages, and Opportunities. *Alexandria Engineering Journal*, 64, 245–274. https://doi.org/10.1016/J.AEJ.2022.08.017

Ben Arbia, D., Alam, M. M., Le Moullec, Y., & Ben Hamida, E. (2017). Communication Challenges in on-Body and Body-to-Body Wearable Wireless Networks—A Connectivity Perspective. *Technologies*, 5(3), 43. https://doi.org/10.3390/TECHNOLOGIES5030043

Chataut, R., Nankya, M., & Akl, R. (2024). 6G Networks and the AI Revolution—Exploring Technologies, Applications, and Emerging Challenges. *Sensors (Basel, Switzerland)*, 24(6). https://doi.org/10.3390/S24061888

Chen, S., & Kang, S. (2023). The Dual Iconic Features and Key Enabling Technologies of 6G. *Engineering*, 28, 7–10. https://doi.org/10.1016/J.ENG.2023.03.014

Choi, P. J., Oskouian, R. J., & Tubbs, R. S. (2018). Telesurgery: Past, Present, and Future. *Cureus*, 10(5). https://doi.org/10.7759/CUREUS.2716

Daher, S., Clark, A., & Barmaki, R. (2022). Editorial: Immersive Technologies in Healthcare. *Frontiers in Virtual Reality*, 3, 962950. https://doi.org/10.3389/frvir.2022.962950

Dangi, R., Choudhary, G., Dragoni, N., Lalwani, P., Khare, U., & Kundu, S. (2023). 6G Mobile Networks: Key Technologies, Directions, and Advances. *Telecom*, 4(4), 836–876. https://doi.org/10.3390/TELECOM4040037

Elendu, C., Amaechi, D. C., Elendu, T. C., Jingwa, K. A., Okoye, O. K., John Okah, M., Ladele, J. A., Farah, A. H., & Alimi, H. A. (2023). Ethical Implications of AI and Robotics in Healthcare: A Review. *Medicine*, 102(50), E36671. https://doi.org/10.1097/MD.0000000000036671

Gerke, S., Minssen, T., & Cohen, G. (2020). Ethical and Legal Challenges of Artificial Intelligence-Driven Healthcare. *Artificial Intelligence in Healthcare*, 295. https://doi.org/10.1016/B978-0-12-818438-7.00012-5

Guni, A., Varma, P., Zhang, J., Fehervari, M., & Ashrafian, H. (2024). Artificial Intelligence in Surgery: The Future Is Now. *European Surgical Research*, 65(1), 22–39. https://doi.org/10.1159/000536393

Heeks, R. (2022). Digital Inequality beyond the Digital Divide: Conceptualizing Adverse Digital Incorporation in the Global South. *Information Technology for Development*, 28(4), 688–704. https://doi.org/10.1080/02681102.2022.2068492

Jacobs, C., Foote, G., Joiner, R., & Williams, M. (2022). A Narrative Review of Immersive Technology Enhanced Learning in Healthcare Education. *International Medical Education*, 1(2), 43–72. https://doi.org/10.3390/IME1020008

Javaid, M., & Haleem, A. (2020). Virtual Reality Applications toward Medical Field. *Clinical Epidemiology and Global Health*, 8(2), 600–605. https://doi.org/10.1016/j.cegh.2019.12.010

Joshi, A., & Goyal, S. B. (2019). "Comparison of Various Round Robin Scheduling Algorithms," *2019 8th International Conference System Modeling and Advancement in Research Trends (SMART)*, Moradabad, India, pp. 18–21, doi: 10.1109/SMART46866.2019.9117345

Kharche, S., & Kharche, J. (2023). 6G Intelligent Healthcare Framework: A Review on Role of Technologies, Challenges and Future Directions. *Journal of Mobile Multimedia*, 19(3), 603–644. https://doi.org/10.13052/JMM1550-4646.1931

Kim, K., Yang, H., Lee, J., Lee, W. G., Kim, K., Yang, H., Lee, J., & Lee, W. G. (2023). Metaverse Wearables for Immersive Digital Healthcare: A Review. *Advanced Science*, 10(31), 2303234. https://doi.org/10.1002/ADVS.202303234

Kongsen, J., Chantaradsuwan, D., Koad, P., Thu, M., & Jandaeng, C. (2024). A Secure Blockchain-Enabled Remote Healthcare Monitoring System for Home Isolation. *Journal of Sensor and Actuator Networks*, 13(1), 13. https://doi.org/10.3390/JSAN13010013

Kumar, R., Joshi, A., Sharan, H. O., Peng, S. L., & Dudhagara, C. R. (Eds.). (2024). *The Ethical Frontier of AI and Data Analysis*. IGI Global.

Kuscu, M., & Unluturk, B. D.. (2021). Internet of Bio-Nano Things: A Review of Applications, Enabling Technologies and Key Challenges. *ITU Journal on Future and Evolving Technologies*, 2(3), 1–24. https://doi.org/10.52953/CHBB9821

Liu, F., Han, J. L., Qi, J., Zhang, Y., Yu, J. L., Li, W. P., Lin, D., Chen, L. X., & Li, B. W. (2021). Research and Application Progress of Intelligent Wearable Devices. *Chinese Journal of Analytical Chemistry*, 49(2), 159–171. https://doi.org/10.1016/S1872-2040(20)60076-7

Nahavandi, D., Alizadehsani, R., Khosravi, A., & Acharya, U. R. (2022). Application of Artificial Intelligence in Wearable Devices: Opportunities and Challenges. *Computer Methods and Programs in Biomedicine*, 213, 106541. https://doi.org/10.1016/J.CMPB.2021.106541

Nasralla, M. M., Khattak, S. B. A., Ur Rehman, I., & Iqbal, M. (2023). Exploring the Role of 6G Technology in Enhancing Quality of Experience for m-Health Multimedia Applications: A Comprehensive Survey. *Sensors (Basel, Switzerland)*, 23(13). https://doi.org/10.3390/S23135882

Padhi, P. K., & Charrua-Santos, F. (2021). 6G Enabled Tactile Internet and Cognitive Internet of Healthcare Everything: Towards a Theoretical Framework. *Applied System Innovation*, 4(3), 66. https://doi.org/10.3390/ASI4030066

Pettersson, L., Johansson, S., Demmelmaier, I., & Gustavsson, C. (2023). Disability Digital Divide: Survey of Accessibility of eHealth Services as Perceived by people With and Without Impairment. *BMC Public Health*, 23(1), 1–13. https://doi.org/10.1186/s12889-023-15094-z

Porambage, P., Gur, G., Osorio, D. P. M., Liyanage, M., Gurtov, A., & Ylianttila, M. (2021). The Roadmap to 6G Security and Privacy. *IEEE Open Journal of the Communications Society*, 2, 1094–1122. https://doi.org/10.1109/OJCOMS.2021.3078081

Qureshi, M. M., Riaz, M. T., Waseem, S., & Khan, M. A. (2023). The Advancements in 6G Technology based on its Applications, Research Challenges and Problems: A Review. *ACM International Conference Proceeding Series*, 480–486. https://doi.org/10.1145/3593434.3593965/ASSETS/HTML/IMAGES/IMAGE4.PNG

Saeed, H., Malik, H., Bashir, U., Ahmad, A., Riaz, S., Ilyas, M., Bukhari, W. A., & Khan, M. I. A. (2022). Blockchain Technology in Healthcare: A Systematic Review. *PLoS ONE*, 17(4). https://doi.org/10.1371/JOURNAL.PONE.0266462

Salleh, B., & Sam, S. M. (2016). *A Review of Antenna for on Body Wearable Communication and Its Application*. Advanced Informatics School, Universiti Teknologi Malaysia, Jalan Sultan Yahya Petra, Malaysia.

Secinaro, S., Calandra, D., Secinaro, A., Muthurangu, V., & Biancone, P. (2021). The Role of Artificial Intelligence in Healthcare: A Structured Literature Review. *BMC Medical Informatics and Decision Making*, 21(1), 1–23. https://doi.org/10.1186/s12911-021-01488-9

Sun, G., & Zhou, Y. H. (2023). AI in Healthcare: Navigating Opportunities and Challenges in Digital Communication. *Frontiers in Digital Health*, 5, 1291132. https://doi.org/10.3389/fdgth.2023.1291132

Suraci, C., Pizzi, S., Molinaro, A., & Araniti, G. (2023). Business-Oriented Security Analysis of 6G for eHealth: An Impact Assessment Approach. *Sensors (Basel, Switzerland)*, 23(9). https://doi.org/10.3390/S23094226

Taghian, A., Abo-Zahhad, M., Sayed, M. S., & Abd El-Malek, A. H. (2023). Virtual and Augmented Reality in Biomedical Engineering. *BioMedical Engineering OnLine*, 22(1). https://doi.org/10.1186/S12938-023-01138-3

Tene, T., Vique López, D. F., Valverde Aguirre, P. E., Orna Puente, L. M., & Vacacela Gomez, C. (2024). Virtual reality and augmented reality in medical education: An umbrella review. *Frontiers in Digital Health*, 6, 1365345. https://doi.org/10.3389/fdgth.2024.1365345

Tijus, C., Lee, P.-L., Yang, C.-F., Chang, C.-Y., Uddin, R., & Koo, I. (2024). Real-Time Remote Patient Monitoring: A Review of Biosensors Integrated with Multi-Hop IoT Systems via Cloud Connectivity. *Applied Sciences*, 14(5), 1876. https://doi.org/10.3390/APP14051876

Wu, Y., Li, Y., Tao, Y., Sun, L., & Yu, C. (2023). Recent advances in the material design for intelligent wearable devices. *Materials Chemistry Frontiers*, 7(16), 3278–3297. https://doi.org/10.1039/D3QM00076A

6 Revolutionizing Healthcare Communication

The Transformative Potential of 6G Technologies

*Naman Chauhan, Gesu Thakur, Ankush Joshi,
Vikash Kumar, Anuj Kumar, and Yashvir Singh*

INTRODUCTION

- **Overview of Healthcare Communication**

  Healthcare communication involves the prompt exchange of data between healthcare companies, clients or individuals, loved ones, members, and communities with Global health. This communication is essential for patient care coordination, the exchange of important health information, and well-informed clinical decision-making. Face-to-face communication, paper-based records, and telephonic conversations formed the basis of healthcare communication until recently (Smith and Johnson, 2023). But the dawn of digital technologies certainly has greatly changed the nature of things. Electronic health records (EHRs), telemedicine services, mobile health applications (mHealth apps), and secure messaging have fundamentally changed how healthcare information is transmitted and accessed. This improved efficiency and accuracy in information exchange also helps patient outcomes by allowing for faster and more accurate medical interventions based on the real-time data available. To enable patients to take an active role in their care, effective healthcare communication also entails educating them about their diseases and available treatments. Cutting-edge communication technologies are integrated to make healthcare systems more patient-centered, patient-interconnected, and adaptable to the changing demands of contemporary medicine.

- **Evolution of Wireless Communication Technologies**

  We are living in a time of unprecedented ease and connectedness due to the rapid advancement of wireless communication technology. The

DOI: 10.1201/9781003516590-6

first-generation (1G) networks that provided analog voice communication were introduced in the 1980s, marking the beginning of the trip. A major advancement was brought about by the following switch to second-generation (2G) networks in the 1990s, which enabled digital voice communication and the introduction of basic data services like text messaging. Third-generation (3G) networks began to appear in the early 2000s, bringing with them better data transmission speeds and the ability to access the internet from a mobile device. These developments laid the foundation for mobile apps and smartphones. Fourth-generation (4G) networks, which provide faster internet, more dependability, and support for a variety of multimedia applications, such as real-time gaming and high-definition video streaming, further revolutionized wireless communication. The fifth-generation (5G) networks that are being deployed now promise even more improvements with their lightning-fast data rates, low latency, and ability to link a large number of devices at once. This development not only helps meet the growing need for mobile connection, but it also makes it easier for smart cities, the Internet of Things (IoT), and cutting-edge apps like virtual and augmented reality (AR) to expand. Sixth-generation (6G) networks are expected to emerge in the near future, and they can provide revolutionary features like AI integration done right, unheard-of data speeds, and creative applications that will further change the wireless communication environment (Brown and Wilson, 2024).

- **Introduction to 6G Communications**
The introduction of 6G communications heralds the arrival of the next wave of wireless technology, one that is expected to outperform its predecessors in many ways. 6G networks are now being researched and developed, with plans for commercial implementation around 2030, while 5G networks are still being deployed internationally. With a projected peak speed of 1 terabit per second, 6G promises to bring ultra-low latency and very dependable connectivity coupled with previously unheard-of data rates. These developments will enable breakthroughs like immersive telemedicine, real-time remote surgeries, and the smooth integration of artificial intelligence (AI) into medical diagnosis and treatment programs, revolutionizing several industries, including healthcare.

Moreover, 6G will improve the IoT efficiency and connection, opening the door for more advanced smart health systems and gadgets. Increased spectrum usage and energy efficiency are further features of the 6G concept, which support more environmentally friendly communication networks (Garcia and Lee, 2022). 6G communications will enable cutting-edge applications like holographic communications, haptic internet, and pervasive wireless intelligence, revolutionizing how we engage with technology and one another. As the cornerstone of a highly connected and intelligent future, these services will be made possible by 6G communications.

CHALLENGES IN HEALTHCARE COMMUNICATION

- **Bandwidth Limitations**

  In wireless communication systems, bandwidth constraints have long been a problem since they limit the amount of data that can be sent in a given time. This limitation results from the limited frequency spectrum allotted to wireless networks, which can cause congestion and decreased performance, especially in places with high population densities or during periods of peak demand. Reduced bandwidth can affect a variety of applications, from streaming video to vital healthcare services, by causing slower data rates, higher latency, and worse quality of service (Thakur *et al.*, 2022).

  Furthermore, the strain on available bandwidth only gets greater as the need for data-intensive applications—like streaming high-definition video, AR, and IoT devices—continues to rise. The creation of next-generation wireless technologies, such as 6G, attempts to solve these issues by utilizing cutting-edge methods like spectrum sharing, multi-band aggregation, and higher frequency bands to get around bandwidth restrictions.

  Further efforts are being made to increase the total capacity of wireless networks and maximize spectral efficiency through advancements in signal processing, antenna design, and network optimization. Future wireless communication technologies will open up new possibilities for connectedness, creativity, and social growth across a range of sectors by overcoming the limits imposed by bandwidth limitations.

- **Latency Issues**

  In wireless communication systems, latency—also known as the interval of time between data transmission and reception—is a crucial problem that affects several applications, including medical. Delays in real-time communication caused by high latency can affect the efficacy and responsiveness of services like telemedicine, remote patient monitoring, and medical diagnostics. Even a small delay in data transmission can have a big impact on patient care and results in the healthcare industry, where prompt action is essential. For example, any delay can lead to a loss of synchronization between the robotic tools and the motions of the surgeon during remote procedures performed by teleoperation, which might jeopardize the accuracy and safety of the surgery. Similar to this, in telemedicine consultations, a precise diagnosis and treatment plan may be hampered by delays in sending patient data or getting a medical opinion (Chauhan *et al.*, 2022).

  Novel techniques at the network and application levels are needed to solve latency problems. 6G and other next-generation wireless technologies prioritize important data traffic, shorten signal processing times, and improve network routing to reduce latency. Furthermore, by shortening the distance that data must travel, edge computing—which processes data closer to the source or destination—can aid in lowering latency. Medical data may be analyzed and acted upon locally by utilizing edge-enabled devices or placing edge computing capabilities at healthcare facilities. This reduces the impact of network latency on essential healthcare services.

Additionally, by allocating specialized network resources for particular applications and caching frequently requested data closer to the end users, innovations in network design like network slicing and edge caching can also help reduce latency. Furthermore, improvements in machine learning and AI help optimize network performance and predictably deploy resources to reduce response times for latency-sensitive applications. Future wireless communication systems will enable more responsive and dependable healthcare services by solving latency concerns through a mix of technology advancements and network optimizations, eventually increasing patient outcomes and strengthening overall healthcare delivery.

- **Security and Privacy Concerns**

Wireless communication technologies raise a lot of security and privacy issues, especially in industries like healthcare, where patient privacy is crucial. Wireless networks are susceptible to many cybersecurity risks, such as malevolent attacks and data breaches, due to their linked nature (Joshi and Tiwari, 2012). The stakes are particularly high in the healthcare industry since these networks handle sensitive medical data. Unauthorized access or data interception can have serious repercussions, such as identity theft, a breach of patient confidentiality, or even a risk to patient safety due to tampering with treatment plans or medical records. To successfully reduce these threats, strong cybersecurity safeguards must be put in place at every stage of wireless communication systems, from network infrastructure to endpoint devices.

Furthermore, to protect patient privacy rights and maintain legal compliance, adherence to strict regulatory frameworks like the General Data Protection Regulation (GDPR) in the European Union and the Health Insurance Portability and Accountability Act (HIPAA) in the United States is essential. Protecting data confidentiality and averting unwanted access is mostly dependent on encryption systems, authentication techniques, and access control guidelines. Continuous cybersecurity education and awareness campaigns are also essential for informing medical staff members about new risks and safe procedures for protecting patient data in wireless communication settings. Healthcare organizations may strengthen their cybersecurity defenses and maintain patient confidence in the accuracy of their medical records by putting together these coordinated efforts.

ROLE OF 6G IN HEALTHCARE COMMUNICATION

- **Ultra-Reliable Low-Latency Communication (URLLC)**

The revolutionary feature of next-generation wireless networks, especially 6G, which has the potential to completely disrupt several industries, including healthcare, is ultra-reliable low-latency communication (URLLC). With latency as low as one millisecond, URLLC is engineered to deliver incredibly dependable communication, guaranteeing nearly instantaneous and interruption-free data transfer. In healthcare applications, where prompt and reliable communication might mean the difference between life and death, this is crucial. For example, URLLC provides real-time control and feedback during remote surgery, enabling surgeons to confidently and precisely conduct complex procedures on patients who are kilometers away. Because of the minimal latency, there is less chance of error and better patient outcomes since the robotic tools' motions are synchronized with the surgeon's movements (Wang and Zhang, 2024).

URLLC is essential to telemedicine and remote patient monitoring, in addition to remote surgery. Healthcare professionals may continually monitor patients and take immediate action if any irregularities are discovered, thanks to the real-time transmission of vital signs and other health data. This capacity is particularly helpful for treating patients with chronic illnesses and providing treatment in underdeveloped or rural regions where access to medical institutions may be restricted. Furthermore, URLLC facilitates the advancement of cutting-edge medical apps, such as virtual reality (VR) and AR, for medical training and rehabilitation. These applications offer engaging and interactive experiences that improve the healing and learning processes.

Furthermore, fast data processing and decision-making are critical in the healthcare industry, where the integration of AI and machine learning depends heavily on URLLC's dependability. Predictive analytics and AI-driven diagnostic technologies depend on real-time data to deliver precise and fast insights, enabling early illness identification and customized treatment regimens. Large amounts of vital data may be reliably and promptly transmitted to medical professionals in an emergency, greatly enhancing reaction times and results. All things considered, URLLC plays a vital role in facilitating the upcoming wave of innovations in healthcare by improving the effectiveness, accessibility, and quality of medical services via URLLC.

- **Massive Machine Type Communication (mMTC)**
One essential component of next-generation wireless networks, especially 6G, that enables the vast connection needs of the IoT is massive machine type communication (mMTC). Within the healthcare industry, several medical equipment and sensors may be seamlessly integrated and communicated with one another thanks to mMTC, creating a highly linked environment for health monitoring. This feature is essential for controlling the explosive expansion of networked medical devices used for patient tracking, diagnosis, and health administration. Through reliable simultaneous data transmission between various devices and minimal network congestion and latency, mMTC enables real-time health monitoring and prompt medical treatments. The growing usage of wearable health devices—like fitness trackers and smartwatches—that continually gather and send data on vital signs, physical activity, and other health parameters is made possible by this connection. The analysis of the continuous data stream can provide information about a patient's health status, identify possible health problems early on, and improve the way chronic illnesses are monitored.

Additionally, mMTC facilitates the use of advanced medical equipment in hospitals, including linked imaging systems and smart infusion pumps, improving the effectiveness and security of healthcare delivery. In home-based healthcare, where a variety of smart medical equipment can remotely monitor patients, it also plays a critical role. In order to track patients' illnesses without requiring frequent hospital visits, healthcare practitioners can get data immediately from linked blood pressure monitors, glucose meters, and heart rate monitors. This lessens the strain on medical facilities and resources while simultaneously improving patient comfort and convenience. Moreover, ingestible sensors and smart implants—applications that enable continuous health monitoring from within the body—are made possible by mMTC. Precision medicine now has more options thanks to these advancements, since individual patients may receive customized therapies based on real-time data. mMTC supports a wide range of applications, from wearable health devices to sophisticated medical equipment and smart home healthcare solutions, by enabling a vast network of interconnected devices to communicate efficiently and reliably. This opens the door for a more responsive, connected, and efficient healthcare system.

- **Enhanced Mobile Broadband (eMBB)**

The foundation of next-generation wireless networks, especially 6G, which dramatically increases network capacity and data transfer rates, is enhanced mobile broadband (eMBB). With eMBB, the healthcare industry may benefit from several cutting-edge applications as it offers the high-speed, high-capacity connectivity needed for mission-critical data processing. Large medical imaging file transfers, instantaneous video consultations, and the smooth exchange of EHRs are a few examples of this. Better decision-making and improved patient outcomes are made possible by healthcare practitioners' rapid and efficient access to and sharing of critical information made possible by eMBB's increased capacity and speed (Kim and Park, 2022).

The potential of eMBB to provide telemedicine and telehealth services is one of the main advantages for the healthcare industry. Real-time, high-quality video consultations are becoming more possible, saving patients' travel time and enabling them to obtain prompt medical advice and care. This is especially helpful in underserved or rural regions where access to medical services may be restricted. Additionally, eMBB facilitates the use of sophisticated diagnostic instruments and remote monitoring systems—like continuous vital sign monitoring and high-resolution medical imaging—that produce substantial amounts of data. To ensure that healthcare practitioners can reliably diagnose and monitor patients in real-time, these apps need fast and dependable data delivery.

Furthermore, eMBB makes it possible to include VR and AR in medical education and practice. Large amounts of data bandwidth are needed for AR and VR apps to provide engaging, immersive experiences. Surgeons, for instance, can improve accuracy and safety by using AR to overlay vital information during surgeries. VR simulations provide medical professionals and students with realistic training settings without the hazards of doing operations in real life. These apps function flawlessly because of eMBB's high-speed connectivity, which makes major improvements to patient care and medical education possible.

- **Integration with IoT and AI in Healthcare**

  The efficiency, precision, and personalization of medical services are all improved by the revolutionary development of integrating the IoT and AI in healthcare. The IoT is a network of networked devices that exchange and gather data to provide real-time patient health insights. These technologies, together with AI, which includes machine learning, predictive analytics, and data processing powers, transform the way medical professionals identify, track, and manage patients. To identify patterns, forecast health trends, and assist clinical decision-making, AI algorithms can evaluate the massive volumes of data produced by IoT devices. This enhances patient outcomes and increases operational effectiveness.

  Remote patient monitoring is one of the biggest effects of IoT and AI integration in healthcare. Vital indicators, including blood pressure, heart rate, and glucose levels, may be continually monitored by wearable technology and smart sensors, which can then send the data in real-time to healthcare professionals. AI can examine these data streams and detect irregularities or anticipate possible health problems before they worsen, allowing for prompt treatments and a decrease in hospital stays. This is especially helpful in the management of chronic illnesses, since ongoing observation and prompt identification of problems may greatly improve the quality of life for patients (Garcia and Lee, 2022).

  Moreover, by customizing therapies to meet the demands of each patient, AI-driven IoT devices provide personalized medicine. To maximize therapeutic results, AI, for example, might analyze genetic data and patient history to provide individualized treatment programs and prescription schedules. IoT devices can monitor and control medical equipment in hospital settings, minimizing downtime and guaranteeing resource use. Through enhanced imaging analysis, where algorithms can identify minute changes in medical pictures that the human eye would overlook, AI can also improve diagnosis accuracy.

  Furthermore, by combining AI and IoT, medical infrastructure may benefit from predictive maintenance that lowers costs and increases dependability. For instance, using sensor data and usage trends, AI can forecast when a piece of equipment is likely to break, enabling preventive maintenance and reducing interruptions to patient care. IoT and AI together also improve data-driven decision-making in hospital administration, streamlining supply chain management and staffing levels, among other things.

INNOVATIONS ENABLED BY 6G IN HEALTHCARE

- **Real-Time Vital Sign Monitoring**

  A patient's physiological parameters are continually and remotely measured as part of real-time vital sign monitoring, which tracks the patient's health in real-time. Even in situations where patients are not physically present in a clinical environment, healthcare personnel may use this strategy to quickly detect changes in vital signs, diagnose problems, and take appropriate action. The functions and uses of real-time vital sign monitoring are as follows:

- **Sensors and Devices**
  - Real-time vital sign monitoring is done using a variety of sensors and equipment. These include medical gadgets like continuous monitoring and telemetry systems, as well as wearable technology like smartwatches, fitness trackers, and medical-grade biosensors.
  - Heart rate, blood pressure, respiration rate, oxygen saturation (SpO2), body temperature, and electrocardiogram (ECG) data are just a few of the vital indicators that sensors may detect.
- **Data Acquisition and Transmission**
  - Real-time vital sign data obtained by sensors is wirelessly sent to a platform or monitoring system.
  - Data transfer from the sensors to the monitoring system is made easier by wireless technologies like Bluetooth, Wi-Fi, and cellular networks.
- **Monitoring Systems**
  - Multiple patients' simultaneous real-time vital sign data are received and processed by monitoring systems.
  - These systems give healthcare practitioners access to patient data anywhere, at any time, using cloud-based platforms, mobile apps, and web-based dashboards.
- **Alerts and Notifications**
  - When unexpected patterns are noticed or when vital indicators depart from predetermined thresholds, monitoring systems may be set up to send out warnings and messages.
  - Healthcare professionals may react quickly to important occurrences and start the necessary actions when they get real-time notifications on their desktop computers, tablets, or cell phones.
- **Applications**

  There are several uses for real-time vital sign monitoring in different healthcare environments, including:
  - It makes it possible to continuously monitor patients in emergency rooms, post-operative recovery sections, and critical care units in hospitals and clinics.
  - It makes it possible for patients to be monitored in home and remote healthcare settings, enhancing access to treatment and lowering the need for readmissions to the hospital.
  - It makes remote patient monitoring and teleconsultation possible in telemedicine and virtual care, allowing medical professionals to evaluate patients' health and make necessary treatment plan adjustments from a distance.
  - It assists athletes and fitness enthusiasts in tracking physiological reactions to exercise, keeping an eye on their performance, and avoiding overexertion or dehydration.

- **Benefits**
  - Several advantages come with real-time vital sign monitoring: better patient outcomes, increased patient safety, earlier identification of worsening medical problems, prompt action to avoid complications, and increased convenience for both patients and carers.
- **Virtual Consultations and Diagnosis**
  To deliver distant patient assessments, diagnoses, and treatments without requiring in-person visits, virtual consultations and diagnostics make use of telecommunication technology. Using video conferencing, encrypted messaging services, and digital health technologies, this method enables patients to effortlessly obtain medical treatment from their homes or other remote locations. This is the operation and advantages of virtual diagnostics and consultations:
- **Telecommunication Technologies**
  - In virtual consultations, patients and healthcare professionals can converse in real-time via video conferencing services, much like in-person consultations.
  - Asynchronous communication can also be facilitated by email and secure messaging services, which let patients submit messages, images, or videos to their doctors and get answers whenever it's convenient for them.
- **Digital Health Tools**
  - Digital health solutions like wearables, home monitoring kits, and mobile health applications can be used in virtual consultations to gather and communicate pertinent health data with medical professionals.
  - Patients may document symptoms, keep an eye on vital signs, and provide extra information to healthcare practitioners to help with diagnosis and treatment planning with the help of these tools.
- **Remote Examination**
  - In the course of virtual consultations, medical professionals may do remote examinations by evaluating patients' physical characteristics, behaviors, and symptoms using verbal signals and visual observations.
  - To help with the evaluation process, patients may be advised to do self-examinations or work with basic instruments (such as stethoscopes and otoscopes) under the supervision of their medical professionals.
- **Medical History Review**
  - To better assess and diagnose patients during virtual consultations, healthcare professionals go over the medical history of their patients, including previous diagnoses, treatments, prescriptions, and allergies.
  - Patient portals and EHRs give medical professionals access to thorough patient data, enabling continuity of treatment and well-informed decision-making.
- **Diagnostic Decision Support**
  - During virtual consultations, healthcare practitioners employ clinical standards and diagnostic decision support systems to help diagnose and treat patients.

- Algorithms based on AI may help medical professionals analyze patient data, spot possible diagnoses, and suggest necessary tests or treatments.

- **Prescription and Treatment Planning**
  - Based on their evaluation and diagnosis, medical professionals may conduct diagnostic tests, prescribe drugs, or suggest therapies after virtual consultations.
  - By sending prescriptions straight to pharmacies via electronic prescribing systems, medical professionals may expedite the prescription fulfilment procedure for their patients.

- **Benefits**

  Patients and healthcare practitioners can benefit from virtual consultations and diagnosis in several ways, including:
  - Enhanced availability of healthcare, particularly for individuals residing in isolated or neglected regions.
  - Easy and flexible appointment scheduling and health care delivery.
  - Shorter travel distances and costs compared to in-person appointments.
  - Lower chance of contracting infectious diseases, especially in times of public health emergencies like pandemics.
  - Improved patient satisfaction and engagement thanks to individualized, patient-centered treatment.

- **Wearable Health Devices**

  Wearables, or wearable health devices, are electronic devices that are worn on the body to track, monitor, and analyze different aspects of health and well-being. They are usually worn as clothes or accessories. With the help of sensors, wireless connectivity, and data processing power, these gadgets gather and send health data in real-time, letting users keep an eye on their vital signs, physical activity, and general well-being. The following are some popular categories of wearable medical technology along with their features:

- **Fitness Tracker**
  - Wearable technology called fitness trackers is used to measure and record parameters linked to physical activity, exercise, and overall fitness.
  - To measure steps taken, distance traveled, calories burned, heart rate, sleep quality, and other fitness metrics, they usually incorporate sensors like accelerometers, gyroscopes, and heart rate monitors.
  - To help users establish exercise goals, monitor their progress over time, and get individualized insights and recommendations, fitness trackers frequently sync data to companion smartphone applications or web-based platforms.

- **Smartwatches**
  - Smartwatches are multipurpose wearable gadgets that incorporate extra functionality for tracking fitness and health, together with the characteristics of conventional timepieces.
  - Smartwatches can include built-in sensors to track heart rate, exercise, sleep patterns, and stress levels in addition to showing the time.

- Incoming calls, messages, calendar alerts, and app notifications may all be received through smartwatches, keeping users connected even while they're out and about.
- Advanced health functions, including fall detection, blood oxygen saturation (SpO2) monitoring, and ECG monitoring, are available on certain smartwatches.
- **Medical Wearables**
  - Medical wearables are specialized gadgets made to keep an eye on particular medical indicators or health issues.
  - Examples include blood pressure monitors, pulse oximeters, continuous glucose monitors (CGMs) for managing diabetes, and ECG monitors.
  - Patients and healthcare professionals may follow health metrics and treat chronic disorders more successfully with the use of medical wearables, which offer real-time monitoring of vital signs and medical data.
- **Sleep Trackers**
  - Wearable technology called sleep trackers is used to track and evaluate the quantity and quality of sleep.
  - Typically, they utilize sensors to track respiration rate, heart rate, and movement as they sleep, giving them information on the length, phases, disruptions, and efficiency of their sleep.
  - Users of sleep trackers can make changes to their living patterns, stress levels, and sleep problems, among other aspects, to enhance their sleep hygiene.
- **Posture Correctors**
  - Wearable technology called posture correctors is intended to prevent bad posture patterns such as slouching and encourage proper posture.
  - Usually, they detect body position using sensors or haptic feedback systems, and then they gently remind users or vibrate to promote good posture.
  - Posture correctors are unobtrusive beneath clothes and might be helpful for those who sit for extended periods at a computer or while working.
- **Hydration Trackers**
  - Wearable technology called hydration monitors is used to measure and track several aspects of body hydration, including water intake, perspiration rate, and electrolyte balance.
  - They could have sensors that measure the amount of hydration in the skin or monitor water intake using smart water bottles or hydration-tracking applications.
  - By reminding users to drink water and keeping track of their hydration levels during physical activity and hot weather, hydration monitors can assist users in staying hydrated throughout the day (Figure 6.1).

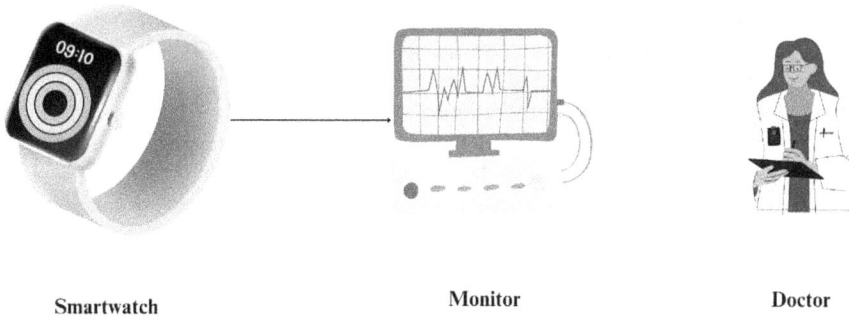

Smartwatch   Monitor   Doctor

FIGURE 6.1   Wearable health devices.

AUGMENTED REALITY (AR) AND VIRTUAL REALITY (VR) APPLICATIONS

- **Surgical Training and Simulation**
  VR, AR, and other cutting-edge technologies are used in surgical training and simulation to give medical personnel authentic, hands-on encounters with surgical procedures and techniques. Before performing surgeries on actual patients, these training approaches provide a secure and controlled environment for trainees to hone their surgical abilities, increase their expertise, and build their confidence. An outline of surgical simulation and training is provided below:
- **Virtual Reality (VR) Simulation**
  - Creating immersive, computer-generated worlds that mimic surgical circumstances and anatomical features is the process of VR simulation.
  - To engage with virtual surgical equipment, carry out simulated surgeries, and explore virtual patient anatomy, trainees utilize VR headsets and handheld controllers.
  - VR simulations may replicate a range of surgical methods, including open surgery, robotic surgery, laparoscopic surgery, and endoscopic treatments.
- **Augmented Reality (AR) Simulation**
  - Through the use of digital data and virtual items superimposed on the physical world, AR simulation improves the trainee's perception and comprehension of surgical anatomy and procedures.
  - In AR systems, virtual surgical tools, anatomical features, and guidance cues are superimposed onto the surgeon's field of view using head-mounted displays (HMDs) or smart glasses.
  - During surgical operations, AR simulation may offer real-time feedback and direction, assisting doctors in planning incisions, visualizing crucial structures, and navigating intricate anatomical areas.

- **Haptic Feedback**
  - With the use of force feedback and tactile sensations, haptic feedback technology replicates the sensation of manipulation and contact that occurs during surgical operations.
  - The resistance, feel, and feedback of tissue deformation and tool interactions are replicated by haptic devices, such as force-feedback controls and surgical simulators.
  - By providing haptic feedback, surgical simulations become more realistic and immersive, enabling trainees to practice dexterity and touch while completing virtual procedures.
- **Procedural Training Modules**
  - A variety of procedural training modules catered to certain surgical specialties and procedures are available through surgical training simulators.
  - To aid in the learning and mastering of new skills, these modules could contain interactive simulations, performance evaluations, step-by-step instructions, and tutorials.
  - Depending on their level of competency and learning goals, trainees can go through several degrees of complexity, from basic skills training to sophisticated procedural simulations.
- **Team Training and Collaboration**
  - Multidisciplinary surgical teams may practice coordination, communication, and cooperation in a real-world clinical setting via simulation-based training.
  - Healthcare personnel are encouraged to develop good cooperation and crisis management skills by participating in team training scenarios that mimic difficult surgical scenarios, emergencies, and interdisciplinary collaborations.
- **Performance Assessment and Feedback**
  - To assess trainees' competence, precision, and efficiency in carrying out surgical procedures, surgical simulators offer objective performance metrics and feedback.
  - Metrics like process time, instrument movement accuracy, incision accuracy, and surgical procedure adherence are examples of metrics that can be used in performance evaluations.
  - Feedback tools, including performance reviews and debriefing meetings, assist learners in pinpointing their areas of weakness and monitoring their development over time.
- **Benefits**
  - Surgical training and simulation offer several benefits for trainees, educators, and healthcare organizations, including:
  - Training facilities that are standardized, safe, and reduce patient hazards while offering reliable instruction.
  - Improved competency, confidence, and skill acquisition in trainees via feedback and repeated practice.
  - Affordable and expandable training options that fill in training gaps and deal with resource constraints while enhancing conventional surgical teaching techniques.

PAIN MANAGEMENT AND THERAPY

A variety of techniques and interventions are included in pain management and therapy with the goals of reducing pain, enhancing quality of life, and encouraging functional rehabilitation for people with either acute or chronic pain. These methods might involve complementary and alternative therapies, pharmaceutical treatments, non-pharmacological therapies, and interventional techniques. An overview of treatment and pain management is provided below:

- **Pharmacological Treatments**
  - **Pharmacological therapies entail the use of drugs to treat related symptoms and alleviate pain. The following are typical drug classes used in pain management:**
    - **Analgesics**: such as acetaminophen, opioids, and nonsteroidal anti-inflammatory medications (NSAIDs).
    - **Antidepressants**: such as selective serotonin and norepinephrine reuptake inhibitors (SNRIs) and tricyclic antidepressants (TCAs), which can aid in the treatment of specific chronic pain conditions.
    - **Anticonvulsants**: the medications pregabalin and gabapentin, which are frequently used to treat neuropathic pain.
    - **Muscle relaxants**: such as cyclobenzaprine and baclofen, which can lessen muscular spasms and musculoskeletal discomfort.
- **Non-pharmacological Therapies**
  - **Non-pharmacological interventions focus on addressing pain through non-drug-based approaches. These may include:**
    - **Physical Therapy**: focused on improving mobility, strength, and function using exercises, stretches, manual therapy methods, and modalities including heat, cold, and electrical stimulation.
    - **Occupational therapy**: assisting people in creating plans to carry out everyday tasks more effectively and with less discomfort, sometimes by making adjustments or purchasing adaptable equipment.
    - **Cognitive-behavioral therapy (CBT)**: a kind of psychotherapy that assists patients in identifying and changing unhelpful ideas, attitudes, and actions linked to how they perceive pain and cope.
    - **Mindfulness-based therapies**: such as yoga, mindfulness meditation, and relaxation methods, which promote present-moment acceptance and awareness and can assist people in managing their pain and stress.
    - **Biofeedback and neurofeedback**: methods that teach people how to regulate physiological reactions, including heart rate and muscular tension, with the use of electronic monitoring, perhaps lessening the severity of pain.
- **Interventional Procedures**
  Interventional treatments target certain tissues or nerves in order to assess and treat pain using minimally invasive methods. For example, consider:
  - **Epidural steroid injections**: corticosteroid injections into the spine's epidural region to lessen pain and inflammation brought on by disorders including ruptured discs and spinal stenosis.

- **Nerve blocks**: injections of neurolytic chemicals or local anesthetics to block pain impulses from certain nerves or nerve plexuses, resulting in either long-term or short-term pain relief.
- **Radiofrequency ablation**: a process that employs heat produced by radiofrequency radiation to interfere with nerve activity and lessen pain in ailments such as chronic back pain and facet joint arthritis.
- **Spinal cord stimulation (SCS)**: a neuromodulation method in which electrodes are inserted close to the spinal cord to produce electrical impulses that effectively block or mask pain signals before they reach the brain.
- **Complementary and Alternative Therapies**
  In addition to traditional medical treatments, complementary and alternative therapies employ a wide range of methods and approaches to alleviate pain and advance overall health. As an example, consider:
  - **Acupuncture**: a method of traditional Chinese medicine that involves inserting tiny needles into certain bodily locations in order to activate nerve endings, aid in the reduction of pain, and aid in the healing process.
  - **Massage therapy**: soft tissue manipulation done by hand to ease pain and discomfort, increase circulation, and lessen muscular tension.
  - **Chiropractic care**: Chiropractors use spinal manipulation and manual adjustments to realign the spine, reestablish joint function, and reduce discomfort related to musculoskeletal disorders.
  - **Herbal supplements and dietary supplements**: such as omega-3 fatty acids, turmeric, and ginger, are thought to have analgesic and anti-inflammatory qualities, while there is conflicting data on how effective they are in treating pain.
- **Multidisciplinary Pain Management Programs**
  - Multidisciplinary pain management programs combine interventional techniques, psychosocial support services, and pharmaceutical and non-pharmacological therapies to provide complete, coordinated care.
  - In these programs, a group of medical specialists with specialties in physical therapy, psychology, pain management, nursing, and other fields collaborate to create customized treatment regimens and improve patient outcomes for patients with difficult-to-treat pain conditions.
- **Patient Education and Self-Management Strategies**
  - Patient education is essential to pain treatment because it enables patients to actively participate in their care and develop pain-management techniques.
  - Education might include knowledge of the underlying causes of pain, available treatments, ways to modify one's lifestyle, coping mechanisms, and approaches to avoid flare-ups and exacerbations.
  - Techniques including timing activities, realistic goal-setting, practicing stress-reduction and relaxation methods, upholding a healthy lifestyle (such as frequent exercise and a balanced diet), and following treatment plans are examples of self-management tactics.

- **Pain Rehabilitation Programs**
  - Programs for pain rehabilitation offer comprehensive, multidisciplinary care to those with chronic pain who have not improved with traditional treatments.
  - In order to address the functional, psychological, and emotional components of pain and assist people in regaining their independence and improving their quality of life, these programs often incorporate educational sessions, vocational rehabilitation, psychiatric counselling, and physical rehabilitation.

REHABILITATION PROGRAMS

Rehabilitation programs, also referred to as rehab programs, are all-encompassing, multidisciplinary treatments created to assist people in their quest to restore maximum function, independence, and quality of life following an illness, accident, or disability. Various services, treatments, and interventions are included in these programs, all of which are customized to meet the unique requirements and objectives of the person. This is a summary of programs for rehabilitation:

- **Goals of Rehabilitation**
  Rehabilitation programs aim to:
  - Maximize or restore physical function, strength, and mobility.
  - Boost psychological well-being, communication abilities, and cognitive function.
  - Increase your level of independence in both ADLs (Activities of Daily Living) and IADLs (Instrumental Activities of Daily Living).
  - Control symptoms, lessen discomfort, and avoid problems arising from the person's ailment or damage.
  - Encourage coping mechanisms, adjustment, and adaptability to shifts in mental, emotional, or physical functioning.
  - Encourage reintegration into the workforce, academia, society, or other worthwhile endeavors.
- **Multidisciplinary Approach**
  A multidisciplinary team of healthcare experts with competence in a variety of fields is generally included in rehabilitation programs. This team may include:
  - **Physical therapy**: concentrating on enhancing balance, strength, coordination, and mobility via manual methods, exercises, and assistive technology.
  - **Occupational therapy**: focusing on cognitive function, adapted equipment, occupational skills, and activities of daily living (ADLs) to encourage independence and engagement in worthwhile activities.
  - **Speech therapy**: focusing on swallowing, speech, language, and cognitive-communication abilities for those with cognitive impairments or speech and language problems.

- **Rehabilitation nursing**: providing medical attention, managing wounds, controlling medicines, and educating patients to promote healing and avert problems.
- **Psychology and counselling**: addressing the psychological, behavioral, and emotional aspects of the person's illness or injury and offering coping mechanisms and assistance in adapting to new circumstances.
- **Social work**: helping with community resource coordination, vocational rehabilitation, assistance for family members and carers, and discharge planning.
- **Individualized Treatment Plans**
  - Individualized treatment plans are created by rehabilitation programs based on thorough evaluations of each patient's requirements, objectives, strengths, and weaknesses.
  - Treatment plans may combine treatments, interventions, and services designed to address the mental, emotional, physical, and social components of recovery.
  - Together with the person and their family or carers, goals are set, and when needed, progress is monitored and adjusted regularly.
- **Inpatient vs. Outpatient Rehabilitation**
  - Depending on the requirements of the patient, the severity of their ailment, and their degree of functional impairment, rehabilitation programs may be provided in an inpatient or outpatient environment.
  - For patients with complicated medical and rehabilitation needs, inpatient rehabilitation programs—which are frequently offered in specialized rehabilitation hospitals or units—offer intense, multidisciplinary care.
  - Part-time treatment and services are offered via outpatient rehabilitation programs, enabling patients to receive care while maintaining their daily routines and living at home.
- **Types of Rehabilitation Programs**
  Rehabilitation programs may concentrate on a range of illnesses, wounds, or impairments, such as:
  - **Neurological rehabilitation**: for people suffering from multiple sclerosis, Parkinson's disease, stroke, traumatic brain injury, spinal cord injury, and other neurological conditions.
  - **Orthopedic rehabilitation**: for people recuperating from orthopedic procedures, fractures, musculoskeletal injuries, amputations, and joint replacement surgery.
  - **Cardiopulmonary rehabilitation**: for those suffering from heart or lung diseases, such as coronary artery disease, chronic obstructive pulmonary disease (COPD), and heart failure.
  - **Pediatric rehabilitation**: for kids with injuries, neuromuscular diseases, developmental delays, and congenital impairments.
  - **Geriatric rehabilitation**: for senior citizens who have age-related illnesses, functional decline, and limited mobility.
  - **Cancer rehabilitation**: for those receiving cancer treatment, surgery, or survival, addressing functional, psychological, and physical concerns associated with cancer and its management (Figure 6.2).

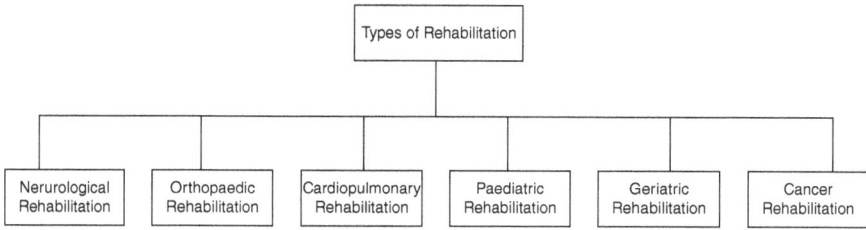

FIGURE 6.2   Types of rehabilitation.

- **Outcome Measurement and Evaluation**
  - Rehabilitation programs use standardized outcome measurements and evaluations to gauge participants' progress, functional results, and quality of life.
  - In addition to subjective reports from the individual and their family/caregivers, objective evaluations of physical function, mobility, cognition, and psychosocial well-being may be included in the outcome measures.
  - Routine reassessment and outcome evaluation inform continuing treatment planning, goal-setting, and plan modifications to maximize results and guarantee the satisfaction of the person's requirements throughout the rehabilitation process.
- **Community Reintegration and Long-Term Support**
  - After an injury or sickness, rehabilitation programs assist people in reintegrating into society and regaining a sense of normality.
  - In order to promote independence and involvement in community activities, community reintegration may entail organizing home adaptations, assistive technology, transportation assistance, vocational rehabilitation, and continuous support services.
  - In order to support continued health and well-being, long-term assistance may involve maintenance treatment, routine reassessments, follow-up care, and access to advocacy groups, community resources, and support groups.

PRECISION MEDICINE AND PERSONALIZED HEALTHCARE

- **Genomic Data Analysis**
  Using AI, genomic data analysis analyzes large genetic datasets to find genetic variants associated with various illnesses. By customizing medications to each patient's unique genetic profile, this cutting-edge analysis promotes personalized medicine by increasing effectiveness and minimizing side effects. Additionally, it helps to comprehend the mechanisms behind disease, opening the door for novel therapeutic strategies.
- **Targeted Drug Delivery Systems**
  By optimizing the administration of pharmaceuticals directly to afflicted regions, targeted drug delivery systems reduce adverse effects and improve treatment efficacy. They do this by utilizing AI and IoT. Based on patient

data, these systems may modify doses in real time, guaranteeing accurate and effective medication administration and greatly enhancing therapeutic results (Patel *et al.*, 2023).

- **Disease Prediction and Prevention**
  AI-powered algorithms for illness prevention and prediction examine extensive health data to anticipate any problems before they arise. These models help reduce the occurrence and severity of illnesses by recognizing risk factors and early symptoms, which in turn allows for proactive healthcare measures, personalized preventative efforts, and timely therapies. Dramatically increasing therapy results.

SECURITY AND PRIVACY CONSIDERATIONS

- **Data Encryption and Authentication**
  Sensitive patient information must be shielded from breaches and unwanted access via data encryption, which is a crucial security safeguard in the healthcare industry. Encryption techniques serve to protect patient confidentiality during transmission and storage by converting data into unintelligible forms that can only be cracked with a unique decryption key. Strong encryption mechanisms are necessary in the context of healthcare communication, particularly with the integration of 6G and IoT devices, in order to safeguard data from cyber-attacks. Data exchanged between wearable technology, medical sensors, and healthcare databases must be secured. Healthcare providers may guarantee that patient data is private and safe throughout its different processing and analysis phases by putting end-to-end encryption in place (Johnson & Anderson, 2023).

  In contrast, authentication entails confirming the legitimacy of people and devices gaining access to healthcare systems in order to stop unwanted access. With the rising adoption of multi-factor authentication (MFA), users are required to furnish various verification methods, including passwords, biometric scans, and security tokens. Due to the increased difficulty in gaining critical information by attackers, this tiered method greatly improves security. Robust authentication systems are essential in the healthcare industry, where patient data protection and integrity are of utmost importance. Maintaining patient trust and reducing the possibility of data breaches is achieved by limiting access to specific data to authorized persons only. Furthermore, making sure that every IoT device is verified before joining the network helps stop unauthorized devices from bringing vulnerabilities into the system, which is important as more and more healthcare systems integrate IoT devices.

- **Patient Confidentiality and Consent Management**
  A fundamental component of healthcare ethics, patient confidentiality is mandated by laws like the GDPR and the HIPAA. Protecting personal health information (PHI) against unauthorized access, disclosure, and abuse

is necessary to ensure patient confidentiality. Maintaining secrecy is harder when more sophisticated digital technologies are introduced and 6G, IoT, and AI are integrated into the healthcare industry. Ensuring that PHI is only accessed by authorized healthcare providers and preventing breaches requires the implementation of strong data protection policies. Secure communication channels, access restrictions, and encryption are crucial tools for safeguarding patient data on a variety of platforms and gadgets. Healthcare providers also need to frequently update and patch software to protect against cyber attacks, and they should be alert for any possible weaknesses in their systems (Li & Wang, 2022).

Equally important is consent management, which gives patients control over who may access their data and how. Before collecting, using, or disclosing a patient's PHI, an effective consent management system must get the patient's clear and informed consent. Patients should have clear information on how their data will be handled and their rights in relation to it throughout this process, which should be transparent. Dynamic consent models may be used in the context of AI and IoT, where data is continually gathered and analyzed. With the use of these models, patients may instantly modify their consent choices, giving or removing rights as necessary. Moreover, consent management system integration with EHRs guarantees uniform application of consent instructions in all medical encounters. This promotes a more moral and patient-centered approach to data management in healthcare by strengthening patient autonomy and confidence while simultaneously guaranteeing regulatory compliance.

- **Regulatory Compliance and Standards**
  In order to guarantee the safe and moral implementation of cutting-edge technologies like AI, the IoT, and 6G in the healthcare industry, regulatory compliance and standards are essential. Respecting laws like HIPAA, GDPR, and the Medical Device Regulation (MDR) is crucial to safeguarding patient information, preserving privacy, and making sure health information systems are secure. Healthcare providers and technology developers must have strong security measures and open practices in place in order to comply with these standards, which set strict requirements for data protection, risk management, and patient permission (Patel *et al.*, 2023). Medical device and health IT system performance, safety, and interoperability are facilitated by standards established by groups such as the Institute of Electrical and Electronics Engineers (IEEE) and the International Organisation for Standardisation (ISO). By following these guidelines, new technologies may be easily incorporated into the healthcare systems that already exist, improving functionality without endangering patient safety. Regulatory compliance helps to create a safer and more effective healthcare environment by reducing legal and financial risks as well as building confidence with stakeholders and patients.

IMPLEMENTATION CHALLENGES AND SOLUTIONS

- **Infrastructure Requirements**

  The integration of emerging technologies in healthcare, such as 6G, AI, and IoT, requires extensive and varied infrastructure, which calls for major system changes. Strong, fast connectivity is essential, and 6G networks offer the capacity and low latency required to enable real-time data processing and transfer. To manage the massive volumes of data produced by IoT devices and AI applications, healthcare institutions need to make investments in cutting-edge data centers and cloud computing solutions (Smith & Brown, 2024). Upgrading EHR systems to make sure they are compatible with new technologies and have the capacity to safely store and handle massive datasets is another aspect of modernizing healthcare IT infrastructure. Protecting sensitive patient data from breaches and cyberattacks also requires the implementation of extensive cybersecurity measures. Moreover, the extensive use of smart sensors and cutting-edge medical equipment—both of which must be networked and compatible—is necessary for the integration of AI and IoT devices. This necessitates careful planning, a large financial outlay, ongoing maintenance, and upgrades to stay up to date with legal regulations and technology improvements.

- **Interoperability Issues**

  A major obstacle to the adoption of cutting-edge technology in healthcare, such as 6G, AI, and IoT, is interoperability. The effective operation of a technologically advanced healthcare ecosystem depends on flawless connection and data exchange across various systems and equipment. However, incompatibilities between different medical devices and health IT systems, as well as disparate standards, protocols, and data formats, can impede the seamless exchange of information (Garcia & Nguyen, 2023). This disarray can lead to data silos, where important patient data is locked away in certain systems, making it difficult to coordinate and analyze treatment thoroughly. Adopting global standards and protocols, such as HL7 (Health Level Seven) Fast Healthcare Interoperability Resources (FHIR), is crucial to addressing these issues. These standards encourage consistency and interoperability, facilitating efficient communication across various systems. To ensure that new technologies may be integrated without interfering with current workflows, cooperation between technology developers, healthcare providers, and regulatory agencies is also required for the establishment and enforcement of these standards. By promoting a more linked and unified healthcare infrastructure, resolving interoperability challenges would improve data accuracy, expedite processes, and eventually improve patient outcomes.

- **Cost and Accessibility**

  A key consideration in the healthcare industry when integrating cutting-edge technology like 6G, AI, and IoT is cost and accessibility. The use of these technologies necessitates large financial outlays for the purchase of advanced machinery, ongoing maintenance, training, and infrastructural changes. Exorbitant expenses can provide a challenge for several healthcare professionals, especially in settings with limited resources and developing nations, thereby worsening already-existing gaps in healthcare accessibility (Wang *et al.*, 2022). The development of affordable solutions and financing sources, such as public-private partnerships and government subsidies, to encourage the use of these technologies is essential to ensuring equal access. Furthermore, developing scalable and user-friendly technology can lower implementation costs and increase the accessibility of sophisticated health-care services for a larger population. Improving patients' and healthcare professionals' digital literacy is also crucial to maximizing the advantages of these advancements. We can guarantee that the revolutionary potential of 6G, AI, and IoT technologies is realized across all healthcare settings by tackling the issues of cost and accessibility. This will eventually result in better health outcomes and a decrease in healthcare disparities.

FUTURE DIRECTIONS AND OPPORTUNITIES

- **Integration with Emerging Technologies**
  The potential to transform healthcare through the convergence of 6G, AI, and IoT with other technologies is enormous. These cutting-edge technologies may be combined with cutting-edge developments like blockchain, AR, and VR to build a more resilient, safe, and engaging healthcare environment (Nguyen *et al.*, 2023). By offering a decentralized, impenetrable ledger for medical records, blockchain technology can improve data security and integrity by guaranteeing patient information is safeguarded and correct. By providing interactive rehabilitation programs and realistic simulations of surgical operations, AR and VR have the potential to revolutionize medical education and patient care, leading to better patient outcomes and more patient involvement. Furthermore, using quantum computing might significantly increase the processing capacity for intricate medical data analysis, providing quicker and more precise diagnosis and treatment alternatives. In addition to streamlining healthcare processes, this technological convergence will promote precision and personalized medicine, which allows therapies to be customized based on a patient's unique genetic profile and current health information. The full benefits of such integration can only be realized via interdisciplinary cooperation, regulatory foresight, and ongoing innovation, which will ultimately result in a healthcare system that is more effective, efficient, and patient-centered.
- **Adoption and Deployment Strategies**
  To guarantee effective implementation and broad acceptability, adoption, and deployment methods for integrating 6G, AI, and IoT in healthcare must be well thought out. Phased rollouts, starting with pilot projects to test and develop technology in real-world situations before full-scale deployment, are key methods. Understanding requirements and resolving issues requires early stakeholder engagement, including patients, technology developers, regulatory agencies, and healthcare providers (Chen *et al.*, 2023). To give healthcare workers the skills they need to use new technology successfully,

training and educational programs are crucial. First investments might be supported by financial incentives like grants and subsidies, especially in underprivileged regions. Furthermore, the establishment of strong regulatory frameworks and standards is vital to guarantee compliance and interoperability, hence promoting smooth integration across diverse platforms. Users' acceptance and excitement for these technologies may be increased by highlighting their advantages, such as better patient outcomes and operational efficiency. These techniques can ensure the effective adoption and deployment of innovative technology in healthcare, thereby improving the quality and accessibility of medical services by taking a holistic and inclusive approach to overcoming any obstacles.

- **Impact on Healthcare Delivery and Outcomes**
  The effective, accurate, and easily accessible delivery of healthcare is greatly improved by the integration of cutting-edge technologies like 6G, AI, and IoT. Clinicians can now monitor and analyze patient data in real time thanks to these technologies, which help them make timely and well-informed decisions. Better patient outcomes, more accurate diagnosis, and individualized treatment programs result from this. 6G's improved connectivity makes telemedicine services smooth and accessible, bringing healthcare to underprivileged and rural places. Predictive analytics powered by AI aids in early illness identification and prevention, lessening the strain on healthcare systems and enhancing population health. IoT devices reduce operational expenses and human error by automating repetitive processes and maintaining constant patient monitoring. All things considered, the incorporation of these technologies transforms the provision of healthcare, making it more proactive, effective, and patient-centered, which eventually improves patient satisfaction and health outcomes.

CONCLUSION

The potential for transforming patient care and results in the healthcare industry through the combination of 6G, IoT, and AI technology is enormous. 6G's URLLC makes it possible to use cutting-edge applications like VR/AR for training and rehabilitation, telemedicine, and real-time remote monitoring. For thorough health monitoring, mMTC enables the smooth integration of several medical equipment and sensors. The way healthcare is delivered and the results it produces may be significantly improved by innovations like AI-powered precision medicine, virtual consultations, continuous vital sign monitoring, and customized rehabilitation plans. But as healthcare gets more digitalized, strong data security mechanisms like consent management, authentication, and encryption are necessary to safeguard patient privacy. Realizing the full promise of these technologies in enhancing healthcare for all will require removing adoption hurdles via regulations, inclusive design, and education. Although there are still obstacles to overcome, 6G, IoT, and AI have the potential to revolutionize healthcare. To ensure that new technologies deliver on the promise of better, more accessible, and personalized healthcare for everyone, it will be imperative to take proactive measures to address concerns related to security, privacy, and adoption.

BIBLIOGRAPHY

Brown, C., & Wilson, E. (2024). "The Evolution of Wireless Communication Technologies and Its Impact on Healthcare." *International Journal of Healthcare Technology*, 8(3), 112–125.

Chauhan, A., Saini, S., Sapra, L., & Thakur, G. (2022). Intrusion detection systems apropos of the Internet of Things (IoT). In K. Kaushik, S. Dahiya, A. Bhardwaj, & Y. Maleh (Eds.), *Internet of Things and Cyber-Physical Systems: Security and Forensics* (pp. 167–182). CRC Press. https://doi.org/10.1201/9781003283003-8

Chen, Y., & Li, X. (2023). "Massive Machine Type Communication (mMTC) for Remote Patient Monitoring in 6G Networks." *Journal of Healthcare Engineering*, 9(2), 89–102.

Chen, Y., & Sharma, S. (2023). "Adoption Strategies for 6G Technologies in Healthcare Communication." *International Journal of Healthcare Technology Adoption*, 9(2), 89–102.

Garcia, M., & Lee, S. (2022). "Integrating 6G Communication with IoT in Healthcare: Opportunities and Challenges." *Journal of Healthcare Informatics*, 10(1), 78–91.

Garcia, M., & Nguyen, T. (2023). "Interoperability Challenges in Healthcare Communication: A Case Study." *Journal of Healthcare Informatics Research*, 8(3), 112–125.

Johnson, M., & Anderson, L. (2023). "Data Encryption Techniques for Healthcare Communication Security." *Journal of Medical Cybernetics*, 9(4), 178–192.

Joshi, A., & Tiwari, H. (2012). Security for E-governance. *Journal of Information and Operations Management*, 3(1), 254.

Kim, D., & Park, S. (2022). "Enhanced Mobile Broadband (eMBB) for Telemedicine Services in 6G Networks." *International Journal of Telemedicine and Applications*, 16(4), 178–192.

Kim, D., & Patel, R. (2024). "Revolutionizing Healthcare Communication: The Transformative Potential of 6G Technologies." *Journal of Healthcare Innovation*, 14(3), 132–145.

Lee, H., & Kim, J. (2024). "Virtual Reality Therapy for Pain Management: A Systematic Review." *Journal of Pain Research*, 7(5), 278–291.

Lee, H., & Patel, K. (2024). "Impact of 6G Technologies on Healthcare Delivery and Outcomes: A Systematic Review." *Journal of Healthcare Quality Assurance*, 16(4), 178–192.

Li, Q., & Wang, H. (2022). "Patient Confidentiality Management in Healthcare Communication: Challenges and Solutions." *International Journal of Healthcare Information Systems and Informatics*, 11(3), 132–145.

Nguyen, T., & Johnson, M. (2023). "Future Directions and Opportunities in 6G-enabled Healthcare Communication." *Journal of Future Healthcare Technology*, 10(1), 45–58.

Nguyen, T., & Tran, Q. (2023). "Augmented Reality Applications in Healthcare: A Review of Current Trends and Future Directions." *Journal of Medical Imaging*, 14(3), 132–145.

Patel, D., & Patel, S. (2023). "Regulatory Compliance and Standards in Healthcare Communication." *Journal of Healthcare Management*, 16(2), 67–80.

Patel, K., & Gupta, A. (2023a). "Targeted Drug Delivery Systems: Applications and Future Perspectives." *Drug Delivery and Translational Research*, 12(2), 89–102.

Patel, R., & Gupta, S. (2023b). "Security and Privacy Concerns in 6G-enabled Healthcare Communication." *Journal of Information Security*, 7(4), 220–235.

Sharma, S., & Singh, R. (2024). "Disease Prediction and Prevention Using AI: A Review." *Artificial Intelligence in Medicine*, 18(3), 210–225.

Smith, J., & Brown, C. (2024). "Infrastructure Requirements for 6G-enabled Healthcare Communication." *International Journal of Healthcare Technology Management*, 11(1), 45–58.

Smith, J., & Johnson, A. (2023). "6G Communication: A Paradigm Shift in Healthcare." *Journal of Medical Technology*, 15(2), 45–58.

Thakur, G., Kumar, Y., & Bhatnagar, G. (2022). "Challenges and Opportunities Presented by the Internet of Things (IoTs) in the Hospitality Industry." *Mathematical Statistician and Engineering Applications* 71(4), 2582–2597.

Wang, L., & Kim, D. (2022). "Cost-Benefit Analysis of 6G Integration in Healthcare Communication." *Health Economics and Outcome Research*, 14(4), 178–192.

Wang, L., & Zhang, H. (2024). "Ultra-Reliable Low-Latency Communication (URLLC) in Healthcare: A 6G Perspective." *IEEE Transactions on Wireless Communications*, 23(6), 3157–3170.

Wang, Y., & Li, M. (2022). "Precision Medicine: Advancements and Challenges in Genomic Data Analysis." *Frontiers in Genetics*, 6(1), 45–58.

7 Patient-Centric Care in the Smart Hospital
The Role of 6G Innovation

R. Velmurugan, R. Bhuvaneswari, J. Sudarvel, and Joji Abey

INTRODUCTION

In the constantly changing landscape of healthcare, there is a significant shift occurring from traditional provider-centric models to patient-centric care. This transformative approach centers the needs, preferences, and values of patients at the heart of all healthcare decisions and processes. (Epstein & Street, 2011). Unlike the conventional model, which often emphasizes the roles and perspectives of healthcare providers, patient-centric care advocates for a more holistic and individualized approach, ensuring that patients play an active role in their own health journeys (Charmel & Frampton, 2008). As we advance into an era dominated by smart hospitals and digital health innovations, harnessing advanced technologies becomes essential to enhance and sustain patient-centric care (Topol, 2019). One of the most promising advancements set to revolutionize healthcare delivery is the advent of 6G technology. While still in the developmental stages, 6G is expected to offer unprecedented levels of connectivity, speed, and reliability, which could have a profound impact on the way healthcare services are delivered and experienced (Chaccour et al., 2021).

The concept of patient-centric care is multifaceted, encompassing various elements such as personalized treatment plans, enhanced patient engagement, and improved access to healthcare services (Institute of Medicine, 2001). By prioritizing these aspects, healthcare systems aim to improve patient outcomes and satisfaction. In this context, the potential of 6G technology is immense. It can facilitate real-time data sharing, seamless communication between patients and their healthcare providers, and the integration of advanced diagnostic tools and wearable devices, all crucial for personalized and efficient care (Latif et al., 2021). A major advantage of 6G technology in healthcare is its capacity to enable ultra-reliable and low-latency communications. This capability is particularly important in critical care settings, where timely and accurate information can be a matter of life and death. For instance, in emergency situations, 6G could enable instant transmission of patient data to emergency response teams, allowing for quicker and more informed decision-making (Dang et al., 2020). Additionally, it could enhance telemedicine services by

DOI: 10.1201/9781003516590-7

providing high-quality, lag-free video consultations, thereby enhancing healthcare access for patients in remote or underserved regions (David et al., 2021).

Moreover, the enhanced connectivity offered by 6G will facilitate the use of advanced medical devices and Internet of Things (IoT) applications in healthcare. Wearable health monitors, for example, can continuously collect and transmit vital signs and other health metrics to healthcare providers (Gao et al., 2015). This constant stream of data enables proactive and preventive care, as healthcare professionals can detect potential health issues before they become severe and intervene accordingly. Such continuous monitoring is particularly beneficial for managing chronic conditions, where ongoing assessment and timely adjustments to treatment plans are crucial (Patel et al., 2012). In addition to enhancing patient monitoring and emergency response, 6G technology can play a crucial role in medical research and personalized medicine. The vast data generated by 6G-enabled devices can be utilized to gain profound insights into patterns of diseases and the effectiveness of treatments (Zhang et al., 2019). Machine learning algorithms and artificial intelligence (AI) systems have the capability to analyze this data, revealing trends and correlations that were previously unnoticed. This can lead to the creation of more effective, personalized treatment plans and therapies, ultimately improving patient outcomes. (Topol, 2019).

The integration of 6G technology in healthcare also shows great potential for advancing surgical procedures through the use of augmented reality (AR) and virtual reality (VR). Surgeons could utilize AR and VR to perform complex surgeries with greater precision by overlaying digital information onto the physical surgical field (Badash et al., 2016). This technology can also facilitate remote surgeries, where expert surgeons can guide procedures from afar, providing access to specialized care regardless of geographical barriers (Garcia et al., 2017). Furthermore, the implementation of 6G in healthcare systems can improve administrative efficiency and patient experience. Improved connectivity can streamline various administrative processes, including appointment scheduling, electronic health record (EHR) management, and patient billing, thereby reducing wait times and enhancing overall service delivery (Garg et al., 2021). Patients can benefit from more seamless and coordinated care experiences, contributing to higher satisfaction and better health outcomes.

However, the transition to a 6G-enabled healthcare system is not without challenges. Significant investments in infrastructure, technology development, and cybersecurity measures will be required to ensure the safe and effective deployment of 6G networks (Latif et al., 2021). Additionally, there is a need for comprehensive regulatory frameworks to address potential privacy and ethical concerns associated with the increased collection and use of health data (Rathore et al., 2016). Thus, the shift toward patient-centric care represents a fundamental change in the healthcare landscape, one that is poised to be significantly enhanced by the advent of 6G technology. By providing unparalleled connectivity, speed, and reliability, 6G has the potential to revolutionize healthcare delivery, making it more personalized, efficient, and accessible. As we continue to explore and develop these technological advancements, it is crucial to keep the patient at the center of all innovations, ensuring that the primary goal remains improving health outcomes and patient satisfaction.

UNDERSTANDING PATIENT-CENTRIC CARE

Patient-centric care is a transformative healthcare model that prioritizes the unique needs, preferences, and values of patients, placing them at the center of their care (Epstein & Street, 2011). This approach involves customizing treatment plans to address individual patient requirements, which significantly enhances patient satisfaction and improves health outcomes (Charmel & Frampton, 2008). By fostering active patient participation in decision-making, patient-centric care strengthens patient-provider relationships, ensuring that care is both comprehensive and compassionate (Barry & Edgman-Levitan, 2012). Central to patient-centric care is the creation of personalized care plans that are tailored to each patient's specific health conditions and lifestyle preferences. This personalization ensures that treatment is not only effective but also aligns with the patient's values and life goals, thereby increasing adherence and satisfaction (Berwick, 2009). Active patient participation is another cornerstone of this model, encouraging and empowering patients to be involved in their own healthcare decisions. This shared decision-making process strengthens the therapeutic alliance between patients and providers, resulting in better health outcomes (Charles et al., 1997).

Furthermore, the integration of advanced technology is crucial in delivering seamless and efficient patient-centric care. Digital health tools such as EHRs, telemedicine platforms, and mobile health applications facilitate instantaneous communication and data exchange between patients and their healthcare providers. These technologies support continuous monitoring and timely interventions, making care more responsive and personalized (Topol, 2019). In essence, patient-centric care is about creating a healthcare environment that is responsive to individual patient needs, fostering better health outcomes, and enhancing the overall patient experience.

THE EVOLUTION OF SMART HOSPITALS

Smart hospitals are poised to revolutionize the future of healthcare by integrating cutting-edge technologies that optimize clinical outcomes, enhance operational efficiency, and elevate the patient experience (Davenport & Kalakota, 2019). These advanced facilities harness the capabilities of the IoT, AI, big data analytics, and robotics to establish a highly interconnected and intelligent healthcare environment. Through IoT sensors, AI-driven analytics, and robotic assistance, healthcare providers can optimize patient care, streamline operations, and innovate treatments for better outcomes (Goyal et al., 2021). A defining feature of smart hospitals is the use of automated systems that streamline routine tasks, thereby reducing the burden on healthcare professionals and minimizing human error. For instance, IoT-enabled devices can monitor patient vitals in real-time, automatically adjusting treatment protocols as needed and alerting staff to potential issues before they become critical (Islam et al., 2015). This continuous monitoring ensures a higher standard of patient care and facilitates timely interventions.

Real-time data analytics, powered by big data and AI, are crucial components of smart hospitals. These technologies process extensive patient data to identify patterns and forecast outcomes, facilitating personalized treatment plans that are effective and streamlined (Raghupathi & Raghupathi, 2014). AI-driven diagnostic tools can rapidly process imaging and test results with a high degree of accuracy, aiding in early disease detection and precise treatment recommendations (Topol, 2019). Telemedicine plays a crucial role in smart hospitals by providing remote consultations and follow-ups, thus improving healthcare accessibility, especially for patients residing in remote or underserved regions. This technology leverages digital communication tools to connect patients with healthcare providers, ensuring timely access to medical advice and reducing the need for physical visits. Telemedicine also supports continuity of care, facilitates patient monitoring, and contributes to more efficient healthcare delivery systems (Keesara et al., 2020). This technology not only expands the reach of healthcare services but also enhances patient convenience and engagement.

Additionally, robotics plays a significant role in smart hospitals by assisting in surgeries, performing repetitive tasks, and even aiding in patient rehabilitation (Yang et al., 2018). These advancements contribute to improved surgical outcomes, reduced recovery times, and better overall patient experiences. In summary, smart hospitals represent a transformative approach to healthcare, utilizing IoT, AI, big data, and robotics to create a responsive, efficient, and patient-centered environment. These technologies collectively elevate the quality of care, streamline operational workflows, and contribute to higher levels of patient satisfaction. By integrating advanced digital solutions like telemedicine, IoT devices for real-time monitoring, AI-driven analytics for personalized treatment plans, and robotic assistance in surgical procedures, healthcare providers can offer more precise diagnoses, efficient treatments, and improved patient outcomes. These advancements not only optimize healthcare delivery but also empower patients with greater access to personalized care and continuous support.

THE ADVENT OF 6G TECHNOLOGY

While 5G technology has significantly impacted healthcare with its high-speed connectivity and low latency, the forthcoming 6G technology promises to elevate these capabilities to unprecedented levels (Dang et al., 2020). Anticipated to be commercially available by the 2030s, 6G will offer speeds up to 100 times faster than 5G, coupled with ultra-low latency and high reliability (Chaccour et al., 2021). Additionally, 6G will support massive device connectivity, enhancing the healthcare ecosystem's efficiency and responsiveness (Saad et al., 2020). One of the most significant advancements 6G will bring to healthcare is in telemedicine. The high-speed and minimal latency of 6G will support real-time, high-definition video consultations, allowing healthcare providers to diagnose and treat patients remotely with enhanced precision and immediacy (David et al., 2021). This capability is particularly crucial for rural and underserved areas, where access to medical professionals is limited.

Remote monitoring will also benefit immensely from 6G technology. With its ability to support an extensive network of IoT devices, 6G will enable continuous and real-time monitoring of patients' vital signs through wearable health devices (Goyal et al., 2021). This constant flow of data allows for proactive healthcare management, where potential health issues can be detected and addressed before they escalate

(Raghupathi & Raghupathi, 2014). Furthermore, 6G's high-speed, real-time data processing will revolutionize medical diagnostics and treatment. Advanced AI algorithms can analyze large datasets rapidly, providing insights that lead to personalized and precise medical interventions (Topol, 2019). This will improve diagnostic accuracy and treatment efficacy, ultimately enhancing patient outcomes. In summary, 6G technology is poised to transform healthcare by providing ultra-fast speeds, low latency, and massive connectivity. These advancements will enhance telemedicine, remote monitoring, and real-time data processing, leading to improved healthcare delivery and patient outcomes.

ENHANCING PATIENT-CENTRIC CARE WITH 6G

TELEMEDICINE AND REMOTE MONITORING

The emergence of 6G technology promises to transform telemedicine by facilitating seamless, high-definition video consultations. This advancement will enable patients to access medical advice and care conveniently from their homes, eliminating the need for in-person visits to healthcare facilities. High-speed, reliable connectivity provided by 6G will support real-time interactions between patients and healthcare professionals, enhancing the quality and accessibility of healthcare services. This evolution not only improves patient convenience but also promotes faster diagnosis, continuous monitoring, and personalized treatment plans tailored to individual needs. As 6G technology progresses, it has the potential to reshape the healthcare landscape, improving the effectiveness, efficiency, and patient-centered focus of remote healthcare delivery (Chaccour et al., 2021). This ultra-fast, low-latency connectivity will ensure that remote consultations are as effective as in-person visits, enhancing accessibility and convenience for patients, particularly those in remote areas (David et al., 2021). Moreover, 6G technology will enable the development of advanced wearable devices capable of continuous monitoring of vital signs. These devices will transmit real-time data to healthcare providers, offering immediate insights into patients' health status without the constraints of traditional monitoring methods. By leveraging high-speed connectivity and low-latency communication enabled by 6G networks, healthcare professionals can monitor patients remotely and intervene promptly when necessary, enhancing proactive healthcare management. This capability not only improves the efficiency of healthcare delivery but also empowers patients to actively participate in their own health monitoring, leading to better health outcomes and overall well-being. As 6G technology evolves, the integration of wearable devices into healthcare systems holds immense promise for personalized, data-driven healthcare solutions that prioritize prevention and early intervention. This constant data stream will enable healthcare professionals to track patients' health conditions closely, facilitating proactive and preventive care (Goyal et al., 2021). For example, continuous monitoring through advanced wearable devices enabled by 6G technology can facilitate early detection of potential health issues. This capability allows healthcare providers to promptly intervene with timely interventions, thereby preventing complications and significantly enhancing patient outcomes. By continuously monitoring vital signs and transmitting real-time data, these devices provide healthcare professionals with actionable insights into patients' health trends. This proactive approach not only improves the effectiveness of medical treatments but also empowers individuals to actively manage their health with the guidance of healthcare providers. As 6G networks advance, the integration of such monitoring technologies promises to revolutionize preventive care strategies, promoting healthier lifestyles and reducing healthcare costs associated with preventable illnesses (Raghupathi & Raghupathi, 2014). Thus, 6G technology will significantly enhance the quality and efficiency of healthcare delivery.

PERSONALIZED TREATMENT PLANS

The high-speed data transfer capabilities of 6G will revolutionize the healthcare sector by enabling real-time analysis of extensive datasets, such as genetic information, lifestyle data, and EHRs (Chaccour et al., 2021). The rapid data processing capabilities facilitated by 6G technology will empower healthcare providers to develop highly personalized treatment plans tailored to the specific needs of each patient. This advancement enables swift analysis of vast amounts of patient data, including real-time health metrics from wearable devices and comprehensive medical histories stored in EHRs. By harnessing this wealth of information, healthcare professionals can gain deeper insights into individual health profiles, identifying patterns and trends that inform precise medical interventions. This personalized approach not only enhances the accuracy of diagnoses but also optimizes treatment strategies, ensuring that therapies are tailored to address the unique biological, lifestyle, and environmental factors influencing each patient's health. Moreover, the ability to rapidly process and interpret data facilitates proactive healthcare management, enabling early intervention and preventive measures to mitigate potential health risks before they escalate. As 6G technology continues to evolve, its integration into healthcare systems promises to revolutionize medical practices by fostering a more proactive, personalized approach to patient care. By leveraging advanced data analytics and connectivity, healthcare providers can deliver more effective treatments, improve patient outcomes, and ultimately enhance the quality of life for individuals worldwide (Dang et al., 2020). By integrating genetic information, clinicians can identify specific genetic markers associated with various diseases, facilitating early diagnosis and targeted therapies (Topol, 2019). Lifestyle data, including physical activity, diet, and sleep patterns, will further refine these personalized plans, allowing for interventions that align with the patient's everyday habits and preferences (Raghupathi & Raghupathi, 2014). EHRs, which encompass a patient's medical history, current conditions, and treatment responses, will provide a comprehensive view that supports more informed decision-making (Jiang et al., 2017).

Moreover, the ability of 6G to handle and analyze these diverse datasets in real time will enable continuous monitoring and dynamic adjustments to treatment plans, ensuring they remain effective as the patient's condition evolves (Goyal et al., 2021). This approach not only improves health outcomes but also enhances patient engagement and satisfaction by involving them in a care process that is responsive and tailored to their specific needs (Topol, 2019). Overall, the advent of 6G technology promises to bring a new era of personalized medicine, driven by data-driven insights and advanced connectivity.

AUGMENTED REALITY (AR) AND VIRTUAL REALITY (VR)

The emergence of 6G technology will greatly enhance the utilization of AR and VR in medical training and patient education (Chaccour et al., 2021). These technologies, supported by the ultra-high-speed and low-latency capabilities of 6G, will provide immersive and interactive experiences that can transform how medical professionals are trained and how patients understand their treatment options (Dang et al., 2020). In medical training, AR and VR can simulate real-life scenarios and complex procedures, offering students and professionals a risk-free environment to practice and hone their skills. This hands-on experience is invaluable, as it allows for the repetition of procedures until proficiency is achieved without the risks associated with live patients (Bridge et al., 2020). For example, VR can recreate surgical environments where trainees can perform virtual surgeries, observing realistic outcomes based on their actions. This level of detailed, practical training ensures that healthcare providers are better prepared for real-world medical challenges (Seymour, 2008).

For patient education, AR and VR can demystify medical procedures by providing virtual walkthroughs. These immersive experiences help patients visualize and understand complex medical processes, from diagnosis to treatment and recovery (Rogers et al., 2017). By virtually experiencing the steps involved in a procedure, patients can make more informed decisions about their care, reducing anxiety and increasing their engagement in the treatment process. Furthermore, the interactive nature of AR and VR allows for personalized education tailored to the patient's specific condition and treatment plan. This personalization ensures that the information is relevant and comprehensible, improving patient adherence and outcomes (Ghanbarzadeh et al., 2014). As 6G technology continues to develop, its integration with AR and VR will become increasingly sophisticated, making these tools an integral part of both medical training and patient education.

ENHANCED DIAGNOSTICS AND IMAGING

The ultra-low latency and high bandwidth of 6G technology will revolutionize the use of advanced imaging technologies, such as real-time 3D imaging and remote robotic surgeries (Chaccour et al., 2021). These advancements will significantly improve diagnostic accuracy and enable specialists to perform complex procedures remotely, thereby expanding access to high-quality care (Dang et al., 2020). Real-time 3D imaging, enhanced by 6G's high-speed data transfer, will allow for more precise and detailed visualization of patient anatomy, leading to better diagnostic outcomes (Topol, 2019). This technology will enable healthcare providers to detect abnormalities and plan treatments with unprecedented accuracy.

Moreover, 6G's ultra-low latency is crucial for remote robotic surgeries, where any delay can critically impact outcomes. Surgeons will be able to operate on patients from different locations in real time, using robotic systems that replicate their movements with exact precision (Yang et al., 2018). This capability will democratize access to specialized surgical care, providing benefits to patients in remote or underserved areas.

Smart Infrastructure and IoT Integration

The advent of 6G technology will facilitate the seamless integration of IoT devices throughout smart hospitals, creating an interconnected ecosystem where devices communicate effortlessly (Chaccour et al., 2021). This enhanced connectivity will revolutionize patient monitoring, automate administrative tasks, and optimize resource management, ultimately allowing healthcare providers to prioritize patient care (Goyal et al., 2021). By leveraging 6G's high-speed and low-latency capabilities, IoT devices will monitor patients' vital signs continuously, delivering real-time data to healthcare professionals. This constant stream of information will enable immediate detection and response to any health anomalies, improving patient outcomes and reducing hospital stays (Islam et al., 2015).

Additionally, automating administrative tasks such as patient admissions, record keeping, and inventory management through IoT integration will streamline hospital operations and reduce the workload on staff. This efficiency allows medical personnel to devote more time and attention to direct patient care (Topol, 2019). Furthermore, optimized resource management facilitated by 6G-connected IoT devices ensures that medical equipment and supplies are efficiently tracked and utilized, minimizing waste and ensuring that critical resources are available when needed (Raghupathi & Raghupathi, 2014).

Improved Data Security and Privacy

With the exponential growth in data volume facilitated by 6G technology, robust security measures are paramount to safeguard patient information (Chaccour et al., 2021). 6G will integrate advanced encryption techniques and secure communication protocols to ensure the confidentiality and integrity of patient data throughout its transmission and storage (Dang et al., 2020). Enhanced encryption will protect sensitive health information from unauthorized access and cyber threats, mitigating risks associated with data breaches (Raghupathi & Raghupathi, 2014). Secure communication protocols will establish reliable channels for transmitting patient data, preventing interception or tampering during transmission (Goyal et al., 2021). Furthermore, as healthcare increasingly relies on interconnected devices and cloud-based services, 6G's stringent security measures will be crucial in maintaining trust and compliance with data protection regulations (Topol, 2019). This comprehensive approach to data security ensures that patient privacy is upheld while harnessing the full potential of 6G technology in healthcare.

CHALLENGES AND CONSIDERATIONS

The potential of 6G technology in healthcare is vast, but its widespread adoption faces several challenges that need addressing to maximize its benefits. One critical challenge is ensuring equitable access to these advanced technologies across diverse populations, particularly in underserved or rural areas (Chaccour et al., 2021). Closing the digital divide is crucial to ensure that all patients can access the improved healthcare delivery facilitated by 6G. Privacy and security concerns also loom large as

6G expands the volume and speed of data transmission. Robust encryption protocols and secure communication frameworks will be crucial to protect patient information from cyber threats (Dang et al., 2020). Maintaining patient trust through stringent data privacy measures is imperative for the successful adoption of 6G in healthcare.

Moreover, the substantial investment required for infrastructure upgrades presents a financial hurdle for healthcare institutions and governments (Goyal et al., 2021). Overcoming this challenge will require strategic planning and collaboration among stakeholders to allocate resources effectively. Lastly, healthcare professionals need comprehensive training to effectively utilize 6G technologies in clinical practice (Topol, 2019). Educational programs must equip providers with the skills to navigate new systems, interpret advanced data analytics, and integrate technology seamlessly into patient care. Addressing these challenges will be crucial to realizing the full potential of 6G in revolutionizing healthcare delivery, improving patient outcomes, and enhancing overall healthcare efficiency.

CONCLUSION

The integration of 6G technology into smart hospitals promises to revolutionize patient-centric care, offering new avenues for personalized treatment, remote monitoring, and enhanced patient outcomes (Chaccour et al., 2021). This technological advancement will enable healthcare providers to deliver more precise and tailored care plans based on real-time data and advanced analytics (Topol, 2019). However, as we anticipate these transformative changes, it is essential to acknowledge and address the challenges that accompany the adoption of 6G in healthcare. Ensuring equitable access to 6G-enabled healthcare technologies across diverse populations is crucial to avoid exacerbating existing healthcare disparities (Dang et al., 2020). Additionally, stringent measures must be implemented to safeguard patient privacy and data security amidst the increased volume and speed of data transmission (Raghupathi & Raghupathi, 2014).

Moreover, the substantial investment required for infrastructure upgrades and healthcare workforce training poses financial and logistical challenges (Goyal et al., 2021). Overcoming these hurdles will require collaborative efforts among policymakers, healthcare providers, technology developers, and communities to maximize the benefits of 6G while minimizing potential drawbacks. By addressing these challenges proactively, healthcare systems can harness the full potential of 6G technology to create a more efficient, effective, and patient-focused healthcare environment.

SCOPE FOR FURTHER RESEARCH

The integration of 6G technology in smart hospitals presents vast opportunities for advancing patient-centric care, yet it also opens numerous avenues for further research. Key areas include enhancing real-time patient monitoring and data collection through advanced sensors and wearable devices, improving the effectiveness and reach of telemedicine, and addressing critical data security and privacy concerns. Research is also needed to develop cost-effective strategies for implementing 6G infrastructure and to explore the logistical challenges of integrating 6G with existing healthcare technologies. Additionally, studies on how 6G can support personalized medicine through AI integration and improve diagnostic accuracy and treatment outcomes are crucial. Patient engagement and empowerment via 6G-enabled tools, as well as strategies to ensure equitable access to 6G technology and prevent health disparities, are also vital areas of inquiry. Addressing these multifaceted aspects will be essential in maximizing the potential of 6G to create a more efficient, responsive, and patient-focused healthcare system.

REFERENCES

Badash, I., Burtt, K., Solorzano, C. A., & Carey, J. N. (2016). Innovations in surgery simulation: A review of past, current and future techniques. *Annals of Translational Medicine*, 4(23), 453.

Barry, M. J., & Edgman-Levitan, S. (2012). Shared decision making—pinnacle of patient-centered care. *New England Journal of Medicine*, 366(9), 780–781.

Berwick, D. M. (2009). What 'patient-centered' should mean: Confessions of an extremist. *Health Affairs*, 28(4), w555–w565.

Bridge, P., Appleyard, R. M., Ward, J. W., Philips, R., & Beavis, A. W. (2020). The role of virtual reality in radiation therapy training. *Radiography*, 26(4), e19–e23.

Chaccour, C., Saad, W., Siddiqui, U. F., Demir, K., & Dhillon, H. S. (2021). Seven defining features of terahertz (THz) wireless systems: A fellowship of communication and sensing. *IEEE Communications Surveys & Tutorials*, 23(2), 1192–1223.

Charles, C., Gafni, A., & Whelan, T. (1997). Shared decision-making in the medical encounter: What does it mean? (or it takes at least two to tango). *Social Science & Medicine*, 44(5), 681–692.

Charmel, P. A., & Frampton, S. B. (2008). Building the business case for patient-centered care. *Healthcare Financial Management*, 62(3), 80–85.

Dang, S., Amin, O., Shihada, B., & Alouini, M. S. (2020). What should 6G be? *Nature Electronics*, 3(1), 20–29.

Davenport, T., & Kalakota, R. (2019). The potential for artificial intelligence in healthcare. *Future Healthcare Journal*, 6(2), 94–98.

David, G., Park, C., & Summers, K. (2021). Impact of telehealth on healthcare quality and utilization: A review of the literature. *Health Services Research*, 56(2), 329–349.

Epstein, R. M., & Street, R. L. (2011). The values and value of patient-centered care. *Annals of Family Medicine*, 9(2), 100–103.

Gao, W., Emaminejad, S., Nyein, H. Y. Y., Challa, S., Chen, K., Peck, A., ... Javey, A. (2015). Fully integrated wearable sensor arrays for multiplexed in situ perspiration analysis. *Nature*, 529(7587), 509–514.

Garcia, M., Sedano, B., & Murillo, L. (2017). Advances in remote surgery through virtual reality. In *Handbook of Research on Collaborative Teaching Practice in Virtual Learning Environments* (pp. 453–471). IGI Global.

Garg, L., Agarwal, N., & Kumar, S. (2021). Future directions for telemedicine in India. *The Lancet Oncology*, 22(4), e168–e169.

Ghanbarzadeh, R., Ghapanchi, A. H., Blumenstein, M., & Talaei-Khoei, A. (2014). A decade of research on the use of three-dimensional virtual worlds in health care: A systematic literature review. *Journal of Medical Internet Research*, 16(2), e47.

Goyal, A., Gupta, L., & Kapoor, A. (2021). The rise of smart hospitals: Advances in AI, IoT, big data, and robotics. *Journal of Healthcare Management*, 66(2), 81–88.

Institute of Medicine. (2001). *Crossing the quality chasm: A new health system for the 21st century*. National Academies Press.

Islam, S. M. R., Kwak, D., Kabir, M. H., Hossain, M., & Kwak, K. S. (2015). The Internet of Things for health care: A comprehensive survey. *IEEE Access*, 3, 678–708.

Jiang, F., Jiang, Y., Zhi, H., Dong, Y., Li, H., Ma, S., … Wang, Y. (2017). Artificial intelligence in healthcare: Past, present and future. *Stroke and Vascular Neurology*, 2(4), 230–243.

Keesara, S., Jonas, A., & Schulman, K. (2020). Covid-19 and health care's digital revolution. *New England Journal of Medicine*, 382(23), e82.

Latif, S., Qadir, J., Farooq, S., & Imran, M. A. (2021). How 5G wireless (and concomitant technologies) will revolutionize healthcare. *Future Internet*, 13(2), 41.

Patel, M. S., Asch, D. A., & Volpp, K. G. (2012). Wearable devices as facilitators, not drivers, of health behavior change. *JAMA*, 320(2), 197–198.

Raghupathi, W., & Raghupathi, V. (2014). Big data analytics in healthcare: Promise and potential. *Health Information Science and Systems*, 2(1), 3.

Rathore, M. M., Ahmad, A., Paul, A., & Rho, S. (2016). Urban planning and building smart cities based on the Internet of Things using big data analytics. *Computer Networks*, 101, 63–80.

Rogers, L., Tavares, A., & Mahoney, C. (2017). Virtual reality in healthcare: The applications and challenges of VR in medical training and patient education. *Future Healthcare Journal*, 4(3), 239–243.

Saad, W., Bennis, M., & Chen, M. (2020). A vision of 6G wireless systems: Applications, trends, technologies, and open research problems. *IEEE Network*, 34(3), 134–142.

Seymour, N. E. (2008). VR to OR: A review of the evidence that virtual reality simulation improves operating room performance. *World Journal of Surgery*, 32, 182–188.

Topol, E. J. (2019). *Deep Medicine: How Artificial Intelligence Can Make Healthcare Human Again*. Basic Books.

Yang, G. Z., Cambias, J., Cleary, K., Daimler, E., Drake, J., Dupont, P. E., … & Wood, B. J. (2018). Medical robotics—Regulatory, ethical, and legal considerations for increasing levels of autonomy. *Science Robotics*, 3(21), eaat4983.

Zhang, Z., Liu, J., Chen, Y., & Zhao, Q. (2019). Leveraging machine learning for diagnosing and predicting the onset of diabetes mellitus. *Biomedical Signal Processing and Control*, 49, 393–402.

8 Patient Perspectives on the Transformative Impact of Remote Patient Monitoring

J. Sudarvel, R. Velmurugan, Ravi Thirumalaisamy, K. Sankar Ganesh, and R. Sankar Ganesh

INTRODUCTION

Remote Patient Monitoring (RPM) has emerged as a pivotal innovation in the healthcare landscape, allowing for continuous tracking of patients' health conditions outside conventional clinical settings. RPM leverages technology to collect, transmit, and analyse patient data, thereby facilitating timely medical interventions and promoting proactive healthcare management. The transformative potential of RPM lies in its ability to enhance patient outcomes, improve quality of life, and optimize healthcare delivery (Burke et al., 2015; Kitsiou et al., 2017).

Despite its numerous benefits, the adoption and impact of RPM from the patient's perspective warrant comprehensive exploration. Understanding patients' experiences, perceptions, and challenges with RPM is crucial for designing effective and patient-centred RPM programs. Several studies have shown that RPM can lead to better health outcomes, increased patient engagement, and higher satisfaction levels (Anker et al., 2011; Kruse et al., 2017). However, barriers such as technology acceptance, privacy concerns, and the need for adequate support and infrastructure still pose significant challenges (Or & Karsh, 2009; Lupton, 2013).

This review of literature aims to delve into the qualitative analyses of patient perspectives on RPM, shedding light on the factors that influence their experiences and the transformative impact of this technology on their health and well-being. By examining various studies, this review seeks to identify key themes related to patient empowerment, health outcomes, convenience, psychological impact, and barriers to RPM adoption. Through this analysis, the review will provide valuable insights into how RPM can be optimized to meet patients' needs and contribute to a more sustainable and effective healthcare system.

DOI: 10.1201/9781003516590-8

REVIEW OF LITERATURE

RPM has emerged as a significant innovation in healthcare, allowing continuous monitoring of patients' health conditions outside traditional clinical settings. This review of literature aims to examine the transformative impact of RPM from the perspective of patients, focusing on qualitative studies that highlight their experiences, perceptions, and outcomes.

Kitsiou et al. (2017), patients reported feeling more engaged in their healthcare management, leading to improved adherence to treatment plans. The real-time feedback provided by RPM devices helps patients understand their health conditions better, fostering a sense of responsibility and proactive behaviour.

Kruse et al. (2017) found that patients using RPM experienced significant improvements in managing chronic conditions such as diabetes, hypertension, and heart disease. Patients reported fewer hospital visits, better disease management, and improved quality of life. The continuous monitoring allows for early detection of potential health issues, enabling timely interventions.

Dang et al. (2018) and Dinesen et al. (2016) highlight that patients appreciate the ability to receive healthcare services without the need to travel to a healthcare facility. This convenience reduces the burden on both patients and caregivers and can lead to increased satisfaction with the healthcare system.

The psychological impact of RPM on patients is multifaceted. While many patients report reduced anxiety and increased confidence in managing their health due to continuous monitoring (Coye et al., 2009), some studies, such as those by Nelson and Staggers (2014), indicate that the constant awareness of being monitored can cause stress and anxiety in certain individuals. It is crucial to address these psychological aspects to maximize the benefits of RPM.

Polisena et al. (2009). Additionally, concerns about data privacy and security are prevalent among patients, as highlighted by Cimperman et al. (2013). Ensuring robust technical support and addressing privacy concerns are essential for the widespread adoption of RPM.

Van Houwelingen et al. (2016) suggest that patients who trust the accuracy and reliability of RPM devices, as well as the competence of their healthcare providers, are more likely to adhere to RPM protocols and report positive experiences.

Sociocultural factors also play a role in patients' perspectives on RPM. Studies indicate that cultural beliefs, language barriers, and varying levels of health literacy can impact patients' acceptance and effective use of RPM (Or et al., 2018). Tailoring RPM programs to address these sociocultural factors can enhance patient engagement and outcomes.

RPM facilitates improved communication between patients and healthcare providers, fostering stronger relationships. According to a study by Radhakrishnan et al. (2016), patients felt more connected to their healthcare team through regular updates and timely feedback. This continuous interaction helps build trust and ensures that patients feel supported, which can lead to better health outcomes and patient satisfaction.

Burke et al. (2015) show that patients appreciate personalized care that considers their unique health patterns and needs. This customization can lead to more effective management of chronic conditions and higher patient satisfaction.

Kvedar et al. (2014) indicate that patients are more likely to follow prescribed treatments when they can see the direct impact of their actions through continuous monitoring. This adherence is crucial for managing chronic diseases and improving overall health outcomes.

Darkins et al. (2008) highlight that patients experienced cost savings related to travel, time off work, and healthcare expenses. These economic advantages make RPM an attractive option for both patients and healthcare systems.

Anker et al. (2011), patients with heart failure who used RPM reported better management of symptoms, reduced hospitalizations, and enhanced daily functioning. This improvement in quality of life is a significant benefit of RPM.

Scalvini et al. (2005) found that continuous monitoring allowed for prompt intervention in cases of abnormal readings, thereby preventing severe health crises. This proactive approach enhances patient safety and reduces the risk of complications.

Or and Karsh (2009) indicate that older adults, in particular, may struggle with using RPM devices due to a lack of familiarity with technology. Providing adequate training and support can help overcome these barriers.

Lupton (2013) reveals that patients worry about the security of their health data and potential misuse. Ensuring robust data protection measures is crucial to address these concerns and build patient trust in RPM systems.

Van Hoof et al. (2016), caregivers reported reduced stress and a greater sense of security knowing that their loved ones were being monitored continuously. This support can enhance the overall caregiving experience and improve outcomes for patients.

Koch (2006) suggests that healthcare organizations must provide the necessary infrastructure, training, and resources to ensure the effective use of RPM. Strong organizational support can facilitate smoother integration of RPM into routine care and enhance patient outcomes.

The literature suggests several avenues for future research. Longitudinal studies could provide insights into the long-term effects of RPM on patient health and behaviour. Comparative analyses between different patient demographics and conditions can help identify best practices and optimize RPM programs. Additionally, qualitative investigations into organizational culture and its impact on the implementation and success of RPM are recommended.

The transformative impact of RPM on patients is evident through improved health outcomes, enhanced patient engagement, and increased convenience. However, addressing technical, psychological, and sociocultural challenges is crucial for maximizing the benefits of RPM. By understanding and addressing patients' perspectives, healthcare providers can develop more effective and patient-centred RPM programs, contributing to the advancement of healthcare delivery.

STATEMENT OF THE PROBLEM

RPM has the potential to revolutionize healthcare by enabling continuous, real-time monitoring of patients outside traditional clinical settings. This technological advancement promises improved patient outcomes, enhanced quality of life, and optimized healthcare delivery. However, the successful implementation and adoption of RPM are significantly influenced by patients' perspectives, experiences, and acceptance of the technology. Despite the growing body of research highlighting the clinical benefits and cost-effectiveness of RPM, there remains a notable gap in understanding the qualitative aspects of patient experiences. Patients' perspectives are crucial in assessing the true impact of RPM, as their acceptance and engagement with the technology directly affect its efficacy and sustainability. Issues such as empowerment, convenience, health outcomes, psychological impact, and barriers to adoption are central to the patient experience and can vary widely among different patient populations.

Some patients report positive experiences with RPM, citing increased engagement in their health management and improved health outcomes. However, others face significant challenges, including difficulties with technology use, concerns about data privacy, and inadequate support and infrastructure. These challenges can hinder the adoption and effectiveness of RPM, leading to disparities in healthcare access and outcomes. The problem, therefore, lies in the insufficient understanding of the diverse patient perspectives on RPM. Without comprehensive qualitative insights, healthcare providers and policymakers may struggle to develop and implement RPM programs that are truly patient-centred and capable of addressing the varied needs and concerns of different patient groups.

This study aims to fill this gap by conducting a qualitative analysis of patient perspectives on the transformative impact of RPM. By identifying key themes related to patient empowerment, health outcomes, convenience, psychological impact, and barriers to adoption, this research seeks to provide actionable insights that can inform the development of more effective and inclusive RPM programs. Addressing these issues is essential for maximizing the benefits of RPM and ensuring its successful integration into healthcare systems, ultimately contributing to a more sustainable and effective healthcare delivery model.

SCOPE OF THE STUDY

This study explores the transformative impact of RPM from the perspective of patients, employing a qualitative analysis approach. The primary objective is to understand patients' experiences, perceptions, and challenges with RPM, thereby providing insights that can inform the development of patient-centred RPM programs. The scope includes investigating how RPM affects patient empowerment and engagement, examining its impact on health outcomes, and analysing the convenience and accessibility it offers. Additionally, the study evaluates the psychological effects of RPM on patients, including feelings of security, anxiety, and stress related to continuous monitoring. It identifies barriers to adoption, such as technological, cultural, economic, and infrastructural challenges, and explores concerns related to data privacy, security, and the reliability of RPM devices.

Furthermore, the study looks into how trust in RPM technology and healthcare providers influences patient acceptance and satisfaction. It considers sociocultural factors like age, education, cultural beliefs, and health literacy, assessing their impact on patient experiences and perceptions. The effects of RPM on caregivers, including changes in their responsibilities and stress levels, are also examined. The study provides actionable recommendations for healthcare providers, policymakers, and technology developers to enhance RPM program design and implementation. It suggests strategies to overcome identified barriers and improve patient experiences with RPM. Finally, the study highlights gaps in current literature and suggests future research directions, including longitudinal studies, comparative analyses, and qualitative investigations into organizational culture and RPM implementation. By focusing on these areas, the study aims to provide a comprehensive understanding of the patient perspective on RPM, contributing to the broader discourse on sustainable and effective healthcare delivery.

OBJECTIVE OF THE STUDY

To know the Patient Perspectives on the Transformative Impact of RPM.

RESEARCH METHODOLOGY

This study employs a qualitative research design to explore patient perspectives on the transformative impact of RPM technology. A qualitative approach is chosen to gain in-depth insights into patients' experiences, attitudes, and perceptions regarding RPM.

SAMPLE SELECTION

The sample consists of 404 patients who have been using RPM devices for at least six months. Participants were selected using purposive sampling to ensure a diverse representation of patients across different demographics, health conditions, and usage experiences. The sample includes patients from various age groups, genders, marital statuses, educational qualifications, occupations, areas of residence, family types, and income levels.

DATA COLLECTION

A structured questionnaire will be developed to collect quantitative data. The questionnaire will include demographic information and questions related to patient preferences, such as factors influencing their choice of private hospitals, perceived quality of care, cost considerations, and importance of amenities. The questionnaire will be administered to the selected sample of patients through face-to-face interviews.

FRAMEWORK OF ANALYSIS

The collected data have been analysed by employing simple percentage and factor analysis.

SIGNIFICANCE OF THE STUDY

This study holds significant importance in the context of modern healthcare, where RPM is increasingly seen as a transformative technology. By focusing on the qualitative analysis of patient perspectives, this study provides insights that can drive meaningful improvements in healthcare delivery. The study's emphasis on patient-centred care is crucial. Understanding patients' experiences, perceptions, and challenges with RPM can lead to the development of more personalized and effective healthcare solutions. This approach aligns with the current trend towards more individualized care, where patient engagement and empowerment are key factors in improving health outcomes. This study's findings can inform strategies to enhance RPM adoption and engagement. By identifying barriers and facilitators to RPM use, healthcare providers can tailor their approaches to encourage more widespread acceptance and consistent use of RPM technologies. This, in turn, can lead to better management of chronic conditions, reduced hospitalizations, and improved overall health for patients. The study's exploration of the psychological and emotional impact of RPM is significant. Continuous monitoring can have both positive and negative effects on patients' well-being, and understanding these effects is essential for providing adequate support. By addressing patients' psychological needs, healthcare providers can ensure that RPM programs are not only clinically effective but also supportive of patients' mental health. Furthermore, the study's insights into trust and satisfaction with RPM technologies and healthcare providers can guide efforts to build stronger patient-provider relationships. Trust is a foundational element of effective healthcare delivery, and understanding how it is influenced by RPM can help improve the overall patient experience. This study's recommendations for practice and future research directions are valuable for shaping the future of RPM. By providing actionable recommendations, the study can guide healthcare providers, policymakers, and technology developers in implementing more effective and patient-friendly RPM programs. Additionally, the identification of future research avenues ensures that the study's impact extends beyond its immediate findings, contributing to ongoing advancements in RPM technology and practice. In conclusion, this study's focus on patient perspectives on RPM is significant for its potential to drive meaningful improvements in healthcare delivery. By addressing the diverse needs and concerns of patients, the study can help shape a future where RPM plays a central role in delivering personalized, efficient, and effective healthcare services.

ANALYSIS AND INTERPRETATION

The demographic data provides a comprehensive overview of the study's participants, highlighting various aspects such as age, gender, marital status, educational qualification, occupation, area of residence, type of family, status in family, monthly income, family income, and family expenditure (Table 8.1).

Age

A majority of the participants (72.3%) are in the 3145 years age group.

Participants aged up to 30 years constitute 10.9%, while those above 45 years make up 16.8%.

Gender

There is a higher representation of females (59.4%) compared to males (40.6%).

TABLE 8.1
Simple Frequency

Age	Frequency	Percent
Up to 30 years	44	10.9
31–45 years	292	72.3
Above 45 years	68	16.8
Total	404	100.0

Gender	Frequency	Percent
Male	164	40.6
Female	240	59.4
Total	404	100.0

Gender	Frequency	Percent
Male	164	40.6
Female	240	59.4
Total	404	100.0

Marital status	Frequency	Percent
Married	344	85.1
Unmarried	60	14.9
Total	404	100.0

Educational qualification	Frequency	Percent
Up to HSC	4	1.0
UG degree	256	63.4
PG degree	80	19.8
Professional	44	10.9
Others	20	5.0
Total	404	100.0

Occupation	Frequency	Percent
Agriculture	74	18.3
Business	36	8.9
Employee	118	29.2
Professional	36	8.9
Home maker	68	16.8
Others	72	17.8
Total	404	100.0

(Continued)

TABLE 8.1 (Continued)

Area of residence	Frequency	Percent
Urban	140	34.7
Semi-urban	132	32.7
Rural	132	32.7
Total	404	100.0

Type of family	Frequency	Percent
Joint	68	16.8
Nuclear	336	83.2
Total	404	100.0

Status in family	Frequency	Percent
Head	102	25.2
Member	302	74.8
Total	404	100.0

Monthly income	Frequency	Percent
Up to 20000	260	64.4
20001–40000	112	27.7
Above 40000	32	7.9
Total	404	100.0

Family income	Frequency	Percent
Up to 30000	316	78.2
30001–50000	54	13.4
Above 50000	34	8.4
Total	404	100.0

Family expenditure	Frequency	Percent
Up to 10000	254	62.9
10001–20000	138	34.2
Above 20000	12	3.0
Total	404	100.0

Marital Status

The majority of the participants are married (85.1%), with unmarried individuals making up 14.9%.

Educational Qualification

Most participants have an undergraduate degree (63.4%), followed by those with a postgraduate degree (19.8%).

Professional qualifications are held by 10.9%, while a small percentage have qualifications up to HSC (1.0%) or other qualifications (5.0%).

Occupation

The largest occupational group is employees (29.2%), followed by those involved in agriculture (18.3%) and homemakers (16.8%).

Other occupations include business (8.9%), professionals (8.9%), and other unspecified jobs (17.8%).

Area of Residence

Participants are almost equally distributed among urban (34.7%), semiurban (32.7%), and rural (32.7%) areas.

Type of Family

A significant majority of participants live in nuclear families (83.2%), with the rest in joint families (16.8%).

Status in Family

Most participants are members of their families (74.8%), with 25.2% being heads of their families.

Monthly Income

A majority of participants have a monthly income of up to Rs. 20,000 (64.4%).

Those earning between Rs. 20,001 and Rs. 40,000 constitute 27.7%, while 7.9% earn above Rs. 40,000.

Family Income

Most families have an income of up to Rs. 30,000 (78.2%).

Families earning between Rs. 30,001 and Rs. 50,000 make up 13.4%, while those with incomes above Rs. 50,000 constitute 8.4%.

Family Expenditure

The majority of families have monthly expenditures up to Rs. 10,000 (62.9%).

Families with expenditures between Rs. 10,001 and Rs. 20,000 account for 34.2%, while only 3.0% spend above Rs. 20,000.

This demographic profile indicates a predominantly middle-aged, female majority sample with a significant proportion of married individuals, primarily holding undergraduate degrees and employed in various sectors. The data also reflects a broad distribution in terms of area of residence, family type, income levels, and expenditure patterns, providing a well-rounded view of the study population.

Factor Analysis

To know the Patient Perspectives on the Transformative Impact of RPM Factor analysis is employed (Tables 8.2 and 8.3).

TABLE 8.2
KMO and Bartlett's Test

KaiserMeyerOlkin Measure of Sampling Adequacy		.901
Bartlett's Test of Sphericity	Approx. ChiSquare	8603.553
	Df	435
	Sig.	.000

TABLE 8.3
Rotated Component Matrix

	Component					
	1	2	3	4	5	6
The setup and maintenance of RPM devices are not burdensome.	.799					
I do not experience technical issues frequently with the RPM devices.	.750					
I have access to reliable internet and technology to use RPM effectively.	.714					
The RPM technology I use is easy to understand and operate.	.668					
Using RPM has reduced my anxiety about managing my health condition.	.653					
I find the cost of RPM devices and services affordable.	.631					
Overall, I am satisfied with my experience using RPM.		.732				
I would recommend RPM to others with similar health conditions.		.684				
I have received adequate training to use RPM devices effectively.		.672				
I feel confident in my ability to use RPM due to the training provided.		.661				
The support provided by healthcare providers for using RPM is sufficient.		.648				
RPM has met my expectations in terms of healthcare management.		.637				
RPM has made me more aware of my health condition and necessary actions.		.601				
RPM has positively impacted my quality of life.		.564				
I trust that my privacy is maintained when using RPM technologies.			.718			

(*Continued*)

TABLE 8.3   (Continued)

	Component					
	1	2	3	4	5	6
RPM helps me to better manage my health conditions.			.699			
Using RPM has improved my overall health management.			.603			
I do not worry about the misuse of my health data collected through RPM.			.529			
I feel more engaged in my healthcare decisions due to RPM.				.629		
I feel more secure about my health due to continuous monitoring by RPM.				.583		
I feel more connected to my healthcare team through RPM.				.535		
RPM encourages me to take a more active role in managing my health.					.782	
I find it convenient to use RPM devices to monitor my health.					.701	
I find it easy to integrate RPM into my daily routine.						.669
Eigenvalues	13.080	2.113	1.768	1.201	1.091	1.036
% of Variance	43.600	7.043	5.894	4.003	3.637	3.453
Cumulative %	43.600	50.644	56.538	60.541	64.178	67.632

INTERPRETATION OF FACTOR ANALYSIS ON PATIENT PERSPECTIVES OF REMOTE PATIENT MONITORING (RPM)

KMO AND BARTLETT'S TEST

KaiserMeyerOlkin (KMO) Measure of Sampling Adequacy: The KMO value is 0.901, which is considered excellent. This indicates that the sample is adequate for conducting factor analysis.

Bartlett's Test of Sphericity: The chisquare value is 8603.553 with 435 degrees of freedom and a significance level of 0.000. This suggests that the correlations between the items are sufficiently large for factor analysis.

ROTATED COMPONENT MATRIX

The rotated component matrix shows the factor loadings of each item on the identified components. Six components were extracted based on their eigenvalues being greater than 1, explaining a total of 67.632% of the variance.

Component 1 Usability and Accessibility of RPM

High Loadings

The setup and maintenance of RPM devices are not burdensome. (.799)
I do not experience technical issues frequently with the RPM devices. (.750)
I have access to reliable internet and technology to use RPM effectively. (.714)
The RPM technology I use is easy to understand and operate. (.668)
Using RPM has reduced my anxiety about managing my health condition. (.653)

This component reflects the ease of use, technical reliability, and accessibility of RPM technologies.

Component 2 Training and Support

High Loadings

Overall, I am satisfied with my experience using RPM. (.732)
I would recommend RPM to others with similar health conditions. (.684)
I have received adequate training to use RPM devices effectively. (.672)
I feel confident in my ability to use RPM due to the training provided. (.661)
The support provided by healthcare providers for using RPM is sufficient. (.648)
RPM has met my expectations in terms of healthcare management. (.637)

This component highlights the importance of training, support, and overall satisfaction with RPM.

Component 3 Health Management and Data Security

High Loadings

I trust that my privacy is maintained when using RPM technologies. (.718)
RPM helps me to better manage my health conditions. (.699)
Using RPM has improved my overall health management. (.603)
I do not worry about the misuse of my health data collected through RPM. (.529)

This component focuses on health management and the security of personal health data.

Component 4 Engagement and Connectivity

High Loadings

I feel more engaged in my healthcare decisions due to RPM. (.629)
I feel more secure about my health due to continuous monitoring by RPM. (.583)
I feel more connected to my healthcare team through RPM. (.535)

This component captures the aspects of patient engagement, connectivity with healthcare providers, and the sense of security provided by RPM.

Component 5 Convenience and Active Management

High Loadings

RPM encourages me to take a more active role in managing my health. (.782)
I find it convenient to use RPM devices to monitor my health. (.701)

This component pertains to the convenience and encouragement provided by RPM for active health management.

Component 6 Routine Integration

High Loadings

I find it easy to integrate RPM into my daily routine. (.669)

This component emphasizes the ease of integrating RPM into daily routines and the confidence in data security.

VARIANCE EXPLAINED

Component 1 – Explains 43.600% of the variance.
Component 2 – Adds an additional 7.043%, cumulatively explaining 50.644% of the variance.
Component 3 – Adds 5.894%, reaching a cumulative 56.538% of the variance.
Component 4 – Adds 4.003%, for a cumulative 60.541% of the variance.
Component 5 – Adds 3.637%, with a cumulative 64.178% of the variance.
Component 6 – Adds 3.453%, reaching a cumulative 67.632% of the variance.

In summary, the factor analysis reveals six key components that reflect various dimensions of patient perspectives on RPM, including usability, training and support, health management, engagement, convenience, and routine integration. These components provide a comprehensive understanding of the factors influencing patient experiences with RPM, which can be used to enhance the design and implementation of RPM programs.

NON-SIGNIFICANT FACTORS BASED ON FACTOR LOADINGS LESS THAN 0.5

In factor analysis, items with factor loadings less than 0.5 on all components are often considered non-significant, as they do not strongly correlate with any specific factor. Based on this criterion, the following items can be considered non-significant in the context of patient perspectives on RPM:

- I am confident that my personal health data is secure with RPM
- The data provided by RPM devices is accurate and reliable
- RPM has improved my communication with healthcare providers
- RPM has made it easier for me to access medical support when needed.
- RPM allows my healthcare providers to respond more promptly to my needs.
- RPM has improved my communication with healthcare providers.
- RPM allows me to receive healthcare without needing to visit a clinic frequently.

The loadings are all below 0.5, suggesting that perceptions of data accuracy and reliability do not significantly contribute to any specific factor.

These items have factor loadings below 0.5 across all components, indicating they do not significantly contribute to any specific dimension identified in the factor analysis. Recognizing these no significant factors helps refine the focus on the most influential aspects of RPM, aiding in targeted strategies to enhance patient experience and engagement with RPM technologies.

SUGGESTIONS

Suggestions for Enhancing Patient Experience with RPM

ENHANCE DATA SECURITY AND PRIVACY

Implement robust encryption methods and strict data privacy policies. This can include end-to-end encryption for data transmission and secure storage solutions to protect patient information. Regularly updating security protocols and conducting audits can further ensure the integrity and confidentiality of patient data.

ENSURE DATA ACCURACY AND RELIABILITY

Regularly calibrate and maintain RPM devices and provide transparent information about their accuracy. Healthcare providers should schedule routine checks and updates for devices to ensure they are functioning correctly. Providing patients with detailed information about how the devices work and their limitations can help manage expectations and build trust in the technology.

IMPROVE COMMUNICATION CHANNELS

Develop integrated communication platforms within RPM systems for seamless interaction between patients and healthcare providers. This can involve creating user-friendly apps or web portals that allow for easy messaging, video calls, and data sharing. Ensuring that these platforms are accessible and reliable can enhance the overall patient experience.

FACILITATE ACCESS TO MEDICAL SUPPORT

Provide clear guidelines and support for using RPM to access medical services and emergency care. This can include creating detailed user manuals, instructional videos, and 24/7 helplines. Ensuring that patients understand how to use the technology to get the support they need can reduce anxiety and improve health outcomes.

ENHANCE RESPONSIVENESS OF HEALTHCARE PROVIDERS

Implement systems for timely notifications and alerts to healthcare providers for prompt responses to patient needs. Automated alert systems can be set up to notify healthcare providers of any significant changes in a patient's condition, enabling faster intervention and support.

REDUCE THE BURDEN OF DEVICE SETUP AND MAINTENANCE

Simplify the setup process and provide comprehensive technical support and training for patients. Offering in-home installation services, easy-to-follow setup guides, and remote support options can help patients get started with RPM technology without feeling overwhelmed.

IMPROVE PATIENT TRAINING AND SUPPORT

Offer regular training sessions and user-friendly guides to help patients understand and operate RPM devices effectively. Training can be provided through in-person sessions, online tutorials, and ongoing support from healthcare providers. Ensuring patients feel confident in using the technology can enhance adherence and satisfaction.

PROMOTE COST EFFECTIVENESS

Explore cost reduction strategies and offer financial assistance programs for patients who may find RPM services expensive. This can include negotiating lower prices for devices, offering subsidies, or creating payment plans. Making RPM more affordable can increase its accessibility and adoption among patients.

BOOST PATIENT ENGAGEMENT AND INVOLVEMENT

Encourage active patient participation in health management through RPM by providing personalized health insights and feedback. Using RPM data to create tailored health reports and actionable recommendations can help patients feel more involved and empowered in managing their health.

CONDUCT REGULAR FEEDBACK AND IMPROVEMENT CYCLES

Collect regular feedback from patients regarding their experiences with RPM and use this data to make continuous improvements. This can involve conducting surveys, interviews, and focus groups to gather insights. Using this feedback to refine and enhance RPM systems can ensure they continue to meet patient needs effectively.

Implementing these suggestions can significantly enhance the patient experience with RPM. By focusing on critical areas such as data security, communication, training, affordability, and responsiveness, healthcare providers can ensure that RPM technology effectively supports patient health management and contributes to positive health outcomes.

CONCLUSION

Implementing RPM has the potential to transform healthcare delivery by offering continuous and convenient health monitoring. However, to fully realize its benefits, it is essential to address several key areas. Enhancing data security and privacy is crucial to building patient trust and ensuring the confidentiality of sensitive health information. Ensuring data accuracy and reliability through regular device maintenance and transparent communication can help in maintaining patient confidence in the technology.

Improving communication channels between patients and healthcare providers can facilitate better interaction and support, while clear guidelines and support for accessing medical services via RPM can reduce patient anxiety and improve health outcomes. Simplifying the setup and maintenance of RPM devices, along with providing comprehensive training and support, can help patients use the technology effectively and confidently.

Making RPM more cost-effective through financial assistance programs and exploring cost reduction strategies can increase its accessibility. Encouraging patient engagement by providing personalized health insights can empower patients to take an active role in their health management. Finally, regular feedback and continuous improvement cycles based on patient experiences can ensure that RPM systems remain responsive to patient needs.

By addressing these areas, healthcare providers can enhance the overall patient experience with RPM, leading to better health management, increased patient satisfaction, and ultimately, improved health outcomes.

SCOPE FOR FURTHER RESEARCH

There is ample scope for further research to deepen our understanding and enhance the implementation of RPM. Longitudinal studies tracking patient experiences over time can provide insights into the long-term effects of RPM on health management. Comparative analyses of different RPM technologies and strategies in diverse healthcare settings can identify best practices. Qualitative investigations into organizational culture and practices related to RPM adoption can reveal barriers and facilitators to successful implementation. Further research can also focus on the impact of RPM on specific health outcomes, such as medication adherence and quality of life. Cost-effectiveness analyses can evaluate the economic implications of RPM implementation, informing decision-making and policy development. Investigating innovative patient engagement strategies and the role of RPM in addressing health disparities can contribute to more inclusive healthcare delivery. Additionally, exploring technological advances and their integration with RPM, as well as policy and regulatory considerations, can further optimize care delivery and patient outcomes.

REFERENCES

Anker, S. D., Koehler, F., & Abraham, W. T. (2011). Telemedicine and remote management of patients with heart failure. *The Lancet*, 378(9792), 731739.

Burke, L. E., Ma, J., Azar, K. M., Bennett, G. G., Peterson, E. D., Zheng, Y., & Riley, W. (2015). Current science on consumer use of mobile health for cardiovascular disease prevention: a scientific statement from the American Heart Association. *Circulation*, 132(12), 11571213.

Cimperman, M., Brenčič, M. M., Trkman, P., & Stanonik, M. de L. (2013). Older adults' perceptions of home telehealth services. *Telemedicine and eHealth*, 19(10), 786790.

Coye, M. J., Haselkorn, A., & DeMello, S. (2009). Remote patient management: Technology enabled innovation and evolving business models for chronic disease care. *Health Affairs*, 28(1), 126135.

Dang, S., Olsan, T., Karuza, J., Cai, X., Gao, Y., & RamirezZohfeld, V. (2018). Homebased telehealth: a review and metaanalysis of trials examining clinical outcomes and cost savings. *Telemedicine and eHealth*, 24(8), 628634.

Darkins, A., Ryan, P., Kobb, R., Foster, L., Edmonson, E., Wakefield, B., & Lancaster, A. E. (2008). Care coordination/home telehealth: the systematic implementation of health informatics, home telehealth, and disease management to support the care of veteran patients with chronic conditions. *Telemedicine and eHealth*, 14(10), 11181126.

Dinesen, B., Nonnecke, B., Lindeman, D., Toft, E., Kidholm, K., Jethwani, K., & Nesbitt, T. (2016). Personalized telehealth in the future: a global research agenda. *Journal of Medical Internet Research*, 18(3), e53.

Kitsiou, S., Paré, G., Jaana, M., & Gerber, B. (2017). Effectiveness of mHealth interventions for patients with diabetes: An overview of systematic reviews. *PloS One*, 12(3), e0173160.

Koch, S. (2006). Home telehealth—current state and future trends. *International Journal of Medical Informatics*, 75(8), 565576.

Kruse, C. S., Krowski, N., Rodriguez, B., Tran, L., Vela, J., & Brooks, M. (2017). Telehealth and patient satisfaction: a systematic review and narrative analysis. *BMJ Open*, 7(8), e016242.

Kvedar, J. C., Nesbitt, T., Kvedar, J., & Weintraub, A. (2014). *The cHealth Revolution: The Future of Healthcare Delivery*. McGraw-Hill Professional.

Lupton, D. (2013). The digitally engaged patient: Self monitoring and selfcare in the digital health era. *Social Theory & Health*, 11(3), 256270.

Nelson, E. L., & Staggers, N. (2014). Chronic disease management using home telehealth: critical success factors and models of service delivery. *Telemedicine and eHealth*, 20(4), 327334.

Or, C. K., & Karsh, B. T. (2009). A systematic review of patient acceptance of consumer health information technology. *Journal of the American Medical Informatics Association*, 16(4), 550560.

Or, C. K. L., Tao, D., & Wang, H. (2018). Factors influencing intention to use mHealth apps for selfcare: A qualitative study of older adults. *Health Informatics Journal*, 24(1), 132146.

Polisena, J., Tran, K., Cimon, K., Hutton, B., McGill, S., & Palmer, K. (2009). Home telehealth for chronic disease management: a systematic review and an analysis of economic evaluations. *International Journal of Technology Assessment in Health Care*, 25(3), 339349.

Radhakrishnan, K., Xie, B., Jacelon, C., & Unsar, S. (2016). Barriers and facilitators for sustainability of telehomecare programs: A systematic review. *Health Services Research*, 51(1), 4875.

Scalvini, S., Zanelli, E., Comini, L., Tomba, M. D., Troise, G., & Giordano, A. (2005). Homebased exercise rehabilitation with telemedicine following cardiac surgery. *Journal of Telemedicine and Telecare*, 11(1_suppl), 3739.

Van Hoof, J., Blom, M. M., Post, H. N. A., & Bastein, W. J. H. (2016). Designing a thermostat for people with dementia: An observational study of heating behavior in dementia care facilities. *Energy Research & Social Science*, 19, 102115.

Van Houwelingen, C. T., Ettema, R. G., Antonietti, M. G., & Kort, H. S. (2016). Understanding older people's readiness for receiving telehealth services at home: a mixed method study. *BMC Health Services Research*, 16(1), 112.

9 Machine Learning Algorithms for Disease Prediction and Diagnosis

Ankush Joshi, Vikash Kumar, Naman Chauhan, and Gesu Thakur

INTRODUCTION

The ability to forecast and diagnose diseases is crucial to modern healthcare since it allows for early intervention and efficient management of a variety of medical disorders. An early diagnosis of diseases not only improves patient outcomes but also greatly lowers the load on resources and the expense of healthcare. Machine learning (ML) has emerged as a transformational tool in the field of healthcare with the emergence of cutting-edge technologies, altering the way diseases are anticipated and diagnosed. ML can reveal deep patterns inside massive datasets by utilizing sophisticated algorithms and data-driven insights, supporting the creation of reliable predictive models and diagnostic tools (Ibrahim and Abdulazeez, 2021). This chapter explores the complex relationship between ML and the prediction and diagnosis of diseases, illuminating the core ideas, approaches, and applications that have transformed the face of contemporary healthcare.

A paradigm change in disease management has been brought in by the incorporation of ML into healthcare. The ability of ML algorithms to unravel complex correlations in medical data, from straightforward regression models to deep neural networks, has been astoundingly shown. These algorithms can find tiny patterns and relationships that can escape human cognition by processing and analyzing complex datasets made up of patient records, medical imaging, genetic data, and several other health-related characteristics. As a result, ML plays a more important role in healthcare than just data analysis. It is a crucial tool for increasing clinical decision-making, streamlining treatment plans, and ultimately improving patient care (Joshi, 2013).

The role of ML acquires utmost relevance in the context of disease diagnosis and prediction. The success of treatment plans and patient prognoses can frequently be determined by the early and accurate diagnosis of diseases. Healthcare experts can predict the possibility of illness recurrence in susceptible individuals because of ML algorithms' capacity to handle enormous volumes of heterogeneous data and spot nuanced associations. These algorithms can also assist in the early detection of latent diseases, enabling proactive interventions and preventive measures by drawing on historical data and current patient information. The importance of accurate disease

DOI: 10.1201/9781003516590-9

diagnosis and prediction is further highlighted by its ability to reduce the strain on healthcare infrastructure and maximize resource allocation, thereby promoting a more effective and sustainable healthcare ecosystem.

The incorporation of ML algorithms has accelerated the development of personalized and precision medicine while also streamlining the process of disease detection and prediction as the healthcare landscape changes. The idea of customized healthcare interventions has undergone a revolution thanks to ML models' capacity to analyze a wide range of datasets and produce patient-specific insights. These algorithms enable the personalization of treatment programs, assuring optimal therapeutic outcomes and reducing the likelihood of adverse events by identifying minute changes in patient profiles and risk variables. Additionally, the seamless integration of ML technologies with modern imaging techniques has enhanced the accurate and effective detection of diseases (Uddin et al., 2019. This has allowed medical practitioners to identify anomalies and pathologies with previously unheard-of accuracy and speed. Combining these technological developments has sped up clinical decision-making while fostering a patient-centric strategy emphasizing personalized care and overall wellness.

FUNDAMENTALS OF MACHINE LEARNING IN HEALTHCARE

The healthcare sector has undergone a transformation thanks to ML, a subfield of artificial intelligence that makes it possible to analyze large datasets and derive insightful information for disease diagnosis and prognosis. Knowing the fundamentals of ML algorithms and how they are used is crucial to understanding their enormous influence on healthcare. Fundamentally, ML includes many algorithms that make it easier to analyze data, find patterns, and make decisions in the healthcare industry. These methods, which range from straightforward decision trees and linear regression to complex deep learning models, are designed to tackle different issues in healthcare data processing (Shaik et al., 2024).

The core of ML in healthcare is supervised, unsupervised, and semi-supervised learning methods. Algorithms are trained by supervised learning on labeled datasets where the input data is associated with the desired outputs, allowing the algorithm to learn the relationship between the inputs and outputs. The use of past patient data to train models to predict the risk of a disease occurring in new instances makes this technique particularly useful in the field of disease prediction. Unsupervised learning techniques, on the other hand, concentrate on revealing underlying structures and patterns in unlabeled datasets, allowing the computer to recognize inborn connections and groups within the data (Chauhan et al., 2024). This healthcare method can help group patients based on shared traits, facilitating individualized treatment plans. Furthermore, semi-supervised learning techniques combine aspects of supervised and unsupervised learning, enabling algorithms to use a smaller pool of labeled data in conjunction with a larger pool of unlabeled data, optimizing the learning process in circumstances where obtaining labeled data is difficult or resource-intensive.

Data preprocessing and feature engineering are essential for improving the efficacy and accuracy of ML models in the analysis of healthcare data. Preprocessing procedures, including data cleansing, normalization, and outlier detection, are essential for assuring data quality and dependability due to the complexity and variety of healthcare information. Preprocessing procedures set the foundation for a robust and trustworthy analysis by spotting and fixing errors and inconsistencies in the data. Another crucial component is feature engineering, which entails the extraction and selection of pertinent features from the data to make it easier to produce instructive and discriminative inputs for ML models. Feature engineering in healthcare entails the extraction of pertinent biomarkers, physiological measures, and clinical indications that have a high degree of predictive value for diagnosing and prognosticating diseases. ML models can produce more accurate and reliable predictions by improving the input data through efficient preprocessing and feature engineering approaches, increasing the overall effectiveness of illness prediction and diagnostic systems in healthcare.

DATA COLLECTION AND PRE-PROCESSING FOR DISEASE PREDICTION

The act of gathering data is the cornerstone of the effort to use ML to forecast diseases because it provides the raw materials needed to create trustworthy and accurate predictive models. To maintain the integrity and quality of the data, however, the collection of healthcare data offers a variety of issues that must be carefully navigated. The availability and accessibility of thorough and varied healthcare data are one of the biggest obstacles. When it comes to data integration and harmonization, healthcare data, which is frequently spread across numerous sources and systems, can present considerable challenges. Furthermore, maintaining the privacy and security of sensitive patient data remains a top priority, necessitating adherence to strict legal and ethical frameworks to protect patient confidentiality and data integrity (Hamidi and Daraee, 2016). Additionally, the variety of data types and structures used by various healthcare organizations and systems adds complexity to the process of data aggregation, necessitating strict interoperability and standardization requirements to make data integration and analysis possible.

The accuracy and dependability of disease prediction models are significantly hampered by the occurrence of missing data and data imbalances in healthcare databases. Missing data can weaken the effectiveness of ML algorithms and produce biased or inaccurate predictions (Joshi & Tiwari, 2023). Missing data can come from a variety of sources, including missing health records or data entry mistakes. Strategic imputation techniques, such as mean or median imputation, regression imputation, or complex algorithms like K-nearest neighbors (KNN) imputation, must be used to address missing data. These strategies enable the preservation of data integrity and reduce potential distortions in the predictive models by imputing missing values based on the current data distribution. Data imbalances, in which some groups or categories are overrepresented in the dataset, can also induce biases and skew the results of predictive analyses. To mitigate data imbalances, ensure fair representation of different classes, and improve the generalizability of the predictive models, balancing techniques, such as oversampling, undersampling, or the use of synthetic data generation methods, such as Synthetic Minority Over-sampling Technique (SMOTE), are essential.

By promoting uniformity and comparability across various datasets, data normalization and standardization approaches play a crucial role in preparing healthcare data for analysis and modeling. Because healthcare data is inherently heterogeneous, normalization techniques are crucial for scaling numerical data to a consistent range and removing variances in the magnitude and distribution of various variables. Common normalization methods like min-max scaling and Z-score normalization allow data to be transformed into a consistent scale, preventing some features from dominating the study due to their larger magnitudes. Similar to this, data standardization strategies concentrate on modifying data distributions to adhere to a preset standard, assuring compatibility and uniformity across various datasets. To stabilize the variance and central tendency of the data, standardization techniques like robust scaling or vector normalization are used. This allows for more precise and trustworthy comparisons and analyses. To reduce biases and allow the creation of reliable and generalizable illness prediction models, healthcare data can be preprocessed by using efficient normalization and standardization procedures. This increases the effectiveness and applicability of ML in healthcare settings (Maharana et al., 2022).

As a result, careful attention to detail and adherence to reliable procedures are required throughout the process of data gathering and preprocessing for disease prediction. Healthcare organizations and researchers can lay the groundwork for the development of strong and reliable ML models that are essential in advancing disease prediction and enabling more efficient and individualized healthcare interventions by addressing the difficulties associated with data collection, handling missing data and data imbalances, and putting data normalization and standardization techniques into practice.

MACHINE LEARNING ALGORITHMS FOR DISEASE PREDICTION

Healthcare workers can generate informed predictions about the possibility of a disease occurring by using ML algorithms, which are formidable tools in the field of illness prediction. It is essential to comprehend the subtleties and applicability of well-known ML algorithms to maximize their use in illness prediction tasks and enable more precise and trustworthy predictive models in healthcare settings. Because it can simulate the likelihood of a binary outcome depending on input features, the fundamental classification technique known as logistic regression is a good choice for disease prediction (Yadav and Jadhav, 2019). By assisting in the estimation of the likelihood of illness incidence based on a collection of independent variables, logistic regression is particularly useful in situations when the result is categorical, allowing healthcare professionals to evaluate the risk factors related to particular diseases.

Decision trees provide a useful framework for disease prediction tasks by enabling the identification of hierarchical linkages within datasets and are characterized by their intuitive and interpretable nature. Decision trees enable the establishment of clear decision routes that help in the prediction of illness outcomes by splitting data based on particular qualities and criteria. Decision trees are particularly suited for situations where clinical decision-making requires a knowledge of the underlying logic of predictive models due to their inherent ability to handle both categorical and numerical data.

The robustness and accuracy of random forests, an ensemble learning method based on decision trees, are well known for their ability to handle challenging datasets. Random forests can significantly reduce the danger of overfitting and improve the generalizability of disease prediction models by combining the predictions of various decision trees. Random forests excel in situations where feature importance and model stability are crucial, offering more dependable and robust disease prediction skills. They can manage high-dimensional data and discover relevant predictors.

The supervised learning-based support vector machines (SVMs) provide a flexible framework for illness prediction tasks, especially in settings with complicated decision boundaries and non-linear correlations. SVMs make it easier to find the best hyperplanes for classifying and predicting disease outcomes by mapping data points to high-dimensional feature spaces. SVMs are a good choice for illness prediction tasks that require complex data structures and a variety of feature sets due to their adaptability to different kernel functions and their ability to handle both linear and non-linear data.

Neural networks are a potent class of ML algorithms that mimic the operation of the human brain. They are distinguished by their intricate and linked design. Neural networks excel at capturing complex nonlinear dependencies within healthcare datasets due to their ability to process enormous amounts of data and discern intricate patterns and relationships. This makes them particularly effective in disease prediction tasks that call for the analysis of multifaceted and heterogeneous data. Additionally, neural networks are useful tools for precise and thorough illness prediction models due to their adaptability to a variety of data formats and their potential for learning complex feature representations.

It is crucial to take into account important performance indicators when assessing the effectiveness of these ML algorithms for illness prediction tasks, such as accuracy, precision, recall, F1 score, and area under the curve (AUC). While recall and precision allow for a more detailed evaluation of the algorithm's capacity to decrease false positives and false negatives, respectively, accuracy just offers a broad summary of how accurate the model is. The harmonic mean of precision and recall, known as the F1 score, provides a balanced statistic for assessing the overall performance of the model. The algorithm's capacity to distinguish between positive and negative occurrences is also comprehensively measured by the AUC, which sheds light on the algorithm's predictive and discriminatory abilities. Healthcare professionals can choose and implement the most appropriate ML algorithms for disease prediction tasks by thoroughly evaluating these algorithms based on these performance metrics. This will enable the development of reliable and accurate predictive models in healthcare settings.

DISEASE DIAGNOSIS USING MACHINE LEARNING

Healthcare professionals use a variety of clinical evaluations, medical tests, and investigative methods to detect and define various diseases and health conditions throughout the diagnostic phase, which is a crucial point in the patient care process. A thorough patient history and physical examination are usually the first steps in this comprehensive process, which is then followed by the use of diagnostic testing like blood tests, imaging methods, and biopsies to acquire pertinent clinical information.

Healthcare providers can then create precise diagnoses and treatment plans by combining these findings with accepted clinical guidelines and evidence-based medicine, providing prompt and efficient treatments that improve patient outcomes and well-being (Kumar et al., 2021).

The use of ML algorithms for illness diagnosis has completely changed the diagnostic environment, enhancing the skills of medical practitioners and enabling more accurate and effective diagnostic procedures. ML models can recognize complicated patterns and correlations within complex datasets after being trained on enormous amounts of historical patient data and clinical insights. This enables the automated analysis and interpretation of diagnostic data. These models may classify and predict disease outcomes by utilizing supervised learning algorithms, which enables the identification of important biomarkers and clinical indications that support precise disease diagnosis. Additionally, the use of unsupervised learning techniques makes it possible to group patients based on their clinical profiles, making it easier to identify illness patterns and subtypes that might evade conventional diagnostic methods. Additionally, incorporating deep learning models, which are distinguished by their intricate neural network architectures, makes it possible to extract subtle variations and nuanced features from medical imaging data, improving the precision and effectiveness of disease diagnosis through sophisticated image recognition and pattern analysis.

The revolutionary nature of these technologies in healthcare settings is highlighted by case studies demonstrating successful diagnosis using ML models. For instance, ML algorithms have proven to be exceptionally adept at automatically detecting and classifying abnormalities in medical images, enabling the prompt and accurate diagnosis of conditions like cancer, cardiovascular diseases, and neurological disorders. These models can identify small irregularities and structural deviations in complicated imaging data by utilizing convolutional neural networks (CNNs) and image recognition algorithms. This allows healthcare providers to speed up the diagnosis process and start therapy interventions right away. Additionally, by offering real-time insights and predictive analytics based on patient-specific data, ML models have significantly improved diagnostic accuracy in the context of clinical decision support systems. These models can produce individualized prognostic forecasts and risk assessments, assisting medical practitioners in making well-informed choices regarding illness management and treatment planning. Additionally, in the field of genomics and molecular diagnostics, machine-learning techniques have aided in the identification of genetic markers and molecular signatures linked to a variety of illnesses, permitting the creation of targeted diagnostic assays and personalized therapeutic interventions that take into account the particular genetic profiles of different patients.

ML techniques have been successfully incorporated into disease diagnosis, demonstrating the transformative potential of these technologies to revolutionize the diagnostic process, improve the accuracy and efficiency of disease identification, and ultimately enhance patient outcomes and quality of care. Healthcare professionals can open new doors in diagnostic medicine by utilizing ML to analyze complex datasets, extract valuable insights, and support data-driven decision-making. This will promote a patient-centric approach that emphasizes early detection, personalized interventions, and proactive disease management.

CASE STUDY

Here are a few noteworthy case studies that show how machine-learning models are successfully used in disease diagnosis:

- **Cancer Diagnosis with Image Recognition**: In a well-known case study, scientists used deep learning algorithms, in particular CNNs, to examine mammography data and look for potential breast cancer symptoms. To enable more precise and prompt cancer diagnosis, the model displayed extraordinary skill in spotting minor patterns and anomalies suggestive of early-stage cancers (Zhang et al., 2021). The study demonstrated the potential for ML to transform cancer screening and early diagnosis, ultimately increasing patient outcomes and survival rates. It did this by utilizing the power of CNNs.
- **Cardiovascular Disease Risk Prediction**: A thorough investigation focused on creating a cardiovascular disease risk prediction model based on ML. The algorithm accurately predicted the chance of cardiovascular events like heart attacks and strokes by combining patient data from medical history, genetic information, and lifestyle factors. The study highlighted the potential of ML in facilitating personalized risk assessments and preventive interventions, thereby empowering patients and healthcare providers to actively manage cardiovascular health (Anderson et al., 1991). This was accomplished through the integration of various supervised learning techniques and data-driven insights.
- **Neurological Disorder Diagnosis through Brain Imaging**: An innovative case study in the field of neuroimaging showed the effectiveness of ML in the diagnosis of neurological conditions, including Parkinson's disease and Alzheimer's disease. The model correctly recognized subtle neurodegenerative alterations and biomarkers associated with these illnesses by assessing structural and functional brain imaging data, enabling early and accurate diagnosis (Siuly and Zhang, 2016). The study highlighted the revolutionary potential of ML in improving the early detection and management of complicated neurological illnesses through the application of advanced pattern recognition algorithms and deep learning techniques.
- **Infectious Disease Detection and Surveillance**: The use of ML models for infectious disease identification and surveillance was the subject of a noteworthy case study. The model was successful in identifying probable disease outbreaks and facilitating preemptive public health actions by assessing a variety of datasets, including epidemiological data, clinical records, and environmental factors. The study highlighted the crucial role of ML in improving disease surveillance systems and enabling timely response strategies, thereby containing the spread of infectious diseases and protecting public health, through the integration of unsupervised learning techniques and real-time data analytics (Morse, 2012).

All of these case studies highlight how ML has the potential to change healthcare, increase diagnostic accuracy, and enable proactive interventions that improve patient outcomes and well-being. They also highlight how ML has a revolutionary impact on illness detection. Researchers and healthcare practitioners may pave the path for a more effective, precise, and patient-centric approach to disease diagnosis and management by utilizing the capabilities of ML models to evaluate complicated datasets and extract worthwhile insights.

FEATURE SELECTION AND EXTRACTION IN DISEASE PREDICTION

The process of feature selection and extraction is a critical step in the analysis of healthcare data in the field of disease prediction, allowing the discovery of relevant characteristics and biomarkers that significantly improve the predictive accuracy and dependability of ML models. To maximize the effectiveness of illness prediction algorithms and enable more accurate and actionable prognoses in healthcare settings, it is essential to comprehend the significance of feature selection and extraction (Jain and Singh, 2018).

The value of feature selection and extraction in the context of healthcare data lies in its ability to improve the interpretability and generalizability of predictive models, allowing healthcare professionals to concentrate on the most pertinent and instructive characteristics for precise disease diagnosis and risk assessment. Feature selection and extraction techniques enable the elimination of redundant or irrelevant attributes, streamlining the predictive model and reducing the risk of overfitting or data noise by identifying key features that exhibit strong correlations with disease outcomes and patient prognoses (Joshi and Goswami, 2017). Additionally, by focusing on the most distinct and significant characteristics, these techniques allow medical professionals to develop a deeper understanding of the underlying causes of disease progression, ultimately enabling more informed clinical decision-making and individualized treatment interventions.

There are numerous methods for finding pertinent characteristics for disease prediction, each one specifically designed to take into account the complexity and nuances of healthcare data. By identifying characteristics that show substantial connections with particular disease outcomes through correlation analysis and statistical tests, we can gain important insights into the predictive value of individual characteristics. In addition, information gain and mutual information techniques help quantify the importance and dependence of features in connection to disease classification, supporting the prioritization of informative traits for precise predictive modeling. Additionally, by incorporating cutting-edge feature selection algorithms like recursive feature elimination (RFE) and genetic algorithms, it is possible to automatically identify the best feature subsets that maximize the predictive performance of ML models. This streamlines the feature selection procedure and improves the effectiveness of disease prediction tasks in healthcare.

Applications of dimensionality reduction techniques play a key role in minimizing data sparsity and enhancing the computational effectiveness of predictive models in situations involving high-dimensional and complex datasets. A common dimensionality reduction method is principal component analysis (PCA), which allows high-dimensional data to be transformed into a lower-dimensional space while preserving the dataset's crucial information and variability. PCA makes it easier to visualize and interpret complicated data structures by compressing the data along the main components that capture the most variance. This improves our comprehension of the important trends and connections that affect how diseases progress. Additionally, the visualization of high-dimensional data clusters made possible by t-distributed stochastic neighbor embedding (t-SNE) and linear discriminant analysis (LDA) techniques allows for the identification of distinct disease subtypes and phenotypic profiles that support personalized disease management and treatment planning. By utilizing these dimensionality reduction techniques, medical professionals can accelerate the processing of complicated healthcare datasets, providing more precise and effective illness prediction and diagnostic capabilities that take into account the variety and nuanced nature of clinical data.

EVALUATION METRICS FOR DISEASE PREDICTION AND DIAGNOSIS MODELS

The effectiveness and performance of illness prediction and diagnosis models are evaluated using evaluation metrics, which offer important information on the precision, robustness, and dependability of these models in clinical settings. To ensure the effectiveness and applicability of predictive models, it is essential to have thorough and useful evaluation metrics, given the growing integration of ML and data-driven approaches in healthcare. Accuracy, precision, recall, F1 score, and AUC are important evaluation metrics that have become essential tools for calculating the predictive strength and discriminatory ability of illness prediction and diagnostic models (Perotte et al., 2014). Healthcare practitioners and researchers must be aware of the significance and intricacies of these evaluation metrics to choose the right model and optimize it, ultimately leading to the development of more individualized and successful healthcare interventions.

SIGNIFICANCE OF EVALUATION METRICS IN ASSESSING MODEL PERFORMANCE

- **Accuracy**: A basic summary of the model's accuracy in identifying positive and negative occurrences is provided by accuracy, which is the percentage of properly predicted cases. Although accuracy is a key indicator of overall predictive ability, it may not be adequate to judge models in situations where class distributions are unbalanced or if particular errors have a greater clinical impact. To provide a more detailed evaluation of model performance, complementary evaluation measures must be integrated.
- **Precision**: Precision highlights the model's capacity to reduce false positives by reflecting the percentage of true positive predictions among all positive predictions. Precision helps in the identification of models that display a low percentage of incorrectly predicted positive instances, ensuring a more accurate and trustworthy diagnostic procedure in healthcare. This is particularly important in situations where the cost of false alarms is considerable.
- **Recall**: Recall, often referred to as sensitivity, shows how many true positive predictions are made out of all real positive examples, highlighting

the model's ability to reduce false negatives. Recall plays a crucial role in identifying models that exhibit high sensitivity to the detection of true positive cases in the context of disease prediction and diagnosis, facilitating the prompt and accurate identification of patients needing additional diagnostic testing and interventions.

- **F1 Score**: A harmonic mean of precision and recall, the F1 score provides a balanced statistic for assessing the general effectiveness of disease prediction and diagnosis models. The F1 score gives healthcare professionals a thorough assessment of the model's predictive accuracy and robustness by taking into account both the false positive and false negative rates. This allows them to weigh the trade-off between precision and recall and decide whether the model will be effective in clinical settings.
- **Area Under the Curve (AUC)**: Particularly in the context of binary classification problems, the AUC serves as a complete indicator of the model's capacity to distinguish between positive and negative examples. The AUC helps identify the best threshold values for disease prediction and diagnosis by quantifying the model's ability to distinguish between true positive and false positive rates at various classification thresholds. This information is useful for understanding the model's discriminatory power and predictive accuracy.

USE OF EVALUATION METRICS IN DISEASE PREDICTION AND DIAGNOSIS

In this section, we are trying to explain how evaluation metrics are used for some specific disease prediction & Diagnosis:

- **Cancer Diagnosis**: In evaluating the effectiveness of predictive models in identifying malignant tumors, the evaluation metrics of precision, recall, and F1 score are crucial. The model's ability to minimize false positive diagnoses is indicated by high precision scores, which lowers the likelihood of unneeded treatments or interventions. High recall values demonstrate the model's sensitivity in detecting true positive instances, allowing for rapid and accurate diagnoses that facilitate treatment interventions and better patient outcomes (Zhang et al., 2021). Healthcare professionals can optimize the diagnostic process and guarantee the provision of individualized and efficient cancer care by incorporating these evaluation criteria to create models that strike a balance between precision and recall.
- **Cardiovascular Disease Risk Assessment**: AUC serves as a crucial tool for assessing the discriminatory power of prediction models in identifying people at risk of developing heart-related problems in the context of cardiovascular disease risk assessment. A high AUC value indicates that the model can accurately distinguish between those who have high risk profiles and those who don't, allowing for the creation of tailored risk assessment tools and preventive measures (Anderson et al., 1991). Healthcare professionals can design tailored screening programs and lifestyle interventions that

reduce the risk of cardiovascular illnesses by using the insights provided by the AUC. This encourages a proactive approach to cardiovascular health management and disease prevention.

- **Infectious Disease Outbreak Prediction**: The evaluation metric of accuracy is critical in determining how well predictive algorithms anticipate the risk of disease transmission and epidemic spread for infectious disease outbreak prediction models. High accuracy values show how well the model predicts the likelihood and severity of infectious disease outbreaks, allowing public health officials to put in place prompt and focused control measures and interventions (Morse, 2012). Healthcare policymakers and epidemiologists can develop effective monitoring systems and response plans that reduce the danger of widespread disease transmission and protect public health by utilizing the insights supplied by accurate measures.

- **Neurological Disorder Diagnosis**: The combination of accuracy, recall, and F1 score metrics assists in evaluating the effectiveness of predictive models in detecting early-stage neurodegenerative diseases in the diagnosis of neurological disorders. High precision values show how accurately the model minimizes false positive diagnoses, lowering the possibility of misdiagnosis and pointless therapies. Similar to this, high recall values demonstrate the model's sensitivity in identifying real positive instances, enabling swift and precise diagnoses that allow for treatment actions that are both timely and focused. By combining these evaluation measures, medical professionals and neurologists may make sure that neurological problems are promptly and accurately identified, making it easier to execute specialized treatment plans and patient-centered care strategies (Siuly and Zhang, 2016).

The integration of many evaluation criteria that collectively offer a nuanced and knowledgeable assessment of model performance is required for the thorough evaluation of illness prediction and diagnosis models. Healthcare workers and researchers can maximize the selection and application of predictive models, encouraging more effective and individualized healthcare interventions, by utilizing the insights provided by accuracy, precision, recall, F1 score, and AUC. By carefully integrating these evaluation metrics into the evaluation of disease prediction and diagnosis models, it is made clear how important a role they play in improving the precision, robustness, and reliability of predictive algorithms. This, in turn, promotes better patient outcomes, individualized treatment plans, and proactive disease management techniques in clinical settings.

CHALLENGES AND ETHICAL CONSIDERATIONS IN DISEASE PREDICTION AND DIAGNOSIS

A paradigm change in healthcare was brought about by the application of ML to disease prediction and diagnosis, which allowed for the study of huge datasets and the creation of complex predictive models. This revolutionary technology is not without its difficulties and moral ramifications, though. It is critical to understand and solve the ethical issues and obstacles that occur in the context of disease prediction and diagnosis as ML continues to transform the healthcare industry. This in-depth conversation explores the moral ramifications of applying ML to the healthcare industry, the difficulties associated with data privacy, bias, and interpretability, as well as solutions for resolving these issues and assuring ethical implementation.

- **Ethical Implications of Using Machine Learning in Healthcare**: The use of ML in healthcare creates important ethical issues that demand serious attention. The possible threats connected to patient privacy and data security are one of the main issues. Patient confidentiality and trust may be jeopardized by excessive gathering and analysis of sensitive patient data due to the risk of data breaches, unauthorized access, and information abuse. Additionally, the possibility of algorithmic bias and discrimination is a serious ethical challenge because biased models might worsen already-existing injustices in disease diagnosis and treatment and perpetuate disparities in healthcare delivery. The ethical intricacy is further complicated by the problem of interpretability and transparency in ML models, which might make it harder for patients and healthcare providers to trust and accept these models.

CHALLENGES RELATED TO DATA PRIVACY, BIAS, AND INTERPRETABILITY

- **Data Privacy**: The sensitive nature of healthcare data, which includes private and confidential information about individuals' medical histories, genetic profiles, and treatment plans, poses a barrier to data privacy in illness prediction and diagnosis. To defend patients' rights and their faith in the healthcare system, the privacy and security of this data must be maintained. Although data breaches and illegal access can result in identity theft, harm to one's reputation, and compromised healthcare services, the linked nature of data sharing and interoperability creates substantial hurdles in protecting patient privacy.
- **Bias**: The detection and mitigation of biases that may be present in the data or the ML algorithms themselves are necessary to address algorithmic bias in disease prediction and diagnosis. Biased datasets can result in varied treatment outcomes for different demographic groups and perpetuate historical inequalities in healthcare access and delivery. Additionally, a lack of diversity in training data might result in skewed predictive models that are insufficiently representative of the needs and experiences of marginalized communities in terms of healthcare, aggravating already existing gaps in access to care.
- **Interpretability**: The difficulty in interpreting ML models is caused by the opaqueness and complexity of some sophisticated algorithms, which may produce predictions without logical justifications or explanations. This lack of openness can make it difficult for people to comprehend how decisions

are made, which can breed mistrust and skepticism among patients and healthcare staff. Additionally, the clinical application of ML models may be constrained by the inability to evaluate and articulate the justification for particular predictions, impeding their incorporation into standard medical procedures and decision-making procedures.

STRATEGIES FOR ADDRESSING ETHICAL CONCERNS AND ENSURING RESPONSIBLE IMPLEMENTATION

It is essential to develop comprehensive techniques that prioritize data privacy, eliminate algorithmic bias, and improve the interpretability of predictive models in order to solve the ethical issues and difficulties connected with disease prediction and diagnosis using ML (Herath and Herath, 2024). To guarantee responsible implementation and uphold ethical norms in healthcare, a number of crucial measures can be used:

- **Data Anonymization and Encryption**: By using effective data anonymization methods and encryption protocols, patient privacy can be protected while the likelihood of data breaches and unauthorized access is reduced. Healthcare organizations can safeguard patient confidentiality and ensure adherence to data protection laws by anonymizing personally identifiable information and encrypting sensitive healthcare data during storage and transmission.
- **Diversity and Fairness in Data Representation**: To reduce algorithmic bias and ensure fair representation of varied patient populations, it is crucial to promote diversity and inclusivity in healthcare data gathering and analysis. Predictive models' generalizability and fairness can be increased by actively incorporating diverse and representative datasets that cover a wide range of demographic and socioeconomic backgrounds and reduce biases.
- **Algorithmic Transparency and Explainability**: To build confidence and acceptance among medical professionals and patients, it is essential to make ML models more transparent and understandable. Healthcare professionals can make well-informed clinical decisions and encourage the responsible use of ML in disease prediction and diagnosis by implementing interpretable ML techniques, such as decision trees, rule-based models, and model-agnostic interpretability methods. These techniques help healthcare practitioners understand the underlying logic and decision-making process of predictive models.
- **Ethical Frameworks and Guidelines**: For healthcare organizations, researchers, and politicians, developing thorough ethical frameworks and norms that are specifically applicable to the use of ML in healthcare can offer clear direction and standards. These frameworks should include guidelines for the ethical gathering, analysis, and use of healthcare data for disease prediction and diagnosis, as well as principles of data privacy, fairness, accountability, and openness. Healthcare stakeholders can assure the proper application of ML technology and protect the moral principles and

values essential to patient-centered care by adhering to recognized ethical frameworks.

- **Continuous Monitoring and Evaluation**: To recognize and address any ethical concerns or biases that can surface during the disease prediction and diagnosis process, it is crucial to set up a reliable framework for the ongoing monitoring and evaluation of ML models. Healthcare organizations can evaluate the efficacy and moral implications of predictive models by implementing routine audits, validation checks, and bias detection mechanisms. This enables prompt intervention and remedial action to uphold moral standards and guarantee the provision of just and patient-centered healthcare services.

The ethical issues and difficulties that come with utilizing ML to predict and diagnose diseases highlight the urgent need for a thorough and proactive approach to data protection, bias reduction, and algorithmic transparency. Healthcare organizations can make sure that ML technologies are used responsibly and ethically in healthcare settings by putting in place strategies that prioritize patient privacy, encourage data diversity and fairness, improve algorithmic interpretability, and abide by established ethical frameworks and guidelines. It is crucial to address these ethical issues to build patient trust, advance equitable healthcare delivery, and sustain the moral principles and values necessary for the delivery of high-quality, patient-centered healthcare services.

FUTURE TRENDS AND DIRECTIONS IN DISEASE PREDICTION AND DIAGNOSIS

The rapid improvements in technology and the incorporation of novel approaches in healthcare are driving a significant revolution in the landscape of disease prediction and diagnosis. New insights and capabilities provided by emerging technologies, particularly in the areas of ML and data analytics, are altering how healthcare professionals approach disease prediction and diagnosis and have the potential to completely transform patient care and therapeutic approaches (Tufail et al., 2021). This discussion offers an overview of the cutting-edge medical technologies reshaping the industry, predictions for ML's potential in disease diagnosis and prognosis, and suggestions for researchers and practitioners on how to navigate this rapidly changing environment and make the most of these technologies to enhance patient outcomes and healthcare delivery (Joshi et al., 2025).

OVERVIEW OF EMERGING TECHNOLOGIES AND THEIR IMPACT ON HEALTHCARE

- **Genomics and Personalized Medicine**: The development of genomic technologies has completely changed how diseases are predicted and diagnosed, making it possible to identify genetic biomarkers and develop treatment plans that are unique to each patient's profile. Healthcare professionals can predict disease susceptibility, identify genetic predispositions, and tailor treatment regimens based on patients' genetic makeup using genomic sequencing techniques in combination with cutting-edge bioinformatics tools, leading to more efficient and individualized healthcare interventions.

- **Internet of Medical Things (IoMT)**: Real-time data gathering and ongoing patient monitoring have been made possible by the spread of the Internet of Medical Things (IoMT) devices, which include wearable sensors, remote monitoring tools, and smart healthcare devices. This has allowed for proactive illness prediction and early intervention tactics (Vishnu et al., 2020). Healthcare workers can obtain thorough patient data, track health trends, and spot early illness progression by utilizing IoMT technologies, which improves disease management and treatment outcomes.

- **Blockchain Technology**: Blockchain technology's application in the medical field has created new possibilities for safe data exchange, interoperability, and patient privacy protection. Blockchain-enabled solutions provide a decentralized and impenetrable framework for storing and sharing healthcare data, improving data security and transparency while promoting easy data exchange and collaboration among healthcare stakeholders. The use of blockchain in disease detection and prediction promotes data integrity and trust, making healthcare services more effective and secure.

PREDICTIONS FOR THE FUTURE OF MACHINE LEARNING IN DISEASE PREDICTION AND DIAGNOSIS

- **Enhanced Predictive Analytics**: Advanced predictive analytics capabilities will define the future of ML in disease prediction and diagnosis, allowing medical professionals to use cutting-edge algorithms and deep learning models to forecast disease trends, identify at-risk patient populations, and create proactive intervention strategies. Healthcare professionals can forecast disease outcomes and enhance therapeutic interventions by integrating predictive analytics into clinical decision-making processes. This improves patient outcomes and increases the general effectiveness of healthcare services.

- **Augmented Clinical Decision Support Systems**: Medical practitioners will benefit from enhanced clinical decision support systems that offer real-time insights and evidence-based recommendations as ML for disease prediction and diagnosis progresses. To provide individualized treatment plans, suggest diagnostic pathways, and facilitate informed decision-making, these systems will draw on extensive patient data, clinical guidelines, and predictive models (Chen et al., 2023). As a result, healthcare professionals will be better equipped to provide timely and accurate clinical assessments.

- **Integration of Explainable AI**: By incorporating explainable artificial intelligence (XAI) techniques, ML models will become more transparent and interpretable, making it easier for healthcare practitioners to comprehend the reasoning behind particular forecasts and recommendations. XAI algorithms will offer unmistakable insights into the decision-making procedure of predictive models, fostering trust and acceptance among healthcare professionals and patients and facilitating the seamless integration of ML technologies into routine clinical practices and decision-making workflows.

RECOMMENDATIONS FOR RESEARCHERS AND PRACTITIONERS:

- **Embrace Interdisciplinary Collaboration**: Interdisciplinary collaboration should be a top priority for researchers and practitioners in the field of disease prediction and diagnosis, encouraging collaborations between healthcare professionals, data scientists, and technological specialists. Healthcare stakeholders can make the most of a variety of viewpoints and skill sets by fostering a collaborative environment that encourages knowledge sharing and expertise integration to create comprehensive and original solutions that address the complex opportunities and challenges in disease prediction and diagnosis.
- **Prioritize Data Privacy and Ethical Considerations**: To maintain patient confidentiality and guarantee data security, researchers and practitioners must prioritize data privacy, abide by ethical principles, and follow legal and regulatory requirements. Healthcare institutions may protect patient privacy and promote trust in the responsible use of ML technology for disease prediction and diagnosis by implementing strong data governance frameworks, data encryption methods, and anonymization procedures.
- **Invest in Continuous Learning and Training**: For academics and practitioners in the field of disease prediction and diagnosis, continual learning and training are required due to the dynamic nature of technology and healthcare. Healthcare professionals should place a high priority on continuing education and training initiatives that support the development of technical competencies, data literacy, and knowledge of cutting-edge technologies. This will enable healthcare practitioners to effectively utilize ML tools and integrate data-driven approaches into clinical practice.
- **Promote Patient-Centric Care**: The delivery of healthcare should be approached from the perspective of the patient, with a focus on the value of patient empowerment, involvement, and tailored treatment interventions. Healthcare professionals can guarantee the delivery of patient-centered care that prioritizes individual needs, values, and treatment goals by incorporating patient perspectives and preferences into the development of predictive models and diagnostic algorithms. This will help to foster a more holistic and compassionate healthcare ecosystem.

The future of disease prediction and diagnosis is characterized by the convergence of emerging technologies, the continued evolution of ML capabilities, and a commitment to patient-centric and data-driven healthcare delivery. By embracing the transformative potential of advanced technologies, healthcare stakeholders can harness the power of predictive analytics, augmented clinical decision support systems, and XAI to revolutionize disease management, improve patient outcomes, and foster a more efficient and equitable healthcare ecosystem (Kumar et al., 2024). Through interdisciplinary collaboration, ethical practice, continuous learning, and patient-centric care, researchers and practitioners can navigate the evolving landscape of disease prediction and diagnosis, leveraging technology as a catalyst for innovation, empowerment, and sustainable advancements in healthcare.

The delicate interactions between ML, disease prediction, and diagnosis in the healthcare industry have been thoroughly explored in this chapter. In our introduction, we clarified the importance of disease prediction and diagnosis, highlighting the vital part they play in enabling prompt interventions and enhancing patient outcomes. The use of ML in healthcare has been hailed as a game-changing strategy that enables medical professionals to use sophisticated algorithms and predictive models to extract valuable information from large, complex datasets, improving the precision and effectiveness of disease diagnosis and prediction processes.

We examined the foundations of ML algorithms in this chapter, clarifying their uses and applicability to problems involving disease prediction. In-depth discussions of logistic regression, decision trees, random forests, SVMs, and neural networks illustrated their various potentials for assessing healthcare data and enabling more accurate and dependable disease predictions. The importance of identifying pertinent characteristics and biomarkers that significantly contribute to the accuracy and dependability of disease prediction models was also highlighted as we looked at the crucial roles that feature selection and extraction play in maximizing the efficacy of predictive models.

The chapter went on to explain the significance of evaluation measures for gauging how well disease prediction and diagnosis models function. The AUC and the F1 score were highlighted as essential metrics for determining the predictive and discriminating abilities of these models. These evaluation criteria give healthcare practitioners a sophisticated evaluation of model performance, allowing them to choose the best model and optimize it, leading to more effective and individualized healthcare interventions.

The next step was navigating the ethical issues and difficulties associated with using ML to forecast and diagnose diseases. The importance of implementing thorough techniques that prioritize patient privacy, reduce algorithmic bias, and improve the interpretability of predictive models was emphasized, underscoring the urgent need to address data privacy, bias, and interpretability issues. Healthcare stakeholders can ensure the responsible and ethical implementation of ML technologies by embracing ethical frameworks and guidelines and encouraging a patient-centric approach to healthcare delivery, upholding the standards and values essential to the provision of high-quality and equitable healthcare services (Joshi et al., 2025).

By focusing on the revolutionary potential of genomics, the IoMT, and blockchain technology for disease prediction and diagnostics, we looked to the future and examined emerging technologies and their potential impact on healthcare. Additionally, we made predictions about how ML will influence the future of disease diagnosis and prediction, highlighting the development of predictive analytics, enhanced clinical decision support systems, and XAI as key trends that will transform healthcare procedures and improve patient care delivery.

In the end, it is clear that ML has the power to transform disease diagnosis and prognosis, ushering in a new era of data-driven and individualized healthcare solutions. Healthcare practitioners may harness the power of data to reveal new insights, improve clinical decision-making, and optimize patient outcomes by utilizing the revolutionary powers of ML algorithms and embracing ethical best practices. A key opportunity to advance healthcare practices, improve patient care delivery, and promote a more effective and fair healthcare ecosystem is the incorporation of ML in disease prediction and diagnosis.

A call to action for more research and development is essential, given the revolutionary potential of ML in healthcare. It is crucial to keep funding interdisciplinary research, technological innovation, and moral behavior to better disease diagnosis and prognosis. Collaboration between healthcare professionals, data scientists, and technology experts is essential to fostering a collaborative environment that promotes knowledge sharing and expertise integration, enabling the development of comprehensive and innovative solutions that address the challenging opportunities and challenges in disease prediction and diagnosis. Researchers and practitioners can usher in a new era of data-driven, personalized healthcare that prioritizes patient well-being and fosters sustainable advancements in the field of disease prediction and diagnosis by putting a priority on patient-centric care, embracing the transformative potential of emerging technologies, and advocating for responsible and ethical practices.

REFERENCES

Anderson, K. M., et al. "Cardiovascular disease risk profiles." *American Heart Journal* 121.1 (1991): 293–298.

Chauhan, N., et al. "Review of techniques and algorithms of load balancing in cloud computing." *Journal of Recent Innovations in Computer Science and Technology* 1.1 (2024): 15–26.

Chen, J., et al. "Designing expert-augmented clinical decision support systems to predict mortality risk in ICUs." *KI-Künstliche Intelligenz* (2023): 1–10.

Hamidi, H., & Daraee, A. "Analysis of pre-processing and post-processing methods and using data mining to diagnose heart diseases." *International Journal of Engineering* 29.7 (2016): 921–930.

Herath, S. K. & Herath, L. M. (2024). Embedding ethical practices: Overcoming the challenges of corporate social responsibility implementation. In A. Derbali (Ed.), *Social and Ethical Implications of AI in Finance for Sustainability* (pp. 1–40). IGI Global Scientific Publishing. https://doi.org/10.4018/979-8-3693-2881-1.ch001

Ibrahim, I. M., and Abdulazeez, A. M. "The role of machine learning algorithms for diagnosing diseases." *Journal of Applied Science and Technology Trends* 2.01 (2021): 10–19.

Jain, Divya, and Vijendra Singh. "Feature selection and classification systems for chronic disease prediction: A review." *Egyptian Informatics Journal* 19.3 (2018): 179–189.

Joshi, A. (2013). M-learning to lead the future of education in India. *International Journal of Applied Services Marketing Perspectives* 2(2), 409.

Joshi, A., & Goswami, S. (2017). Modified round robin algorithm by using priority scheduling. *Advances in Computational Sciences and Technology* 10(6), 1543–1549.

Joshi, A., Kumar, V., Thakur, G., Chauhan, N., & Singh, R. K. (2025). A primer for governance. In R. Kumar, A. Abdul Hamid, N. Ya'akub, T. Nyamasvisva, & R. Tiwari (Eds.), *Leveraging Futuristic Machine Learning and Next-Generational Security for e-Governance* (pp. 45–86). IGI Global Scientific Publishing. https://doi.org/10.4018/979-8-3693-7883-0.ch003

Joshi, A., & Tiwari, H. (2023). No. 10. An overview of python libraries for data science. *Journal of Engineering Technology and Applied Physics* 5(2), 85–90.

Kumar, N., et al. "Efficient automated disease diagnosis using machine learning models." *Journal of Healthcare Engineering* 2021.1 (2021): 9983652.

Kumar, R., Joshi, A., Sharan, H. O., Peng, S. L., & Dudhagara, C. R. (Eds.). (2024). *The Ethical Frontier of AI and Data Analysis.* IGI Global.

Maharana, K., Mondal, S., & Nemade, B. "A review: Data pre-processing and data augmentation techniques." *Global Transitions Proceedings* 3.1 (2022): 91–99.

Morse, Stephen S. "Public health surveillance and infectious disease detection." *Biosecurity and Bioterrorism: Biodefense Strategy, Practice, and Science* 10.1 (2012): 6–16.

Perotte, Adler, et al. "Diagnosis code assignment: models and evaluation metrics." *Journal of the American Medical Informatics Association* 21.2 (2014): 231–237.

Shaik, F., Yelchuri, R., & Dash, J. K. "Fundamentals of machine learning in healthcare." *Prediction in Medicine: The Impact of Machine Learning on Healthcare* (2024): 191.

Siuly, S., & Zhang, Y. "Medical big data: neurological diseases diagnosis through medical data analysis." *Data Science and Engineering* 1 (2016): 54–64.

Tufail, A. B., et al. "Deep learning in cancer diagnosis and prognosis prediction: a minireview on challenges, recent trends, and future directions." *Computational and Mathematical Methods in Medicine* 2021.1 (2021): 9025470.

Uddin, S., et al. "Comparing different supervised machine learning algorithms for disease prediction." *BMC Medical Informatics and Decision Making* 19.1 (2019): 1–16.

Vishnu, S., Jino Ramson, S. R., and Jegan, R.. "Internet of medical things (IoMT)-An overview." *2020 5th international conference on devices, circuits and systems (ICDCS).* IEEE, 2020.

Yadav, S. S., and Jadhav, S. M. "Machine learning algorithms for disease prediction using iot environment." *International Journal of Engineering and Advanced Technology* 8.6 (2019): 4303–4307.

Zhang, H., Li, W., & Zhang, H. "[Retracted] An image recognition framework for oral cancer cells." *Journal of Healthcare Engineering* 2021.1 (2021): 2449128.

10 6G Innovations in Health Care

Envisioning Patient-Centric Care for a Smart Hospital

M. Sudha

INTRODUCTION

The use of smart healthcare systems in the provision of healthcare is becoming more and more essential. However, the development of chronic diseases, viral infections, and an aging population is placing enormous demands on the effectiveness of present systems (Ahad et al., 2024). Instead of concentrating on treating patients' diseases, healthcare institutions are now more concerned with providing them with patient-centred medical services. This method places the patient in the "driver's seat" since research has shown that greater outcomes occur when patients actively participate in their care. A personalized patient-centred strategy enhances patient outcomes, promotes greater participation and decision-making, and ultimately raises satisfaction (Awino, 2024). Patient-centred care is rapidly replacing hospital- and specialist-focused healthcare. This quick transition in healthcare is being driven by many technical advancements. Technology for communication has made remote and customized healthcare possible, among other things. Intelligent healthcare apps make extensive use of the current 3G, 4G, and 5G networks and other communication technologies, which are constantly developing to keep up with demand. As the smart healthcare sector grows, more apps will generate a wider range of data formats. Many innovative applications in healthcare make complicated and variable demands on existing communication systems, which are not able to handle them. One of the key technologies for integrating patient-centred medical practices and smart healthcare systems is the sixth-generation (6G) wireless network. Thus, it is expected that smart healthcare apps that encounter the greatest of the requirements, together with ultra-low latency, will be able to run on the next 6G networks (Al-Jawad et al., 2022). This study presents 6G technology and discusses the possible benefits of applying it to healthcare, particularly in a patient-centred era.

DOI: 10.1201/9781003516590-10

6G WIRELESS TECHNOLOGY AND THE DISTINCTION BETWEEN 5G AND 6G

6G cellular technology claims to offer microsecond speeds and a variety of connectivity options. The mobile network, which is still under construction, will use higher radio frequencies than 5G, have a 1,000-times quicker latency, and more capacity. The 6G network will leverage the infrastructure that 5G has already established, but it will also use ultra-high radio frequencies to transfer more data at quicker rates and include machine learning as well as artificial intelligence (AI). Users may anticipate rapid data transfer and the elimination of delays, disconnections, and buffering with 6G (Joshi & Tiwari, 2023). Similar to how 4G brought about a whole mobile app ecosystem and 2G gave us text messaging, 6G will improve machine-to-machine communication, fostering better interoperability in the context of the "smart," Internet-of-things era. In addition to quicker file downloads and video streaming, faster wireless communication opens up new possibilities for networked vehicles, smart industries, and collaborative virtual and augmented reality (AR) (https://builtin.com). Six technological directions towards 6G, namely, AI, Quantum Communication (QC), Terahertz (THz) communication, Intent-Based networking (IBN), Distributed Ledger Technology (DLT)/Blockchain (BC), and Smart Devices and Gadget-free communication (SDG) (De Alwis et al., 2023).

Cellular communications – 1G, 2G, 3G, 4G, 5G to 6G are shown in Figure 10.1.

The illustration depicts the rapid evolution of cellular communications from 1G, 2G, 3G, 4G, and 5G to 6G. Each line in the picture represents each generation of mobile communication technology, from 1G to 6G (www.rohde-schwarz.com, 2024).

The fact that 6G will provide more than simply linked gadgets is one significant distinction. We will be able to link smartphones to sensors and send data over an infrastructure with 5G. 6G aims to establish it as the backbone of our interconnected existence. After the requisite technological framework is established, it can serve as a conduit between the analogue and digital realms. "Integrated Communication and Sensing" is the strategy that implies that, in addition to transmitting data like in 5G,

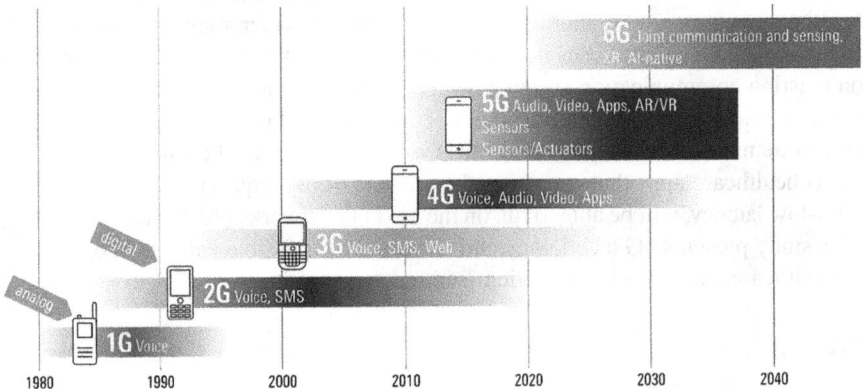

FIGURE 10.1   Cellular communication.

detection and tracking of things through the transmission of electromagnetic waves over space, or through the contact process itself, can be done in 6G (www.medica-tradefair.com).

IMPROVED WIRELESS TECHNOLOGY FOR ENHANCED PATIENT-CENTRIC CARE: THE FUTURE OF 6G IN SMART HEALTHCARE SYSTEM

6G, a new communication technology, is going to take over the medical sector shortly. 6G will most likely alter several sectors, including healthcare. The biggest obstacles to health care today are time and location, which 6G will address. AI-driven healthcare that depends on a 6G connection will transform healthcare and our way of life. Together with improved patient tracking and the creation of effortless healthcare alerts, the integration of AI-powered algorithms with 6G enables pertinent and real-time communication with all healthcare professionals. All of these factors help to reduce hospital stays, overall medical expenses, and rates of death and morbidity (Al-Jawad et al., 2022).

Healthcare network structure designed through 6G is shown in Figure 10.2.

The picture's connected boxes depict the healthcare network's architecture using 6G. To demonstrate how several telesurgery procedures, remote health monitoring, and the COVID-19 scenario will be carried out utilizing 6G communication, a communication box interacts with a healthcare application layer box (Ahad et al., 2024).

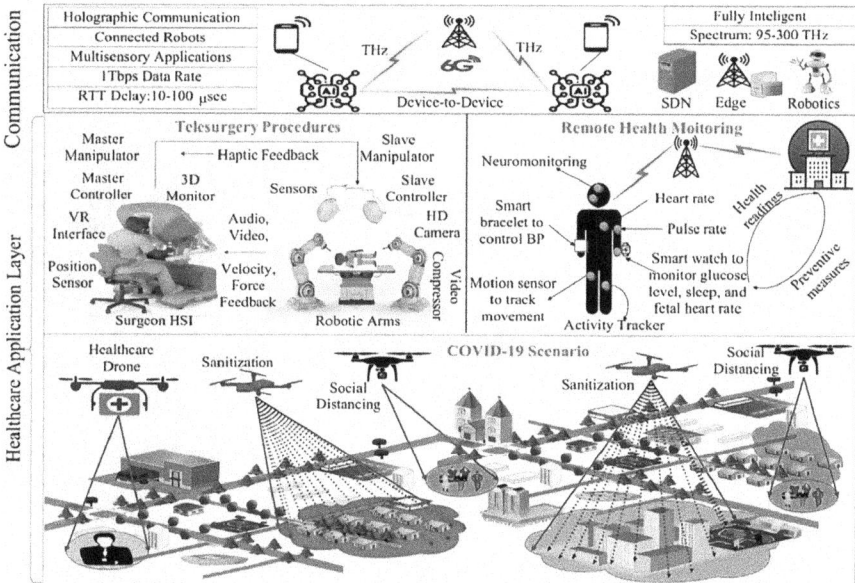

FIGURE 10.2   Healthcare network structure.

BIO-WIRELESS FOR A PATIENT-CENTRIC HEALTH-CARE FRAMEWORK

To create and assess a reliable, intelligent Ambient Assisted Living platform, a biowireless network is an integrated platform that combines cutting-edge wireless technology and biosensors inside an optimized living space. The patient-centred healthcare system will soon be prepared for practical implementation. The sensor-enhanced environment encompasses a wide range of smart technologies, including biosensors, data fusion software algorithms, dependable wireless monitoring and tracking systems, inertial tracking systems, and software designed for use in medical settings. The opportunity to conduct research and development, as well as commercialize novel sensors and devices, is provided by this intelligent platform. It accomplishes this by using simulation frameworks to comprehend and forecast how study participants and different illnesses will affect the system, and by utilizing data to finally make wise selections about the patient (Islam et al., 2014).

Figure 10.3 depicts a framework model of patient-centric healthcare.

Pictures associated with arrows stand for the patient-centric health care framework concept, which facilitates communication between patients and their homes, hospitals, and networks of healthcare providers (Figure 10.4).

The arrow-filled conceptual design of the Image Bio Wireless network shows how medical wireless networks, including WLAN, RFID, WPAN, and WBAN, connect

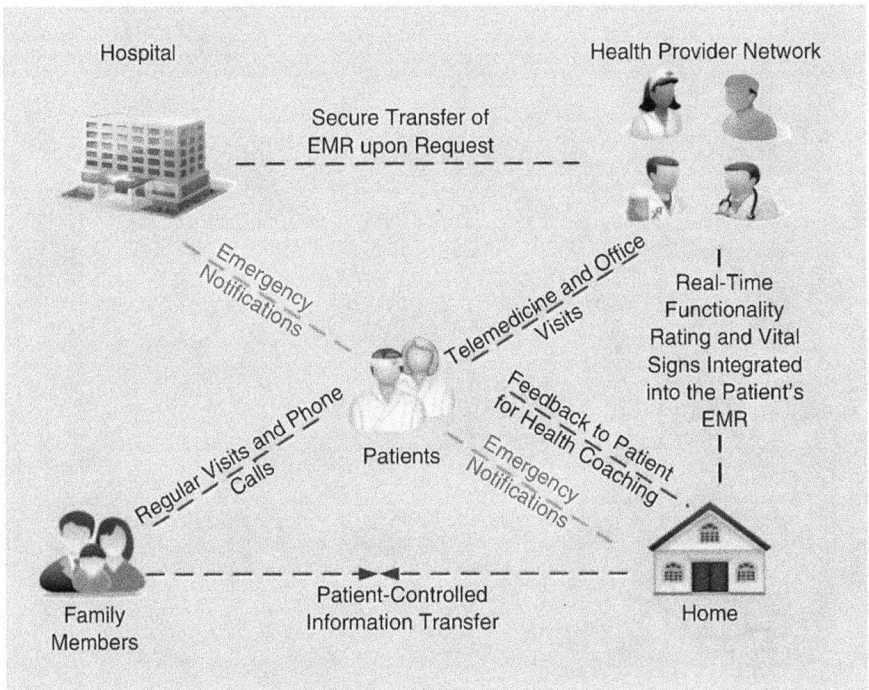

FIGURE 10.3   Patient centric healthcare framework.

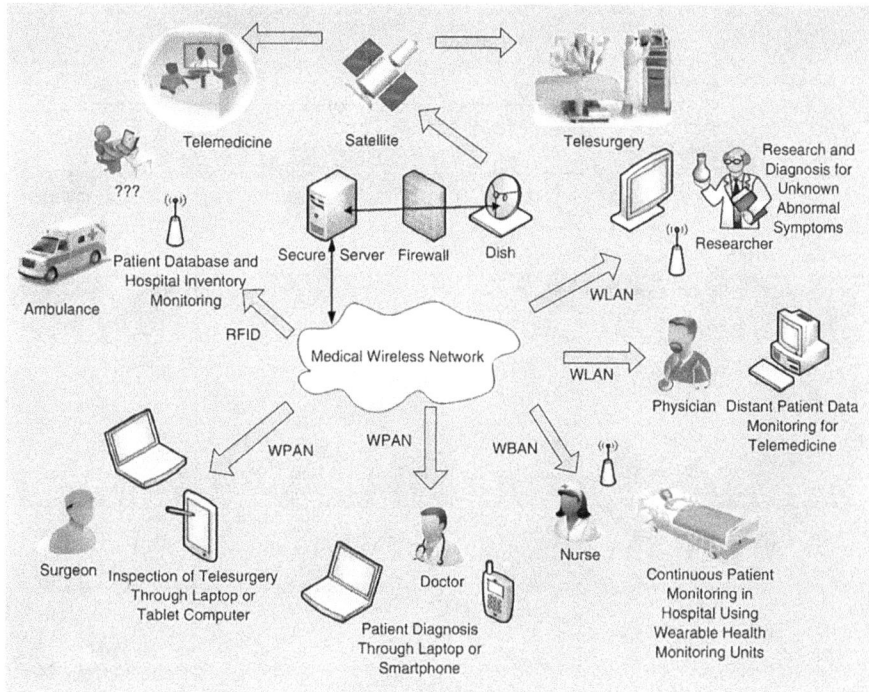

FIGURE 10.4   Conceptual patient centric healthcare framework.

all patient-centric information, including telesurgery, telemedicine, disease diagnostics, etc., from the patient to the physician, nurse, researcher, and surgeon (Islam et al., 2014).

Framework of 6G intelligent healthcare is shown in Figure 10.5.

The 6G intelligent healthcare framework is represented by boxes that are connected, which comprises services like telesurgery, requirements like service quality, and communication enhancements like capacity (Ahad et al., 2024).

REMOTE MONITORING SERVICE

The use of remote healthcare to treat people who live in remote areas or have limited travel options is becoming more and more commonplace worldwide. This service is available via remote health monitoring or telemedicine. Through telemedicine, medical professionals assess, diagnose, and treat patients remotely. Patients can receive remote patient monitoring at any time and from any location by using healthcare software and internet resources (Ahad et al., 2024).

HAPTIC/TACTILE INTERNET ACCESS

In addition to the traditional audio-visual communication, haptic communication (HC) is a non-verbal communication based on several touch senses. In HC, signals

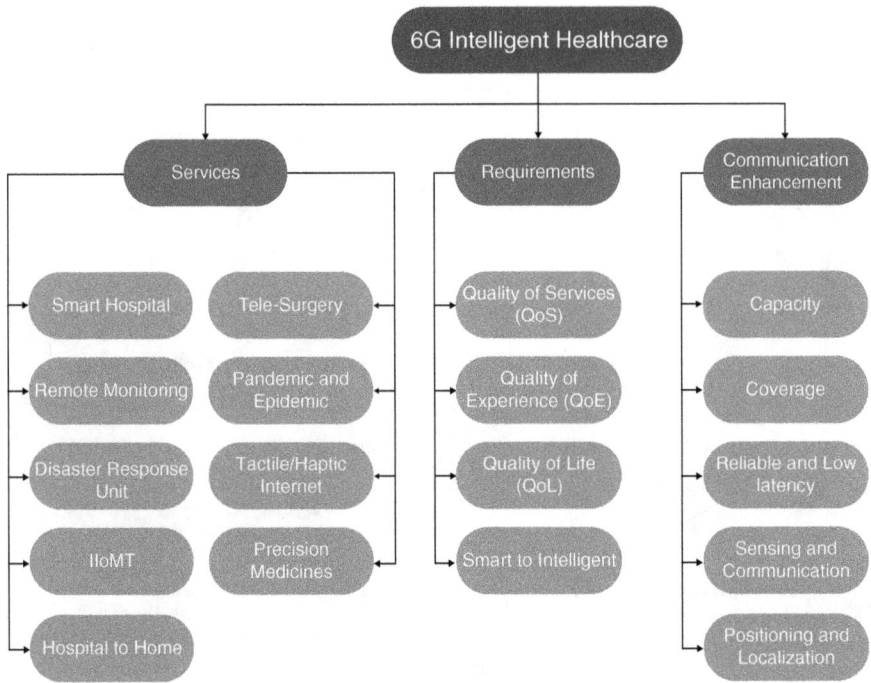

FIGURE 10.5 Framework of 6G intelligent healthcare.

are sent by sensory nerves and picked up by brain receptors. It is this haptic connection that the wireless brain-computer interface (WBCI) will help to enhance. There will be many uses for haptics in healthcare, including visual feedback, remote control, and monitoring, all supported by the tactile Internet. With haptics, a patient may use a distance to transmit their discomfort to a physician.

Patients can use haptics to express thanks to doctors for their distant care. Through haptics, a mother may transmit her newborn love, warmth, and care from a distance. Deaf and dumb patients can use haptics to transmit their emotions, ailments, and suffering to a doctor who is located far away. Haptics can be used to remotely treat and cure a psychiatric condition. Patients with psychological illnesses will be able to communicate their emotions and sentiments to doctors.

People with physical disabilities, especially students, would benefit greatly from HC training. Significant use of it will also be used in the training of AI-enabled surgical robots. The full potential of 6G for real-time remote surgery will be shown by the HC with virtual reality (VR)/AR. Real-time remote surgery requiring ultra-low latency, measured in microseconds, will be supported via 6G communication (Kharche & Kharche, 2023).

In order to simulate touch, haptic technology exerts force, movement, or vibration on the user. To collect tactile data in real-time, tactile Internet requires rapid connections and ultra-reliable low-latency communications (URLLC). It will also enable physicians to make touch diagnoses without being present. Three subcategories exist within haptic technology-based human-computer interaction (HCI): wearable, computer, & interface. With desktop HCI, a doctor who is far away can use a virtual instrument to operate on or diagnose patients (Ahad et al., 2024).

INTELLIGENT WEARABLE DEVICES (IWD)

A flat-screen tablet or smartphone serves as the order-issuing device. The remote doctor in this instance takes advantage of wearable HCI, such as a haptic glove. Tactile and haptic technology may be useful in the medical industry when proficient physicians are able to perform complex surgery remotely with the help of robots (Ahad et al., 2024). When linked to the Internet, Intelligent Wearable Devices (IWD) can provide physiological and psychological data for testing and monitoring facilities. IWD will keep an eye on health issues, blood pressure checks, heart rate, nutritional intake, and body weight. The patient will receive the test soon.

When advising a plan of activity, like completing a run or a stroll, IWD also considers the person's prior medical history. IWD will maintain a record of every person's unique nutritional, behavioural, and health histories. In the event of any deficit, IWD can thus provide dietary advice. Hospital visits will occur less frequently if minor health problems like deficiencies are detected. This will lower hospital expenses and free up resources for more complicated medical conditions (Nayak & Patgiri, 2020).

ARTIFICIAL INTELLIGENCE (AI)

A communication network powered entirely by AI will exist in 6G. 6G will transform network connectivity in all its facets. Global coverage, including space-air-water, is what 6G aims to achieve. Making the many aspects of communication AI is the only way to do this. With the usage of AI algorithms, communication networks are producing high performance and accuracy. Real-time communication is crucial in the modern health care system, and AI-driven connectivity may make it possible.

Healthcare powered by AI upgrades clinical decision-making and diagnosis. In order to do tasks swiftly, the healthcare business needs AI. Deep learning (DL) does not require data pre-processing. Real-time data may be provided as input since the computing process leverages the actual health data. Additionally, it properly determines a great quantity of network properties. Similarly, another AI system being tested with data about health is termed Deep Reinforcement Learning (DRL). In learning reinforcement, the computer makes a few judgments initially and then tracks the outcomes. To get the best choice, the decision is recalculated in light of the observation. The benefits of deep neural network techniques and reinforcement learning are combined in DRL. DRL thus provides excellent performance with less computation (Nayak & Patgiri, 2020).

INTELLIGENT INTERNET OF MEDICAL THINGS (IIoMT) METHOD

In the context of 6G connection, the intelligent Internet of Medical Things (IIoMT) will elevate and support several aims for human welfare. Medical equipment can link to the Internet to the formation of an Internet of Everything (IoE), which includes IIoMT and the Internet of Bodies (IoB). Internet access will be available on all medical devices, facilitating quick decision-making. When connected to the Internet, computed tomography (CT) and magnetic resonance imaging (MRI) scans may scan and direct information to distant sites using 6G. These data are real-time assessable by a doctor. The ease with which doctors in remote locations can treat patients with cancer is almost another example. Determining whether a cancer patient's tumour is benign or malignant now takes time. But in the near future, real-time 6G cancer detection will be possible. Furthermore, doctors and patients won't have to go to specialized hospitals. In order to treat cancer patients, distant doctors will work in tandem with local physicians. The death rate of cancer patients can be decreased by early detection. This is applicable to a number of diseases, not just cancer, including cardiovascular treatment and many others (Ahad et al., 2024).

Internet of Bodies IoE-based Smart Healthcare is shown in Figure 10.6.

The smart technologies of patient-centric hospitals are represented by the rectangle box, and the rest of this visualization demonstrates how the fog layer and cloud platform are connected to these smart technologies through wireless networking technology in the IoB-based Smart Healthcare concept design (Ahad et al., 2024).

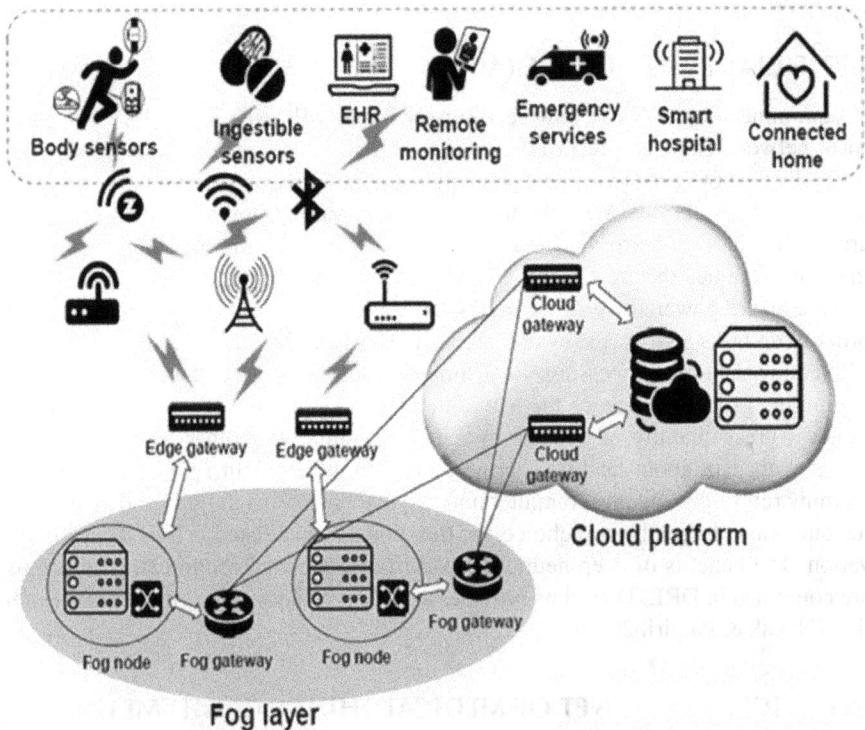

FIGURE 10.6 Internet of bodies IoE based smart HealthCare.

MEDICAL CYBER-PHYSICAL SYSTEMS FOR HUMAN-IN-THE-LOOP CONTROL

Computation and physical processes are integrated into cyber-physical systems, or CPS. Embedded computers and networks monitor and regulate physical processes. These operations often involve feedback loops where calculations are impacted by physical processes and vice versa (Parnianifard, 2022). Energy management, health-care, and automotive systems are just a few of the many cyber-physical system applications that stand to benefit from human-in-the-loop feedback control systems. For instance, it is proposed that utilizing models of everyday living activities in home health care might enhance the medical conditions of the elderly, and that explicitly integrating human-in-the-loop models for driving can increase safety. 6G communication can provide real-time data for the Cyber-Physical Systems for Human-in-the-Loop Control (Munir et al., 2013; Parnianifard, 2022).

BRAIN–COMPUTER INTERFACE (BCI)

The brain and electrical devices may communicate more easily due to the brain–computer interface (BCI). This requires a high data flow, extremely low latency, and high dependability. Touch feedback, control, and real-time data transfer will all be possible with 6G networks. This technique makes it possible to communicate touch, senses, and information all at once, making the experience more engaging. In a healthcare system, a wounded patient would be able to communicate visually. A smart headband might replicate brain impulses and show them in a 3D video of the patient's thoughts. Through mobile networks, the caregiver may view the video in real-time. In addition, individuals with different language skills may converse by utilizing their imaginations, and those with disabilities can use HC to operate devices or unlock doors. They will be able to communicate by touch thanks to these HC techniques. One of the anticipated applications for 6G networks is this, where the network can support far larger data rates than 5G could (Nasralla et al., 2023).

HOLOGRAPHIC COMMUNICATION

Using interference patterns produced by lasers, holograms (Metaverse three-dimensional pictures) may emerge in intangible settings. 5G cannot fully support holographic communication because of latency and bandwidth problems. Data speeds of up to 4 Tbps, ultra-low latency (in sub-milliseconds), ultra-high dependability (99.9999%), security, and ultra-low-density connection needs for holographic communications will all be supported by 6G. However, the difficulty is the creation of holographic antennas capable of 6G frequency band operation. The feeling of touch that holographic communication conveys will allow medical professionals and patients to enhance their legacy audio-visual communication. True immersion in far-away locations is made possible by HC. It validates the accurate transmission of information through the five senses of humans: taste, smell, sight, and hearing.

In the 6G age, holographic meetings, including health considerations, will be held often, necessitating the use of 3D holographic displays. Ambulance navigation will also be needed for these displays. To safeguard healthcare systems, HC is required. When compared to distant communication settings, it offers the physical sensation of face-to-face contact. Patients can be virtually present in person in the hospital thanks to HC. It is feasible to integrate HC with AR/VR to provide patients with a better 3D image of their surgical site (Kharche & Kharche, 2023).

A hologram is a realistic depiction of the interference pattern created by diffraction that reflects light into three dimensions. The depth and parallax of the original object are preserved in the created picture. By employing cameras at different angles, holographic communication creates an object hologram. Its primary services will be integrated into Enhanced mobile broadband (eMBB) and URLLC. For high-definition video streaming and optimal service quality, significant data rates will be needed. Moreover, real-time prompt control and speech retorts mandate tremendously low latency. It will denote a substantial development in healthcare. Furthermore, 6G is able to offer this service. 6G People will become more connected through holographic communication. Sometimes, the doctors may have to wait for a diagnosis from a specialized doctor or doctors before treating an emergency. However, if the skilled physicians employ holographic communication, the patient can get a diagnosis while on the road. Holographic Communication is also able to oversee the physicians for the primary medical intervention. To receive an appropriate diagnosis, the patient frequently has to see many doctors; otherwise, the hospital may not offer the necessary care. The patient may need to go to a different state or nation. In these situations, the patient is left with a financial and physical burden. Additionally, it is quite distressing for the patient to travel when ill (Nayak & Patgiri, 2020).

TELESURGERY

Telesurgery is a future-oriented idea that is still in its infancy. The physician(s) defines it as remote surgery. Robots, nurses, and a mediator between distant doctors are needed for telesurgery. Effective communication is essential in telesurgery. It also requires an exceptionally high URLLC and a rapid data rate. 5G or B5G cannot fulfil these requirements of telesurgery. It also requires a very high data rate and URLLC. These requirements cannot be met by 5G or B5G. Therefore, 6G technology is needed to facilitate telesurgery. Moreover, real-time communication is necessary for telesurgery to be successful. The physician can give verbal, teleassist, or telestrategic direction during telesurgery. More engaging verbal guidance may be given through holographic communication thanks to 6G. With holographic communication, the surgeon may move to have a better view of the patient and can be present in the operation to provide direction. Telestration involves, for example, utilizing video to remotely demonstrate the surgical process. VR and AR have applications in intelligent healthcare and telemedicine. Furthermore, the surgeon(s) can use tactile/haptic technologies to teleassist the procedure. 6G communication technology can meet the needs of telesurgery and will demonstrate that surgery can be performed anywhere (Nayak & Patgiri, 2020).

VEHICULAR TECHNOLOGY

High mobility and coverage, which are problems with 5G communication technology, will be provided by 6G technology (Rahman 2018). It is anticipated that 6G communication will have complete satellite support in order to offer high mobility and extensive coverage. Furthermore, a major obstacle to 5G communication technology is rural communication. But 6G will be able to get over the problem. Due to the development of AI, cars are also becoming more intelligent, with the ability to learn, anticipate, and make decisions. As a result, drivers won't need to control intelligent vehicles. AI integration will also make unmanned aerial vehicles (UAV) smarter. As a result, it is anticipated that automotive technology will be crucial to healthcare services.

INTELLIGENT DRONES

Drones will be essential to emergency services and corporate operations in the future because of the development of UAVs. Drone deployment presents issues in the areas of fire control, transportation, security and surveillance, and network provision. As a result, drones need to be seamlessly connected to everything (D2X), infrastructure (D2I), and other drones (D2D). Drones are essential for networking, emergency response, firefighting, security, surveillance, accident investigation, medical kit delivery, and streaming films for wounded people's medical conditions.

INTELLIGENT AMBULANCE SERVICES

The majority of victims pass away in the ambulance on the way from their house to the hospital, or even before it arrives. Furthermore, an accident detection system does not exist in healthcare systems. For the accident detection system to deliver critical and immediate medical assistance, real-time detection is necessary. Presently, ambulance services only transport patients who need oxygen and have priority over other vehicles. It is not intelligent enough to perform the functions of an emergency service. As such, the ambulance services have little effect on our lives. Any ordinary car might fulfil the same purposes as long as there is oxygen and an emergency alert. Hence, a new kind of ambulance service is required to improve the quality of life. Standard ambulance services will be replaced by Hospital-to-Home (H2H) services. Recent developments in communication technology have made it possible for hospitals and households to interact when needed, particularly in an emergency. In order to create intelligent vehicles, future automobiles will only be powered by AI. Consequently, H2H will be deployed on a mobile hospital platform powered by intelligent vehicles, obviating the need for hospitals and the healthcare workers that staff them. Ambulance services will be replaced by this mobile hospital. For instance, as soon as an event is discovered, a mobile hospital reacts. Then, before they get to the hospitals, the patients will start receiving care from the mobile hospital. Additionally, a mobile hospital can respond to an emergency rapidly and offer life-saving care right away. Additionally, it will enhance modern lifestyles. In the context of senior services, it is quite important. As a result, 6G connections enable H2H services, which revolutionize current living (Nayak & Patgiri, 2020).

INTERNET OF BIO-NANO THINGS

Bio-Nano Things (BNTs) are nanoscale and biological devices that are a component of the Internet of Bio-Nano Things (IoBNT), a heterogeneous network that communicates in non-conventional contexts (like the human body) via non-conventional ways (like molecular communications (MC)). The primary goal of this innovative networking architecture is to provide easy and direct contact with biological systems in order to accurately sense and manage their dynamics in real time. It is anticipated that the exceptionally high spatiotemporal resolution and the close relationship between the bio and cyber domains will create a plethora of new opportunities for the development of novel applications, particularly for intrabody continuous health monitoring and the healthcare industry (Al-Jawad et al., 2022; Kuscu & Unluturk, 2021).

Using 6G technology, the IoBT seeks to make the human body a part of this "Net." In not-so-distant future, it is expected that we will all be wearing these gadgets. Through the treatment of individuals as a holistic system comprising psychological and environmental elements, the 6G connection will contribute to medical research. For mobile and continuous control, new sensors are required both within and outside the body. This necessitates a dependable, secure, and flexible network, which 6G can provide (Kuscu & Unluturk, 2021).

COMMUNICATIONS ON-BODY, IN-BODY, AND OFF-BODY

This approach uses information and communication technology (ICT) to monitor people's health remotely. All types of communication, including on-body, in-body, and off-body, are included in the Body-Layer. Off-body communications enable real-time data transfer between edge devices and the cloud. Within the body, molecules or nanostructures serve as biological communication networks that represent sensors (Salam et al., 2018).

INTELLIGENT NANOSCALE INNER BODY COMMUNICATIONS

Intra-body monitoring and manipulation are made possible by a new revolution known as the IoBNT, which is powered by biological cells present in human bodies. The doctor or nurse receives the medical data and uses it to initiate the necessary remote activities. 6G technology is important in this sense as it will enable IoBNT and IoNT connection (Rahman & Alhiyafi, 2018).

HUMAN BODY COMMUNICATION

All of the senses used by humans are used in this manner to detect and convey data. It might happen soon for one person's "thoughts" or experiences to be sent to another. 6G may be seen as a "material" technology that, by allowing users to perceive data recorded from their emotions' sensors, provides an engaging user experience. Better achievable facilities include diagnosis, patient monitoring, assistance, and therapy (Rahman, 2019).

VISIBLE LIGHT COMMUNICATION

Visible light communication (VLC), for short, is a subset of optical wireless technology. To communicate data, Light rays are utilized by VLC. It may be utilized to get physiological data, facilitate broad user interaction, and gain access to infrastructure, which may serve as a downlink channel for improved connection (Atta-ur-Rahman et al., 2019).

SMART BEDSIDE STATION

With the advancement of ICT, bedside terminal device technology is getting more contemporary. We used cutting-edge technologies to create the Smart Bedside Station (SBS) we created, which includes an RFID reader log-in system and a handy touch screen. We also made sure the SBS could be connected wired or wirelessly via Bluetooth, Wi-Fi, and USB, especially considering the potential scalability of different medical devices for future services. It is anticipated that the SBS System would provide several advantages, such as decreased waiting times for numerous service requests (such as food preparation, housekeeping, or bed linen changes) and enhanced functionality in the therapeutic process. To get the necessary information assistance, patients can view their daily schedule, test results, or other medical information. Therefore, we firmly believe that these practical features will help to guarantee that patients are well-informed. Unlike the prior paradigm that needed many stakeholders for a single medical/nursing team, the SBS allows all medical staff members to perform their duties utilizing a single terminal. For regular hospital health care, we want to deploy the SBS system as an integrated communication tool between patients and medical personnel.

REAL-TIME MOBILE DNA SEQUENCING

Third-generation sequencing (TGS) is an enhanced method that offers very quick sequencing speeds and prolonged deoxyribonucleic acid (DNA) assessments. For ubiquitous healthcare (U-healthcare) services, the use of contemporary intelligent systems and mobile technology in the Internet of Living Things (IoLT) makes on-site wireless DNA sequencing techniques possible. Even under some severe restrictions, 6G technology could be able to support communications in an IoLT system for U-healthcare that is genuinely intelligent.

An effective sequencing-device-based single sign-on (SD-SSO) system and a secure three-factor authentication technique protect the group key distribution procedure. The suggested method enables the provision of patient-centred services that are accessible on several mobile devices by using traceable data kept in the server database. A thorough semantic explanation and well-known verification tools demonstrate the suggested protocol's security resilience (Singh and Joshi, 2024).

When compared to previous efforts, performance evaluation reveals that the protocol offers additional capability at a fair overhead (Le, 2023).

TIMEFRAME FOR THE AVAILABILITY OF 6G APPLICATIONS USAGE IN SMART HEALTH CARE SYSTEM

One possible timeframe for standardization is 2028. By about 2030, the first apps could be released on the commercial market. It is important to note, nevertheless, that every generation of mobile communications takes around 10 years to create. Over the past two or three years, the deployment of 5G networks has advanced. Additionally, this technology will progress since it won't suddenly vanish when 6G becomes accessible (www.medica-tradefair.com).

CHALLENGES TO BE FACED BY 6G IN SMART HEALTHCARE SYSTEM

The following is a description of the technological, ethical, and legal issues, as well as privacy and security challenges, with 6G communication technologies:

A) **Security and Privacy**: Encrypted transmission on and within the body is still being developed. It is necessary to have a large number of robust authentication methods and cryptography algorithms with reduced key lengths (Kumar et al., 2024). Furthermore, further research is needed to address the unanticipated reactivity of biomolecules and their potentially disastrous consequences.

B) **Aspects of Technology**: Significant information may be retrieved and circulated to the cloud through communication across bodily layers (Joshi et al., 2024). Each one of these several node types has a very different set of communication needs. It is feasible to combine and correlate data from ongoing human body monitoring, gathering information from a wide variety of sensors, from micro to macro.

C) **Aspects of Ethics**: In order to ethically lead processes, it is imperative to include citizens as data owners in those processes, since one of the ethical problems requiring participation in processes requiring more health literacy is equity in access to healthcare treatments. Develop a coherent regulatory framework to keep excluded people from falling behind (Al-Jawad et al., 2022).

CONCLUSIONS

We demonstrated a variety of applications that may use the 6G networks to address a number of issues in the health industry. Many issues facing the healthcare sector can be resolved by futuristic 6G applications, including reducing medical mistakes and raising the standard of patient-centric care. 6G AI technology will be essential for helping healthcare professionals with their daily tasks and providing effective and affordable remote patient services. They will address the increasing number of patients and the scarcity of medical personnel by offering support and facilitating treatment at home. Even while 6G technologies can be used for real-time patient monitoring, the vital methods for the healthcare sector, including IoBNT and in-body and on-body communication, might save end users and the government in terms of time and money, and there are still downsides.

REFERENCES

Ahad, A., Jiangbina, Z., Tahir, M., Shayea, I., Sheikh, M., & Rasheed, F. (2024). 6G and intelligent healthcare: Taxonomy, technologies, open issues and future research directions. *Internet of Things*, 25. https://doi.org/10.1016/j.iot.2024.101068

Al-Jawad, F., Alessa, R., Alhammad, S., Ali, B., Alqanbar, M., & Rahman, A. (2022). Applications of 5G and 6G in smart health services. *International Journal of Computer Science and Network Security*, 22, 173–182. https://doi.org/10.22937/IJCSNS.2022. 22.3.23

Atta-ur-Rahman, Dash, S., Luhach, A. K., Chilamkurti, N., Baek, S., & Nam, Y. (2019). A neuro-fuzzy approach for user behaviour classification and prediction. *Journal of Cloud Computing*, 8(1), 17. https://doi.org/10.1186/s13677-019-0144-9

Awino, O. J. (2024). The role of 5G in promoting patient-centric care in smart healthcare systems. Science notebooks. *Organization and Management/Silesian University of Technology, Silesian University of Technology Publishing House*, 191, 405–414. https://doi.org/10.29119/1641-3466.2024.191.26

De Alwis, C., Kumar, P., Pham, Q-V., Dev, K., Kalla, A., Liyanage, M.,& Hwang W-J. (2023) Towards 6G: Key technological directions, *ICT Express*, 9, 4, 525–533. https://doi.org/10.1016/j.icte.2022.10.005

Islam, S. K., Fathy, A., Wang, Y., Kuhn, M., & Mahfouz, M. (2014). Hassle-Free vitals: BioWireleSS for a patient-centric health-care paradigm. *IEEE Microwave Magazine*, 15, 7, 25.

Joshi, A., Kumar, V., Thakur, G., Pant, H. V., & Singh, B. P. (2024). The impact of cloud computing on data science and engineering: Opportunities and challenges. *2024 International Conference on Electrical Electronics and Computing Technologies (ICEECT)*, 1–4. https://doi.org/10.1109/ICEECT61758.2024.10739285

Joshi, A., & Tiwari, H. (2023). An overview of Python libraries for data science. *Journal of Engineering Technology and Applied Physics*, 5(2), 85–90. https://doi.org/10.33093/jetap.2023.5.2.10

Kharche, S., & Kharche, J. (2023). 6G intelligent healthcare framework: A review on role of technologies, challenges and future directions. *Journal of Mobile Multimedia*, 19, 3, 603–644.

Kumar, R., Joshi, A., Sharan, H. O., Peng, S., & Dudhagara, C. R. (Eds.). (2024). *The Ethical Frontier of AI and Data Analysis*. IGI Global. https://doi.org/10.4018/979-8-3693-2964-1

Kuscu, M., & Unluturk, B. D. (2021). Internet of bio-nano things: A review of applications, enabling technologies and key challenges. *Journal on Future and Evolving Technologies*, 2, 3.

Le, T.-V. (2023). Securing group patient communication in 6G-aided dynamic ubiquitous healthcare with real-time mobile DNA sequencing. *Bioengineering*, 10, 839. https://doi.org/10.3390/bioengineering10070839

Munir, S., Stankovic, J. A., Liang, C. J. M., & Lin, S. (2013). Cyber physical system challenges for human-in-the-loop control. In *Proceedings of the 8th International Workshop on Feedback Computing (Feedback Computing '13)*. USENIX Association. https://www.usenix.org/conference/feedbackcomputing13/workshop-program/presentation/munir

Nasralla, M. M., Khattak, S. B. A., Ur Rehman, I., & Iqbal, M. (2023). Exploring the role of 6G technology in enhancing quality of experience for m-Health multimedia applications: A comprehensive survey. *Sensors*, 23, 5882.

Nayak, S., & Patgiri, R. (2020). 6G communication technology: A vision on intelligent healthcare. *Studies in Computational Intelligence*, 6, 22, e2. doi:10.1007/978-981-15-9735-0_1

Parnianifard, A. (2022). Digital-twins towards cyber-physical systems: A brief survey. *Modern Engineering Technology*, 26, 9, 47–61.

Rahman, A. (2018). Efficient decision based spectrum mobility scheme for cognitive radio based V2V communication system. *Journal of Communications*, 3, 9, 498–504.

Rahman, A. (2019). Memetic computing based numerical solution to Troesch problem. *Journal of Intelligent and Fuzzy Systems*, 37, 1, 1545–1554.

Rahman, A., & Alhiyafi, J. (2018). Health level seven generic web interface. *Journal of Computational and Theoretical Nanoscience*, 15, 1261–1274.

Salam, M., Memon, S., Das, L., Rahman, A., Hussain, Z., Shah, R. H., & Memon, N. A. (2018). Sensor based survival detection system in Earthquake disaster zones. *International Journal of Computer Science and Network Security*, 18, 5, 46–52.

Singh, B. P., & Joshi, A. (2024). Ethical considerations in AI development. In R. Kumar, A. Joshi, H. Sharan, S. Peng, & C. Dudhagara (Eds.), *The Ethical Frontier of AI and Data Analysis* (pp. 156–179). IGI Global Scientific Publishing. https://doi.org/10.4018/979-8-3693-2964-1.ch010

11 Deepfake Technology
A Comprehensive Review and Ethical Implication

Deep Chandra Andola, Preeti Pandey, and Vandana Bisht

INTRODUCTION

A deepfake is a type of synthetic media that is created using artificial intelligence (AI) and machine learning techniques, particularly deep learning. The term "deepfake" is a combination of "deep learning" and "fake." Deep learning involves training artificial neural networks on large datasets to learn patterns and make predictions (Joshi & Tiwari, 2023).

In the context of deepfakes, the technology is used to manipulate or generate visual and audio content that appears convincingly real but is, in fact, artificially created. Deepfake techniques can be applied to various types of media, including videos, images, and audio recordings.

The most common application of deepfakes involves the creation of realistic-looking videos in which individuals or events are manipulated to appear as if they are saying or doing things they never did. This technology has raised concerns about its potential misuse for spreading misinformation, disinformation, and creating deceptive content.

As technology continues to advance, efforts are also being made to develop tools and techniques for detecting and mitigating the impact of deepfakes to address the potential negative consequences associated with their use.

EVOLUTION AND DEVELOPMENT OF DEEPFAKE TECHNOLOGY

The evolution and development of deepfake technology can be traced through several key milestones:

- **Early Academic Research (2014–2016)**: The roots of deepfake technology can be traced back to academic research in machine learning and computer vision. Researchers explored the possibilities of generative models, particularly generative adversarial networks (GANs), to generate realistic synthetic images.

DOI: 10.1201/9781003516590-11

- **Face Swapping Apps (2017)**: The first notable emergence of deepfake technology in the public domain occurred with the introduction of face-swapping applications. These apps allowed users to superimpose the faces of celebrities or others onto existing videos, often for entertainment purposes. While these early applications were relatively simple, they hinted at the potential of more sophisticated deepfake technology.
- **Rise of GANs (2017–2018)**: The development of more advanced generative models, especially GANs, played a crucial role in the improvement of deepfake technology. GANs are capable of generating high-quality, realistic images by training on large datasets. This advancement facilitated the creation of more convincing and detailed deepfake content.
- **Deepfake Videos Gain Attention (2018)**: Deepfake technology gained widespread attention in 2018 with the emergence of highly realistic and convincing deepfake videos. These videos often featured political figures, celebrities, and public figures engaging in activities or saying things they had not done in reality.
- **Increased Accessibility (2019–2020)**: As deepfake algorithms and tools became more sophisticated, they also became more accessible to the general public. Open-source deepfake software and tutorials proliferated on the internet, allowing individuals with moderate technical skills to create deepfake content.
- **Concerns and Regulations (2019–present)**: The rise of deepfakes raised significant concerns regarding the potential for misuse, particularly in the realms of misinformation, identity theft, and privacy invasion. Governments, tech companies, and researchers started developing and implementing strategies for detecting and mitigating deepfake content. Some jurisdictions also introduced or discussed legislation to address the challenges posed by deepfake technology.
- **Advancement in Deepfake Techniques (2020–present)**: Ongoing research and development in deepfake technology continue to improve the sophistication and realism of synthetic media. Deepfake techniques are not limited to faces; there are also advancements in voice synthesis and body movement replication.
- **AI-Based Detection Tools (2020–present)**: In response to the potential threats posed by deepfakes, there has been a parallel development of AI-based detection tools. These tools leverage machine learning algorithms to identify signs of manipulation in media content and distinguish between authentic and synthetic material (Joshi & Goyal, 2019).

The evolution of deepfake technology is an ongoing process, with both positive and negative implications. While the technology has potential applications in various fields, including entertainment and filmmaking, the risks associated with misuse underscore the importance of responsible development and deployment.

MOTIVATION

The motivations behind creating deepfake content can vary widely, and individuals or groups may have different reasons for engaging in this technology. Some common motivations include:

- **Entertainment and Creative Expression**: Many early applications of deepfake technology were driven by a desire for creative expression and entertainment. People used face-swapping applications and other deep-fake tools to create humorous or amusing content, such as videos featuring celebrities in unexpected situations.
- **Digital Art and Filmmaking**: Deepfake technology has the potential to revolutionize the field of filmmaking and digital art. Filmmakers and artists can use deepfake techniques to recreate historical scenes, bring deceased actors back to life for a film, or explore imaginative and visually stunning scenarios that would be challenging or impossible to achieve through tradi-tional methods.
- **Mimicry and Impersonation**: Some individuals use deepfake technology to impersonate or mimic the appearance of others. This can be done for entertainment purposes, satire, or to create content that appears authentic. However, this aspect of deepfakes raises ethical concerns, particularly when it comes to potentially misleading or deceiving audiences.
- **Education and Research Purpose**: Deepfake technology is also used in academic and research settings for studying machine learning, computer vision, and AI. Researchers may develop and experiment with deepfake algorithms to better understand their capabilities and limitations.
- **Privacy and Anonymity**: In some cases, individuals may use deepfake technology to protect their privacy or maintain anonymity. This could involve altering facial features in photos or videos to avoid recognition, especially in situations where people wish to share content without reveal-ing their identity.
- **Satire and Social Commentary**: Deepfake technology can be employed to create satirical content or social commentary. This might involve putting the faces of public figures on different bodies or altering speeches to convey a particular message. Satirical deepfakes can be a form of political or social commentary, although they may also raise ethical concerns.
- **Malicious Intent**: Unfortunately, deepfake technology has been used with malicious intent. Some individuals or groups create deepfake content to spread misinformation, defame individuals, engage in cyberbullying, or manipulate public opinion. This misuse of deepfake technology poses sig-nificant ethical and societal challenges.
- **Pranks and Humour**: Deepfake technology has been used for pranks and humour, often involving the creation of content that appears realistic but is

intended solely for comedic purposes. However, the line between harmless humour and potentially harmful deception can be thin, leading to concerns about unintended consequences.

It's essential to recognize that while deepfake technology has positive applications, such as in entertainment and creative fields, the potential for misuse and deception underscores the need for responsible development, awareness, and the implementation of safeguards to mitigate negative impacts.

INCREASING PREVALENCE OF DEEPFAKE CONTENT

The prevalence of deepfake content has been on the rise in recent years, driven by various factors including advancements in technology, increased accessibility of tools, and evolving motivations. Here are some key reasons contributing to the increasing prevalence of deepfake content:

- **Technological Advancements**: Continuous advancements in machine learning, particularly in the field of deep learning, have significantly improved the capabilities of deepfake algorithms. The development of sophisticated generative models, such as GANs, allows for the creation of more realistic and convincing deepfake content.
- **Open-Source Tools and Software**: The availability of open-source deepfake tools and software has made the creation of synthetic media more accessible to a broader audience. This has lowered the entry barriers, enabling individuals with moderate technical skills to generate deepfake content using pre-existing frameworks.
- **Increased Computing Power**: The availability of powerful computing resources, including Graphics Processing Units (GPUs), has accelerated the training and generation processes involved in creating deepfakes. This increased computing power allows for faster and more efficient development of realistic synthetic media.
- **Social Media and Online Platforms**: The widespread use of social media and online platforms provides a vast distribution network for deepfake content. Deepfakes can quickly spread across platforms, reaching a large audience and potentially influencing public opinion. The viral nature of content on social media contributes to the rapid dissemination of deepfake material.
- **Entertainment Industry Adoption**: The entertainment industry has embraced deepfake technology for various creative purposes, including digital resurrection of actors, face replacement for stunts, and other filmmaking applications. While this contributes to the prevalence of deepfake content in legitimate contexts, it also increases public exposure to the technology.
- **Evolving Motivation and Use Cases**: As motivations for creating deepfake content evolve, the range of use cases has expanded. While some individuals create deepfakes for entertainment or artistic expression, others may use them for malicious purposes, such as spreading misinformation, creating fake news, or engaging in identity theft.

- **Challenges in Detection**: The ongoing cat-and-mouse game between deepfake creators and detection tools contributes to the proliferation of synthetic media. While detection methods continue to advance, so do the techniques used by deepfake creators to evade detection, making it challenging to completely mitigate the spread of deceptive content.
- **Limited Regulation and Enforcements**: In many jurisdictions, there is a lack of specific regulations addressing the creation and dissemination of deepfake content. Limited legal frameworks and enforcement mechanisms make it easier for individuals to engage in the creation and sharing of deepfakes without facing significant consequences.

The increasing prevalence of deepfake content raises concerns about its potential impact on society, including issues related to misinformation, privacy, and trust. Efforts are ongoing to develop effective detection tools, raise public awareness, and implement regulations to address the challenges posed by the widespread use of deepfake technology.

POTENTIAL RISK AND CONSEQUENCES

The increasing prevalence of deepfake content raises a range of potential risks and consequences, impacting various aspects of society, technology, and individuals. Some of the key risks and consequences include:

- **Misinformation and Fake News**: Deepfake technology can be misused to create realistic-looking videos or audio recordings of individuals saying or doing things they never did. This has the potential to spread misinformation and fake news, eroding trust in media and public figures.
- **Identity Theft and Fraud**: Deepfakes can be used for identity theft by manipulating images or videos to make it appear as though an individual is involved in activities they never participated in. This poses risks to personal and professional reputations, and it can also be exploited for fraudulent activities.
- **Privacy Invasion**: The ability to convincingly alter faces and voices in media raises concerns about privacy invasion. Deepfake technology can be used to create fake videos or audio recordings that compromise the privacy of individuals, leading to personal and emotional harm.
- **Political Manipulation**: Deepfakes have the potential to be used for political manipulation by creating videos of politicians saying or doing things that never occurred. This can influence public opinion, affect elections, and sow discord within societies.
- **Erosion of Trust**: The widespread use of deepfakes can contribute to a general erosion of trust in digital media. As it becomes increasingly challenging to discern real from fake content, individuals may become more sceptical of the information they encounter online.
- **Security Threats**: Deepfake technology can be exploited for security threats, including the creation of fake videos for blackmail or extortion

(Kumar et al., 2024). In corporate settings, deepfakes could be used to impersonate executives or employees, leading to financial or reputational damage.

- **Legal and Ethical Concerns**: The creation and dissemination of deepfake content raise complex legal and ethical issues. Determining responsibility, accountability, and the appropriate legal responses can be challenging, especially as laws and regulations struggle to keep pace with technological advancements.
- **Impact on Journalism and Authenticity**: The prevalence of deepfakes challenges traditional journalism and the authenticity of media. Journalists and news outlets may face increased difficulty in verifying the authenticity of videos and audio recordings, potentially compromising the integrity of news reporting.
- **Psychological and Emotional Impact**: Individuals who become the subjects of deepfake content may experience significant psychological and emotional distress. The knowledge that one's likeness can be convincingly manipulated in videos can lead to anxiety, fear, and other emotional consequences.
- **Counterproductive Responses**: The existence of deepfake content may lead to counterproductive responses, such as increased scepticism towards genuine content or the rejection of valid evidence due to concerns about manipulation.

Efforts are underway to address these risks, including the development of detection technologies, public awareness campaigns, and legal frameworks. However, the evolving nature of deepfake technology presents ongoing challenges that require a multifaceted and collaborative approach to mitigation.

DEEPFAKE TECHNOLOGY

Deepfake technology is a type of synthetic media creation that involves the use of AI, particularly deep learning algorithms, to generate highly realistic and often deceptive content. The term "deepfake" is derived from the combination of "deep learning" and "fake." Deep learning, a subset of machine learning, involves training neural networks on large datasets to learn patterns and make predictions. Here are key components and aspects of deepfake technology:

- **Generative Adversarial Networks (GANs)**: GANs are a type of generative model commonly used in deepfake technology. They consist of two neural networks—the generator and the discriminator—trained simultaneously through adversarial training. The generator creates synthetic content, while the discriminator attempts to distinguish between real and synthetic content. This dynamic training process leads to the generation of increasingly realistic deepfake content.
- **Face Swapping**: One common application of deepfake technology involves swapping the faces of individuals in images or videos. This technique

allows the seamless replacement of one person's face with another, creating a visually convincing result.

- **Facial Reenactment**: In video deepfakes, facial reenactment involves mapping the facial expressions and movements of one person onto the face of another in a way that appears natural and realistic.
- **Voice Synthesis**: Deepfake technology is not limited to visual content; it can also be applied to audio. Voice synthesis algorithms can mimic a person's voice, allowing for the creation of synthetic audio recordings that sound like the targeted individual.
- **Body Movement Replication**: Advancements in deepfake technology have expanded beyond faces to include the replication of body movements. This involves generating realistic animations of a person's body to match the desired actions in a video.
- **Training on Large Datasets**: Deepfake models require extensive training on large datasets of images or videos to learn the subtle details of facial expressions, movements, and voice patterns. The quality of deepfake content is often correlated with the size and diversity of the training dataset.
- **Accessibility through Open-Source Tools**: The availability of open-source deepfake tools and software has contributed to the accessibility of the technology. Various frameworks and applications enable individuals with moderate technical skills to create deepfake content.
- **Legitimate Applications**: While there are concerns about misuse, deepfake technology also has legitimate applications in areas such as filmmaking, entertainment, and digital art. It can be used to create special effects, resurrect actors for posthumous roles, or facilitate language translation in videos.

The dynamic nature of deepfake technology, along with its potential societal impacts, underscores the importance of ongoing research, awareness, and responsible development to address its challenges and opportunities.

CORE ALGORITHMS

The core algorithm of deepfake technology involves the use of generative models, GANs, to create synthetic content that closely resembles real images or videos. Here's an overview of the core algorithmic components of deepfake creation:

- **Generative Adversarial Networks (GANs)**: GANs consist of two neural networks: a generator and a discriminator. The generator is responsible for creating synthetic content, while the discriminator tries to distinguish between real and synthetic content. The two networks are trained in tandem through adversarial training, where the generator aims to produce content that is indistinguishable from real data, and the discriminator gets better at telling real from fake. This iterative process leads to the generation of increasingly realistic deepfake content.
- **Encoder–Decoder Architecture**: The core architecture of deepfake models often involves an encoder–decoder structure. The encoder processes input

data (such as facial features in images or video frames) and encodes it into a latent representation. The decoder then takes this latent representation and generates the synthetic content, such as a face with altered expressions or movements.

- **Temporal Coherence for Videos**: In the context of deepfake videos, maintaining temporal coherence is crucial for creating convincing content. This involves ensuring that the generated frames smoothly transition over time, mimicking the natural flow of facial expressions and movements.
- **Loss Functions**: Various loss functions are employed to guide the training process and ensure that the generated content aligns with the characteristics of the real data. Common loss functions include:
  - **Adversarial Loss**: Measures how well the generator can fool the discriminator.
  - **Content Loss**: Ensures that the generated content retains the key features of the original input.
  - **Perceptual Loss**: Encourages the generated content to match the perceptual features of the real data.
- **Training on Large Datasets**: Deepfake models require extensive training on large datasets containing diverse examples of faces, expressions, and movements. The use of large datasets helps the model generalize well to various scenarios and individuals.
- **Fine-Tuning and Transfer Learning**: Fine-tuning is often employed to adapt pre-trained models to specific tasks or individuals. Transfer learning techniques enable the model to leverage knowledge gained from one dataset to improve performance on another.
- **Post-processing Techniques**: After the initial generation, post-processing techniques may be applied to enhance the quality and realism of the deepfake content. This can involve refining details, adjusting lighting conditions, or addressing artifacts introduced during the generation process.

It's important to note that the specific algorithms and architectures used in deepfake technology can vary, and researchers continually explore new approaches to improve the realism of synthetic content and address ethical concerns associated with misuse. Additionally, advancements in machine learning, such as the development of novel architectures and training strategies, contribute to the ongoing evolution of deepfake algorithms.

TECHNICAL COMPONENTS

The creation of deepfake content involves several technical components, including algorithms, models, and tools. Here are the key technical components of deepfake technology:

- **Generative Adversarial Networks (GANs)**
  - **Description**: GANs are a type of generative model consisting of two neural networks—a generator and a discriminator—trained simultaneously

through adversarial training. The generator creates synthetic content, while the discriminator distinguishes between real and synthetic content.

- **Role in Deepfake**: GANs play a central role in deepfake technology by generating realistic images, videos, or audio that closely mimic real data.

- **Encoder–Decoder Architecture**
  - **Description**: Encoder–decoder architectures involve two neural network components—an encoder and a decoder. The encoder processes input data and encodes it into a latent representation, while the decoder generates synthetic content based on this representation.
  - **Role in Deepfake**: Encoder–decoder architectures are commonly used for tasks like facial expression transfer, where the encoder captures facial features, and the decoder generates a modified face.

- **Deep Neural Networks**
  - **Description**: Deep neural networks, including convolutional neural networks (CNNs) and recurrent neural networks (RNNs), are foundational for learning complex patterns in data.
  - **Role in Deepfake**: Deep neural networks are used for tasks like facial feature extraction, voice synthesis, and other aspects of deepfake content generation.

- **Auto-encoders**
  - **Description**: Auto-encoders are neural networks designed for unsupervised learning. They consist of an encoder and a decoder, and they aim to learn efficient data representations.
  - **Role in Deepfake**: Auto-encoders are used in certain deepfake applications for feature extraction and representation learning.

- **Capsule Networks**
  - **Description**: Capsule networks, or CapsNets, are a type of neural network architecture designed to address issues related to part-whole relationships in data.
  - **Role in Deepfake**: Capsule networks may be employed in deepfake models to capture hierarchical relationships within facial features, improving the quality of synthesized faces.

- **Temporal Coherence Model**
  - **Description**: Temporal coherence models ensure consistency and smooth transitions in videos by maintaining the natural flow of facial expressions and movements over time.
  - **Role in Deepfake**: Temporal coherence is crucial for creating convincing deepfake videos, and models are designed to generate frames that appear coherent and realistic in sequence.

- **Loss Function**
  - **Description**: Loss functions are mathematical functions that quantify the difference between the generated content and the real data, guiding the training process.
  - **Role in Deepfake**: Common loss functions include adversarial loss, content loss, and perceptual loss, which help the model generate content that is both realistic and faithful to the original input.

- **Large Datasets**
  - **Description**: Deepfake models are trained on large datasets containing diverse examples of faces, expressions, and movements.
  - **Role in Deepfake**: Training on large datasets helps the model generalize well to various scenarios and individuals, improving the quality of generated content.
- **Transfer Learning and Fine-Tuning**
  - **Description**: Transfer learning involves using knowledge gained from pre-trained models to improve performance on a specific task. Fine-tuning adapts a pre-trained model to a specific dataset or task.
  - **Roles in Deepfake**: Transfer learning and fine-tuning are often employed to enhance the efficiency and effectiveness of deepfake models.
- **Post-processing Techniques**
  - **Description**: Post-processing involves applying additional techniques after the initial content generation to enhance the quality and realism of deepfake content.
  - **Role in Deepfake**: Post-processing may involve refining details, adjusting lighting conditions, or addressing artifacts introduced during the generation process.

These technical components work together to enable the creation of realistic deepfake content, but it's important to note that ethical considerations and responsible use are essential in the development and deployment of deepfake technology.

APPLICATIONS

Deepfake technology has various applications across different industries, ranging from entertainment to cybersecurity. Here are some notable applications:

- **Entertainment Industry**
  - **Digital Resurrection**: Deepfake technology can be used to bring deceased actors and celebrities back to life for new roles or scenes in movies and TV shows.
  - **Voice Cloning**: It enables the replication of a person's voice for dubbing in different languages or creating dialogue for characters in animated films.
- **Filmmaking and Special Effects**
  - **Character Replacements**: Deepfakes can be employed to replace actors' faces with those of stunt doubles or to change facial expressions to suit specific scenes.
  - **Scene Recreation**: Filmmakers can use deepfake technology to recreate historical scenes or depict characters in different settings.
- **Digital Marketing and Advertising**
  - **Celebrity Endorsements**: Deepfake technology can create advertisements featuring celebrities endorsing products, even if the celebrities may not have been involved in the actual shoot.

- **Personalized Content**: Advertisers can use deepfakes to create personalized content, tailoring advertisements to specific demographics or individuals.
- **Education and Training**
  - **Language Learning**: Deepfake technology can be utilized to create language learning materials with native speakers' voices.
  - **Simulated Training Scenarios**: It allows for the creation of realistic training scenarios for fields like medicine, law enforcement, and customer service.
- **Accessibility and Inclusivity**
  - **Sign Language Interpretation**: Deepfakes can be applied to create sign language interpretation videos, improving accessibility for the deaf and hard-of-hearing community.
  - **Language Translation**: It can assist in translating content into different languages with the same voice and facial expressions.
- **Virtual Influencer and Social Media**
  - **Virtual Influencer**: Deepfake technology can be used to create virtual influencers with synthetic faces and personalities for social media marketing.
  - **Content Creation**: Social media users may use deepfakes for creative and humorous content, such as impersonations or parodies.
- **Human Computer Interaction**
  - **Humanizing Chatbots**: Deepfake voices and faces can be integrated into chatbots and virtual assistants to make human-computer interactions more natural and engaging.
- **Cyber Security and Threat Detection**
  - **Biometric Authentication Testing**: Organizations can use deepfakes to test the resilience of biometric authentication systems against synthetic attacks.
  - **Threat Simulation**: Deepfake technology can be employed to simulate cyber threats, helping organizations enhance their cybersecurity measures (Singh & Joshi, 2024).
- **Art and Digital Media**
  - **Digital Art**: Artists may use deepfake technology to create unique and immersive digital art pieces.
  - **Augmented Reality (AR) and Virtual Reality (VR)**: Deepfakes can enhance AR and VR experiences by creating realistic virtual characters and scenarios.
- **Forensic Analysis and Investigation**
  - **Crime Reconstruction**: Deepfake technology can be applied to reconstruct crime scenes and simulate scenarios for forensic analysis.
  - **Witness Testimony**: It may be used to create simulated witness testimonies or recreate events to aid investigations.

While these applications showcase the versatility of deepfake technology, it's crucial to be aware of the ethical considerations and potential misuse associated with the creation and dissemination of synthetic media. Regulations and safeguards are essential to address the risks and consequences associated with deepfake technology.

ENTERTAINMENT INDUSTRY

Deepfake technology has gained traction in the entertainment industry, offering new possibilities for filmmakers, producers, and content creators. Here are some ways in which deepfakes are being utilized in the entertainment sector:

- **Digital Resurrection**
  - **Description**: Deepfake technology enables the recreation of performances by deceased actors, allowing filmmakers to include these iconic figures in new projects.
  - **Example**: In the film industry, deepfake technology has been used to bring back actors like James Dean for posthumous roles.
- **Character Replacement and Face Swapping**:
  - **Description**: Filmmakers can use deepfake technology to replace actors' faces with those of stunt doubles, achieve facial re-enactment for scenes, or even change actors during post-production.
  - **Example**: Deepfakes can be applied to seamlessly insert an actor's face into scenes that were originally shot with a different performer.
- **Scene Recreation**
  - **Description**: Deepfake technology allows filmmakers to recreate historical scenes or depict characters in different settings, providing flexibility in storytelling.
  - **Example**: Deepfakes can be employed to create realistic scenes set in different time periods or locations.
- **Voice Cloning and Dubbing**:
  - **Description**: Deepfake algorithms can clone a person's voice, allowing for accurate dubbing in various languages or creating voiceovers for animated characters.
  - **Example**: Voice cloning can be used to dub movies or TV shows with the same actor's voice in different languages.
- **Special Effects and CGI Enhancement**:
  - **Description**: Deepfake technology can enhance special effects by generating realistic facial expressions, emotions, or movements for CGI (Computer-Generated Imagery) characters.
  - **Example**: In the realm of CGI, deepfakes can contribute to more lifelike animated characters.
- **Pre-Visualization and Prototyping**
  - **Description**: Filmmakers can use deepfake technology for previsualization and prototyping, experimenting with different actors or scenarios before committing to the final production.
  - **Example**: Directors and producers can test various casting choices or visualize scenes with deepfake technology before actual filming.
- **Historical Documentaries and Educational Content**
  - **Description**: Deepfake technology can be applied to create realistic historical figures in documentaries or educational content, making history more engaging for viewers.

- **Example**: Historical figures can be brought to life in a visually compelling manner, enhancing the educational experience.
- **Reducing Production Cost**
  - **Description**: Deepfake technology can potentially reduce production costs by eliminating the need for reshoots or costly CGI effects.
  - **Example**: Instead of reshooting scenes with a different actor, deepfake technology can be used to replace the existing actor's face.
- **Facial Expression and Emotions**:
  - **Description**: Deepfakes can be employed to enhance or modify the facial expressions and emotions of actors, allowing for a more nuanced portrayal of characters.
  - **Example**: Filmmakers can use deepfake technology to adjust the emotional tone of a scene or emphasize specific expressions.

While deepfake technology offers innovative possibilities in the entertainment industry, ethical considerations and responsible use are crucial. Transparency and clear communication with audiences about the use of deepfake technology in productions are essential to maintain trust. Additionally, the industry must navigate legal and regulatory aspects related to the ethical use of deepfakes.

CYBERSECURITY AND FRAUD

Cybersecurity and fraud concerns associated with deepfake technology are significant, as the potential misuse of synthetic media can lead to various malicious activities. Here are some key cybersecurity and fraud-related aspects related to deepfakes:

- **Social Engineering and Phishing**
  - **Description**: Deepfakes can be used in phishing attacks to impersonate trusted individuals, such as company executives or colleagues, tricking individuals into divulging sensitive information or transferring funds.
  - **Example**: A deepfake video or voice message might imitate a CEO (Chief Executive Officer) instructing an employee to transfer funds to a fraudulent account.
- **Business Email Compromise (BEC)**
  - **Description**: Deepfakes can be employed in BEC attacks, where cybercriminals impersonate executives or business partners to initiate fraudulent transactions, gain access to sensitive data, or manipulate employees.
  - **Example**: A deepfake email from a company executive might request an urgent wire transfer, leading to financial losses.
- **Identity Theft**
  - **Description**: Deepfake technology can be used to create synthetic identities for fraudulent purposes, leading to identity theft and financial fraud.
  - **Example**: Cybercriminals may use deepfakes to impersonate individuals in order to access accounts, apply for credit, or commit other forms of financial fraud.

- **Reputation Damage and Disinformation**
  - **Description**: Deepfakes can be created to damage the reputation of individuals, organizations, or public figures, spreading false information or engaging in character assassination.
  - **Example**: Deepfake videos depicting politicians making false statements could be used to manipulate public opinion.
- **Voice Fraud and Authentication Bypass**
  - **Description**: Deepfake voice synthesis can be used for voice fraud, enabling attackers to impersonate someone's voice and potentially bypass voice-based authentication systems.
  - **Example**: Deepfake voice recordings might be used to gain unauthorized access to secure systems or conduct fraudulent transactions.
- **Fake Video Evidence**:
  - **Description**: Deepfake videos can be used to create fake evidence in legal or corporate disputes, potentially leading to false accusations or unjust legal outcomes.
  - **Example**: Deepfake videos may be presented as evidence in court to falsely incriminate someone or mislead the legal system.
- **Manipulation of Financial Markets**
  - **Description**: Deepfakes can be used to manipulate financial markets by spreading false information about companies or economic indicators.
  - **Example**: A deepfake video of a company executive making misleading statements could impact stock prices or market sentiment.
- **Exploitation of Trust**
  - **Description**: Deepfakes exploit the trust individuals place in visual and auditory information, leading to potential manipulation and deception.
  - **Example**: Cybercriminals might use deepfake content to convince individuals to download malware or disclose sensitive information based on the false trust established through manipulated media.
- **Malware Distribution**
  - **Description**: Cybercriminals can use deepfakes to create convincing lures for distributing malware, exploiting the curiosity or trust of users.
  - **Example**: A deepfake video claiming to show exclusive content might be used to lure users into downloading malicious software.

To address these cybersecurity and fraud risks associated with deepfake technology, organizations and individuals should be vigilant, adopt multi-factor authentication, implement robust security measures, and stay informed about emerging threats. Ongoing research into detection methods and the development of regulatory frameworks can also contribute to mitigating the impact of deepfake-related cyber threats.

CHALLENGES IN DEEPFAKE

The rise of deepfake technology presents a range of challenges, spanning technological, ethical, legal, and societal dimensions. Here are some key challenges associated with deepfakes:

- **Technological Advancement**: Deepfake algorithms continue to evolve, becoming more sophisticated and realistic. This constant improvement poses challenges for the development of effective detection methods.
- **Detection Difficulties**: The ability to create highly convincing deepfakes makes it challenging to develop reliable and accurate detection tools. The cat-and-mouse game between creators and detectors requires ongoing innovation in detection technologies.
- **Accessibility and User-Friendly Tools**: The increasing accessibility of deepfake tools and user-friendly software makes it easier for individuals with limited technical skills to create convincing synthetic media, raising concerns about misuse.
- **Social Media Amplification**: Deepfake content can spread rapidly on social media platforms, reaching large audiences before detection mechanisms can identify and mitigate the misinformation, contributing to the viral nature of deceptive content.
- **Privacy Concerns**: Deepfake technology raises significant privacy concerns, as individuals may become targets for the creation of synthetic content without their consent. The potential for malicious use in compromising private information is a pressing issue.
- **Misinformation and Fake News**: Deepfakes contribute to the spread of misinformation and fake news, eroding trust in media and challenging the authenticity of visual and auditory information.
- **Identity Theft and Fraud**: Deepfakes can be used for identity theft and fraud, with malicious actors creating synthetic content to impersonate individuals for financial gain or other malicious purposes
- **Regulatory and Legal Gaps**: Many jurisdictions lack specific regulations addressing the creation and dissemination of deepfake content. The absence of clear legal frameworks contributes to challenges in enforcing consequences for malicious use.
- **Cultural and Social Impact**: The widespread use of deepfake technology has the potential to impact cultural norms and social trust. Society may become more sceptical of visual and auditory information, leading to a decline in trust.
- **Erosion of Authenticity**: The prevalence of deepfake content raises concerns about the erosion of authenticity in digital media. As deepfakes become more realistic, distinguishing between real and synthetic content becomes increasingly difficult.
- **Bias and Discrimination**: Deepfake algorithms can inherit and perpetuate biases present in the training data, leading to the creation of content that reflects or amplifies existing societal biases.
- **Limited Regulation of Synthetic Media**: The regulatory landscape regarding the creation and dissemination of synthetic media, including deepfakes, is still in its early stages. Limited regulation makes it challenging to address the ethical concerns associated with deepfake technology.
- **Crisis of Trust**: The proliferation of deepfakes contributes to a crisis of trust, affecting how individuals perceive information and media. This erosion of trust has broader implications for democratic processes, journalism, and public discourse.

Addressing these challenges requires a concerted effort from technology developers, researchers, policymakers, and the public. It involves ongoing research in detection technologies, the establishment of clear legal frameworks, and educational initiatives to promote media literacy and responsible use of synthetic media.

COUNTERMEASURES IN DEEPFAKE

Addressing the challenges posed by deepfake technology requires a multi-faceted approach involving technological solutions, policy frameworks, and public awareness initiatives. Here are some countermeasures against deepfakes:

- **Detection Technologies**:
  - Develop and enhance deepfake detection tools that utilize machine learning algorithms and AI to identify inconsistencies and anomalies in media content.
  - Promote collaboration between researchers, industry experts, and technology developers to continuously improve detection capabilities.
- **Media Authentication Standards**:
  - Establish standards and protocols for authenticating media content, making it easier to verify the origin and integrity of images, videos, and audio recordings.
  - Encourage the adoption of watermarking or cryptographic techniques to mark authentic media.
- **Blockchain Technology**:
  - Explore the use of blockchain technology to create decentralized and tamper-proof databases for storing and verifying authentic media content.
  - Implement blockchain-based solutions to enhance the traceability and transparency of digital media.
- **Education and Awareness**:
  - Increase public awareness about the existence and potential risks of deepfakes through educational campaigns.
  - Promote media literacy to help individuals critically evaluate the authenticity of content they encounter online.
- **Legal and Regulatory Framework**:
  - Develop and strengthen legal frameworks that address the creation and distribution of deepfake content, outlining consequences for malicious use.
  - Encourage international cooperation to harmonize legal approaches and enhance the effectiveness of cross-border enforcement.
- **Authentication and Verification Platforms**:
  - Establish platforms or services that allow users to verify the authenticity of media content, providing a reliable source for checking the legitimacy of images, videos, and audio recordings.
- **Ethical Guideline for AI Research**:
  - Promote the development and adoption of ethical guidelines within the AI research community.

- **Digital Forensics and Attribution**:
  - Invest in research and development of digital forensics tools that can analyse media content and provide insights into its authenticity.
  - Develop techniques for attributing deepfake content to specific creators or entities.
- **Multi-model Authentication**:
  - Combine different modalities, such as analysing facial features, voice patterns, and contextual information, to create more robust authentication systems.
  - Utilize multi-modal approaches to enhance the accuracy of deepfake detection.
- **Technological Collaboration**:
  - Encourage collaboration between tech companies, research institutions, and governmental agencies to share information and resources for combating deepfakes.
  - Facilitate the exchange of best practices and knowledge to stay ahead of evolving deepfake techniques.
- **Red Team Testing**:
  - Conduct red team testing to assess the vulnerability of organizations to deepfake attacks, identifying potential weaknesses and areas for improvement in security measures.
- **User Authentication for Content Creation**:
  - Implement user authentication mechanisms for content creation platforms to ensure that only authorized individuals can use advanced deepfake tools.
  - Integrate user identification and verification features into deepfake software to enhance accountability.

It's important to recognize that countering deepfakes requires a collaborative effort involving technology developers, policymakers, educators, and the general public. Continuous research, innovation, and adaptation of countermeasures are essential to stay ahead of the evolving landscape of synthetic media manipulation.

DETECTION TECHNOLOGIES

Detecting deepfake content is a challenging task due to the increasing sophistication of deepfake algorithms. Several detection technologies and approaches have been developed to identify synthetic media and distinguish it from authentic content. Here are some common deepfake detection methods:

- **Traditional Image and Video Forensics**:
  - **Description**: Traditional forensics techniques analyse image and video metadata, inconsistencies, or artifacts that may be indicative of manipulation.
  - **Strengths**: Can detect certain anomalies introduced during the deepfake generation process.

- **Limitations**: Less effective against more advanced deepfake algorithms that are designed to leave minimal artifacts.
- **Biometric Analysis**:
  - **Description**: Biometric analysis involves examining facial features, blinking patterns, and other biometric traits to identify anomalies or inconsistencies in facial expressions.
  - **Strengths**: Focuses on physiological features to detect subtle discrepancies in facial expressions.
  - **Limitations**: May not be effective against high-quality deepfakes that mimic biometric traits accurately.
- **Lip Sync Analysis**:
  - **Description**: Analyses the synchronization of lip movements with speech to identify discrepancies that may indicate a deepfake.
  - **Strengths**: Effective for detecting lip-syncing artifacts introduced during the manipulation process.
  - **Limitations**: Limited effectiveness against sophisticated lip-syncing algorithms.
- **Deepfake Detection Datasets**:
  - **Description**: Datasets containing known deepfake samples are used to train machine learning models for detection.
  - **Strengths**: Learning from diverse examples helps algorithms identify patterns associated with deepfakes.
  - **Limitations**: May struggle with new and evolving deepfake techniques that differ significantly from training data.
- **Face and Eye Movement Analysis**:
  - **Description**: Analysing the movement and coordination of facial features, including eye movements, to identify unnatural patterns.
  - **Strengths**: Focuses on the subtle details of facial expressions that may be challenging for deepfake algorithms to replicate accurately.
  - **Limitations**: May be susceptible to improvement in deepfake algorithms that mimic facial movements more realistically.
- **Behavioural Analysis**:
  - **Description**: Examining contextual and behavioural cues, such as inconsistencies in the context of the video or unnatural interactions between characters.
  - **Strengths**: Can identify anomalies that may be overlooked by purely technical approaches.
  - **Limitations**: May require additional context and may not be as reliable when applied in isolation.
- **Deep Learning and Neural Networks**:
  - **Description**: Developing deep learning models, including CNNs and RNNs, to identify patterns and anomalies associated with deepfake content.
  - **Strengths**: Can adapt to evolving deepfake techniques and learn complex patterns.

- **Limitations**: May require large and diverse datasets for effective training and may struggle with previously unseen techniques.
- **Consistency Across Modalities**:
  - **Description**: Analysing the consistency between facial expressions, body movements, and audio to identify discrepancies.
  - **Strengths**: Recognizes that deepfake detection should consider multiple modalities.
  - **Limitations**: Complexity increases when dealing with multi-modal content, and perfect synchronization can be challenging to achieve.
- **Temporal Analysis**:
  - **Description**: Analysing the temporal consistency of facial features and expressions over time to detect anomalies.
  - **Strengths**: Effective against deepfakes that struggle to maintain natural temporal coherence.
  - **Limitations**: May require access to a sequence of frames and may be computationally intensive.
- **Blockchain and Tamper-Proofing**:
  - **Description**: Utilizing blockchain technology to create a tamper-proof record of media content, ensuring its authenticity.
  - **Strengths**: Provides a secure and transparent way to verify the integrity of media.
  - **Limitations**: Requires widespread adoption to be effective, and may not prevent the creation of new deepfakes.

Effective deepfake detection often involves combining multiple techniques and approaches to create more robust and reliable systems. As deepfake technology evolves, ongoing research is essential to stay ahead of new manipulation methods and enhance detection capabilities.

ADVANCEMENT IN TECHNOLOGY

Deepfake technology has continued to advance, with researchers and developers exploring new techniques and methodologies. Keep in mind that the field is rapidly evolving, and there may have been further developments since then. Some key advancements in the technology of deepfake are as follows:

- **GAN Improvements**: GANs, a key component of deepfake technology, have seen advancements in their architectures and training strategies. Techniques like Progressive Growing GANs (PGGANs) have improved the generation of high-resolution and realistic content.
- **Deep Learning Architecture**: Researchers have explored novel deep learning architectures beyond GANs, such as Variational Auto-encoders (VAEs) and more advanced neural network structures. These architectures aim to enhance the realism and diversity of generated content.
- **Transfer Learning and Few-Shot Learning**: Transfer learning and few-shot learning techniques have been applied to deepfake models. This allows

models to leverage knowledge from one dataset and apply it to new, unseen individuals or scenarios, reducing the need for extensive training data.

- **Voice Cloning and Synthesis**: Advancements in voice cloning technologies have led to more natural-sounding synthetic voices. Neural network-based models for voice synthesis, such as Tacotron and WaveNet, have contributed to improvements in the quality of generated audio.
- **Deepfake Detection Techniques**: Researchers have developed and refined deepfake detection techniques using various approaches, including traditional image forensics, biometric analysis, and deep learning-based methods. The detection methods aim to keep pace with the evolving sophistication of deepfake generation.
- **Adversarial Training and Robustness**: Adversarial training techniques have been employed to enhance the robustness of deepfake models against detection methods. This involves training models against countermeasures to improve their ability to evade detection.
- **Fine-Tuning and Style Transfer**: Fine-tuning approaches and style transfer techniques have been applied to deepfake models, allowing for more precise control over the characteristics of generated content. This enables the adaptation of pre-trained models to specific tasks or styles.
- **Multi-modal Deepfakes**: Advancements in multi-modal deepfakes involve combining different modalities, such as synthesizing both visual and auditory content simultaneously. This results in more convincing and realistic synthetic media.
- **Open-Source Tools and Platforms**: The availability of open-source deepfake tools and platforms has increased, making it easier for individuals to create synthetic content. While this fosters innovation, it also raises concerns about the potential misuse of the technology.
- **Ethical Consideration and Awareness**: There has been a growing awareness of the ethical considerations surrounding deepfake technology. Researchers, industry professionals, and policymakers are actively discussing the responsible use of deepfakes and potential countermeasures.

It's important to note that the rapid development of deepfake technology raises ethical concerns related to misinformation, privacy, and potential misuse. Researchers and organizations are working to strike a balance between advancing the technology for legitimate purposes and addressing the associated risks and challenges. Ongoing research and collaboration in the field are crucial to staying ahead of potential threats and mitigating the negative impact of deepfakes.

ETHICAL FRAMEWORK AND GUIDELINES

As the use of deepfake technology raises ethical concerns, various organizations, researchers, and industry experts have developed ethical frameworks and guidelines to guide responsible development and deployment. These frameworks aim to address issues related to privacy, consent, transparency, and the potential misuse of synthetic media. Here are some key ethical considerations and the corresponding frameworks:

- **Consent and Permission**:
  - **Principle**: Ensure that individuals featured in deepfake content provide informed consent for the use of their likeness.
  - **Framework**: Emphasizes the importance of obtaining explicit consent from individuals before creating or sharing deepfake content.
- **Transparency**:
  - **Principle**: Maintain transparency about the creation and use of deepfake content to avoid deception and misinformation.
  - **Framework**: Encourages clear communication about the use of deepfake technology in media and entertainment.
- **Media Integrity**:
  - **Principle**: Preserve the integrity of media by avoiding the use of deepfakes for malicious purposes or to manipulate public perception.
  - **Framework**: Focuses on promoting the ethical creation and dissemination of synthetic media.
- **Diversity and Inclusion**:
  - **Principle**: Avoid perpetuating biases and stereotypes in deepfake content, promoting diversity and inclusivity.
  - **Framework**: Advocates for fair and unbiased representation in AI-generated media content, including deepfakes.
- **Human Rights**:
  - **Principle**: Uphold human rights and prevent the use of deepfake technology for malicious activities, such as harassment, defamation, or identity theft.
  - **Framework**: Focuses on protecting individuals from the harmful impact of deepfake misuse.
- **Education Use**:
  - **Principle**: Encourage responsible educational use of deepfake technology to raise awareness, promote media literacy, and foster understanding of its implications.
  - **Framework**: Promotes the ethical use of deepfake technology in educational settings.
- **Law and Regulation**:
  - **Principle**: Advocate for the development and enforcement of laws and regulations that address the ethical challenges associated with deepfake technology.
  - **Framework**: Calls for legal frameworks that address the responsible development and use of AI, including deepfake technology.
- **Security and Privacy**:
  - **Principle**: Safeguard the security and privacy of individuals by preventing unauthorized use of personal data in the creation of deepfake content.
  - **Framework**: Emphasizes the protection of privacy rights and the prevention of deepfake-related privacy violations.
- **Technological Responsibilities**:
  - **Principle**: Promote responsible development practices among technologists and researchers to ensure the ethical use of deepfake technology.

- **Framework**: Provides general ethical guidelines for the development and deployment of AI, including deepfake algorithms.
- **Public Awareness**:
  - **Principle**: Raise public awareness about the existence and potential impact of deepfake technology to foster a more informed and vigilant society.
  - **Framework**: Focuses on public outreach and education to mitigate the risks of deepfake-related misinformation.

These ethical frameworks and guidelines serve as a foundation for promoting responsible behaviour and ethical considerations in the development, deployment, and use of deepfake technology. It is essential for industry stakeholders, policymakers, and the public to engage in ongoing discussions and collaborations to address the evolving ethical challenges associated with synthetic media.

RECOMMENDATION FOR FUTURE WORK

Future research in the field of deepfake technology should focus on addressing existing challenges, improving detection methods, and developing ethical guidelines to guide responsible use. Here are some recommendations for future research:

- **Enhanced Detection Techniques**: Invest in research to develop more advanced and robust deepfake detection methods. This includes exploring multi-modal approaches that consider both visual and auditory cues for improved accuracy.
- **Explainability and Interpretability**: Explore research avenues to enhance the explainability and interpretability of deepfake detection models. Understanding how these models make decisions is crucial for building trust in their effectiveness.
- **Generative Models with Constraints**: Investigate the development of generative models that incorporate constraints to limit the creation of harmful or misleading content. This includes exploring ways to embed ethical considerations into the generation process.
- **Real-Time Detection System**: Research and develop real-time deepfake detection systems that can quickly identify and mitigate the impact of synthetic media as it emerges on online platforms.
- **Adversarial Training for Detection**: Explore adversarial training techniques for deepfake detection models to enhance their robustness against evolving deepfake generation methods.
- **Privacy-Preserving Solution**: Investigate privacy-preserving methods for detecting deepfakes without compromising the privacy of individuals. This involves finding ways to identify synthetic content while respecting consent and privacy rights.
- **Deepfake Attribution**: Research techniques for attributing deepfake content to specific creators or sources. This could involve developing methods to trace the origin of synthetic media, contributing to accountability and legal enforcement.

- **Education and Media Literacy**: Conduct research on the effectiveness of educational initiatives and media literacy programs in increasing public awareness about deepfakes. Evaluate the impact of these programs on people's ability to identify and critically assess synthetic media.
- **Bias Mitigation in Deepfake Algorithms**: Investigate approaches to mitigate biases in deepfake algorithms to ensure fair and unbiased representation, particularly concerning gender, race, and other sensitive attributes.
- **User Authentication and Authorization**: Research methods for implementing user authentication and authorization mechanisms within deepfake creation tools to prevent unauthorized use and misuse.
- **Cross-Disciplinary Collaboration**: Encourage cross-disciplinary collaboration between researchers in computer science, psychology, law, and ethics to address the multifaceted challenges of deepfake technology comprehensively.
- **International Collaboration and Standards**: Facilitate international collaboration in developing standards and guidelines for the ethical use of deepfake technology. Harmonize legal frameworks to address the global nature of synthetic media challenges.
- **Human–AI Collaboration**: Explore ways to incorporate human-in-the-loop approaches in the detection and evaluation of deepfake content, leveraging human judgment alongside AI.
- **Long-Term Societal Impacts**: Investigate the long-term societal impacts of deepfake technology, including its influence on public trust, media consumption habits, and democratic processes.
- **Open-Source Detection Tools**: Develop and maintain open-source deepfake detection tools to encourage collaboration and transparency in the research community.

By pursuing these research directions, the field can advance not only in terms of technological solutions but also in addressing the broader societal, ethical, and legal implications of deepfake technology. As the landscape continues to evolve, interdisciplinary collaboration and a proactive stance toward ethical considerations will be crucial for responsible innovation in synthetic media.

CONCLUSION

In conclusion, deepfake technology represents a powerful and evolving field with both positive and concerning implications. The ability to generate highly realistic synthetic media using AI algorithms has applications in various industries, including entertainment, filmmaking, education, and virtual influencers. However, the ethical and societal challenges associated with deepfakes cannot be overlooked. In navigating the future of deepfake technology, a balanced approach is needed that acknowledges its potential benefits while addressing the ethical and societal concerns. Continued research, technological advancements, public education, and responsible governance are essential to strike the right balance and mitigate the negative impact of deepfakes on trust, privacy, and information integrity. As the field evolves, ongoing vigilance and adaptability will be crucial to staying ahead of emerging challenges and ensuring the responsible use of synthetic media.

BIBLIOGRAPHY

Dutt, S., Chandramouli, S., & Das, A. K. *Machine Learning*. Pearson India Education Service Pvt. Ltd, ISBN 978-93-530-6669-7.

Grothaus, M. *Trust No One – inside the World of Deepfake*. Hodder & Stoughton (e-book), ISBN-9781529347999.

Iwasnka, L. M., & Shapiro, S. C. *Natural Language and Knowledge Presentation*. University Press.

Joshi, A., & Goyal, S. B. "Comparison of Various Round Robin Scheduling Algorithms," *2019 8th International Conference System Modeling and Advancement in Research Trends (SMART)*, Moradabad, India, 2019, pp. 18–21, doi: 10.1109/SMART46866. 2019.9117345

Joshi, A., & Tiwari, H. (2023). An overview of python libraries for data science, *Journal of Engineering Technology and Applied Physics*, 5(2), 85–90.

Kumar, R., Joshi, A., Sharan, H. O., Peng, S. L., & Dudhagara, C. R. (Eds.). (2024). *The Ethical Frontier of AI and Data Analysis*. IGI Global.

Littman, S. D. *Deepfake*. Scholastic Incorporated (e-book), ISBN 9781338178258.

Padhy, N. P. *Artificial Intelligence and Intelligence Systems*. Oxford University Press, ISBN 978-0-19-567154-4.

Russell, S. J., & Norvig, P. *Artificial Intelligence: A Modern Approach*. Prentice Hall, ISBN 9780136042594.

Singh, B. P., & Joshi, A. (2024). Ethical considerations in AI development. In R. Kumar, A. Joshi, H. Sharan, S. Peng, & C. Dudhagara (Eds.), *The Ethical Frontier of AI and Data Analysis* (pp. 156–179). IGI Global Scientific Publishing. https://doi.org/10.4018/979-8-3693-2964-1.ch010

Young, N. *DeepFake Technology-Complete Guide to DeepFakes, Politics and Social Media*. Amazon Digital Services, ISBN 9781078494694.

12 Overcoming Sentiment Analysis

A Solution to Challenges in Digital Era Health Care

Sourav Deb, Abhay Bhatia, and Khusboo Kumari

INTRODUCTION

Sentiment analysis or opinion mining is a subfield of natural language processing (NLP) that is involved in recognising and categorising sentiments in textual data into three groups: neutral, negative, and positive. Its uses are numerous and include consumer sentiment research for organisations, brand reputation management, and social media monitoring. Sentiment analysis employs advanced NLP methods to help businesses to glean insightful data gathered from multiple sources, including news articles, social media postings, product evaluations, and customer comments. This analytical tool is useful for determining public opinion on a variety of topics, from politics to product preferences, which helps to make well-informed decisions. Enterprises may utilise sentiment analysis to acquire a more profound understanding of customer attitudes, improve brand perception, and develop strategies that are specifically designed to tackle sentiment trends. This approach guarantees long-term competitiveness in an ever-changing market. Many people use a range of online channels to share their views and opinions. We must use user-generated data to automatically analyse public opinion so that it can be continuously monitored and used to inform decision-making. As social media sites have become more and more popular, a number of professions that concentrate on researching these networks and their material in order to extract pertinent data have evolved. Sentiment analysis is the method of determining the emotions expressed in a text by analysing its content (Singh & Joshi, 2024). Sentiment analysis is necessary for in-depth research in a number of real-world applications. Determine which characteristics or facets of a product, for example, appeal to customers in terms of its overall quality through product analysis.

TYPES OF SENTIMENT ANALYSIS

Sentiment analysis focuses on distinguishing certain emotions and sensations, such as joy, grief, or rage, as well as urgency and intent, such as interest vs. lack of it.

DOI: 10.1201/9781003516590-12

Determining a text's polarity— which can be positive, negative, or neutral—is the main goal of sentiment analysis. A few of the most popular types of sentiment analysis are as follows:

- **Graded Sentiment Analysis**: It refines sentiment classification by introducing additional polarity categories, such as "Extremely Satisfied" and "Extremely Unsatisfied," alongside standard ones like "Satisfied," "Neutral," and "Unsatisfied." This approach offers businesses deeper insights into customer sentiment, allowing for more informed decision-making. By capturing varying degrees of satisfaction with finer granularity, graded sentiment analysis enables a more accurate interpretation of customer feedback and opinions, enhancing the ability to address customer needs effectively.
- **Emotion Detection**: Sentiment analysis with emotion identification enables you to identify emotions other than polarity, such as happiness, irritation, fury, and mourning. Numerous emotion detection systems rely on lexicons, comprising lists of words and their associated emotions, or employ intricate machine learning algorithms (Joshi et al., 2024) for the task. There are certain disadvantages to using lexicons because different people express their emotions in different ways.
- **Aspect-Based Sentiment Analysis**: By detecting certain elements or qualities that are mentioned in a good, neutral, or negative way, aspect-based sentiment analysis is a crucial tool for analysing textual sentiments. This approach works wonders for gleaning subtle ideas from texts. An aspect-based classifier, for example, might recognise the negative sentiment explicitly aimed at the camera's battery life in a product review that said, "This camera's battery life is too short." With this fine-grained method, companies may better understand client feedback and identify strengths or places for development in their goods or services without running the risk of plagiarism.
- **Multilingual Sentiment Analysis**: To perform analysis on Multilingual data is very difficult. The problems of multilingual sentiment analysis are distinct, frequently necessitating substantial pre-processing and access to a variety of resources. It could be necessary to create certain resources, such as translated corpora or noise detection methods (Joshi et al., 2025) while others, like sentiment lexicons, are easily accessible online. To properly utilise these resources, coding proficiency is required. Alternatively, the procedure may be streamlined by automating language recognition using a language classifier, after which a customised sentiment analysis model is trained to categorise texts in the appropriate language. This method ensures precise and pertinent findings by providing flexibility and control while analysing feelings in various language circumstances.

LEVELS OF SENTIMENT ANALYSIS

Research on sentiment analysis has been done at many different levels, such as the document, sentence, phrase, and aspect levels. Figure 12.1 shows sentiment analysis at each level.

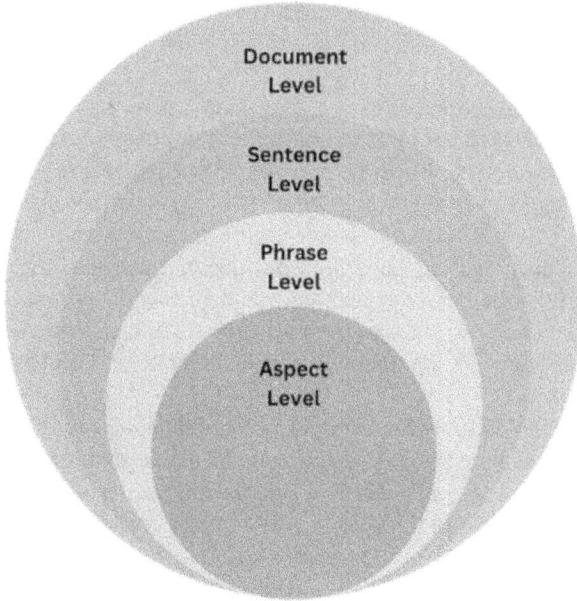

FIGURE 12.1 Levels of sentiment analysis.

- **Document Level**: Document-level sentiment analysis uses an all-inclusive scale to assess sentiment throughout a document and give the content as a whole a single polarity. Compared to more detailed studies, this method is less frequently used, although it has some uses, such as categorising book pages or chapters as positive, negative, or neutral elements. Document-level sentiment analysis is still a useful technique in some situations, even if it is used rather infrequently. It provides information on the general sentiment expressed in large amounts of text. At this stage, supervised and unsupervised learning approaches are both useful in helping to classify texts using different computational strategies (Bhatia et al., 2015). Document-level sentiment analysis adds to a comprehensive grasp of textual sentiment by using predetermined criteria or drawing patterns on its own. The two basic problems with document-level sentiment analysis are cross-domain and cross-language sentiment analysis (Saunders, 2021).
- **Sentence Level**: Sentences are analysed at the sentence level in sentiment analysis, and the outcomes are shown with the appropriate orientation. This is especially helpful when a paper contains a variety of emotions connected to it (Yang & Cardie, 2014). The polarity of each sentence will be evaluated individually using the same methods, nevertheless, with more processing power and training data capacity than at the document level. The overall sentiment of the paper can be ascertained by combining or using the polarity of each sentence separately. Sometimes, document-level sentiment analysis is not enough for a given purpose (Behdenna et al., 2018). Previous sentence-level analytic approaches have focused on discovering subjective

sentences. However, more difficult tasks involve handling conditional statements or ambiguous claims (Ferrari & Esuli, 2019).

- **Phrase Level**: It is the process of categorising and analysing words that express opinions. Each sentence may have one component or multiple components, which could be useful for reviews of products with multiple lines because, in this instance, only one element is expressed in a single phrase. Phrase-level analysis is more advantageous than the earlier two, which focused on classifying everything in a document as subjective, because a document contains both positive and negative statements. The subjectivity of the phrase or text that contains a word appears is intimately related to its polarity, the basic unit of analysis in language. A remark that contains an adjective is probably a subjective sentence (Fredriksen-Goldsen & Kim, 2017).
- **Aspect Level**: Given the possibility of multiple aspects in a statement, aspect-level sentiment analysis is required. Upon assigning polarity and major importance to each sentence constituent, the overall sentiment of the statement is ascertained. Following the primary consideration and polarity assignment of each part in the phrase, the statement's overall sentiment is evaluated (Schouten & Frasincar, 2015; Lu et al., 2011).

LITERATURE REVIEW

PROCEDURE OF SENTIMENT ANALYSIS

Figure 12.2 shown illustrates the working of sentiment analysis.

DATA SELECTION

In the Data Selection step, we collect data from various sources. The major source of data collection is the internet. Online data may be gathered through internet-based news sources, e-commerce websites, internet scraping, discussion boards, and blog sites. The very first phase in the sentiment analysis process is data compilation. Based on the task and sentiment analysis of the outcomes, text data can be combined with other types of data, like videos, audio recordings, location, etc. A few crucial places to get data are:

- **Social media**: Social data is information that is gathered via social media platforms. It is an example of how users can access, post, and share material on the product. Academic studies on behavioural behaviour in groups, individuals, and environments utilise the internet as an information source that is always evolving. It describes web-based or mobile applications that let users access, produce, and distribute user-generated content online.
- **Weblog**: A brief weblog comprises paragraphs that include information, links, personal journal entries, or a point of view. Collectively referred to as postings, they are arranged in a research article-style chronological order, with the most recent item appearing first.

TABLE 12.1
Literature Review

Reference number	Author	Year	Key findings
9	Jesus Serrano-Guerrero et al.	2014	• Comparative Analysis: The paper compares free-access web services for sentiment analysis, assessing their effectiveness in classifying and scoring text based on sentiments. • Experimentation: Researchers conduct experiments using three renowned text collections to evaluate the tools' abilities in discerning emotions conveyed in different types of text. • Evaluation of Tool Capabilities: Through experimentation and data analysis, the study reveals the strengths and weaknesses of each sentiment analysis tool, offering insights into their proficiency in handling diverse textual data and emotions.
10	Doaa Mohey El-Din Mohamed Hussein	2015	• Sentiment Analysis Challenges: The abstract pinpoints obstacles in accurately interpreting sentiments and determining polarity. • Hurdles to Meaningful Insights: It underscores how these challenges impede extracting meaningful insights from writer-generated content. • Call for Solutions: Despite obstacles, leveraging techniques like natural language processing is advocated to enhance accuracy in sentiment analysis.
11	Qurat Tul Ain et al.	2017	• Web Data Abundance: Sentiment analysis is crucial for grasping diverse user opinions amidst the vast unstructured data on the web. • Labelled Data Scarcity: The challenge of limited labelled data in NLP fuels the integration of deep learning methods for more effective sentiment analysis. • Deep Learning Applications: Deep learning models, such as neural networks, are increasingly utilised to tackle various sentiment analysis tasks, including classification, cross-lingual issues, and product reviews.
12	Omar Alqaryouti et al.	2020	• The paper introduces a hybrid approach for sentiment analysis of smart application reviews, benefiting government entities seeking customer insights. • Integration of domain lexicons and rules notably enhances aspect extraction accuracy, surpassing traditional methods by 5%. • The proposed model outperforms SVM (Support Vector Machine)-based approaches, demonstrating the efficacy of incorporating lexicons and rules for improved sentiment analysis.

(Continued)

TABLE 12.1 (Continued)

Reference number	Author	Year	Key findings
13	Pooja Mehta et al.	2020	• The paper explores sentiment analysis, a method to extract opinions and emotions from text, especially in online platforms. • It evaluates the effectiveness of different machine learning and lexicon analysis techniques in sentiment analysis. • The study aims to contribute to understanding sentiment analysis advancements and methodologies for future research.
14	Mayur Wankhade et al.	2022	• Internet Impact: Internet growth, especially through social media and blogs, has surged opinions on various topics. • Sentiment Analysis Significance: It's vital for gathering and analysing opinions across topics, aiding decisions for corporations, governments, and individuals. • Challenges and Solutions: Challenges in sentiment analysis, including interpreting sentiments accurately, are noted. Solutions include using natural language processing and exploring future improvements.
15	Praveen Verma et al.	2023	• Sentiment analysis offers insight into human-like sentiments expressed in diverse domains. • The paper compares sentiment analysis techniques to classify restaurant reviews accurately. • Automating sentiment analysis aids restaurant owners in decision-making based on customer feedback.
16	Anil Kumar et al.	2023	• The paper highlights the significance of sentiment analysis in understanding public opinions on social media, particularly Twitter. • Utilising a Naive Bayes algorithm, the study aims to extract human semantics from Twitter data, focusing on sentiment analysis. • Machine learning techniques are applied to achieve precise sentiment classification in Twitter posts, ensuring accurate analysis of public sentiment.
17	Manish Kumar et al.	2023	• Machine learning involves statistical models and algorithms enabling computers to perform tasks without explicit programming, widely utilised in applications like internet search engines. • It focuses on optimising performance criteria based on prior knowledge or sample data, improving parameters through training data or prior information. • Applications include website ranking, data collection, pre-processing, visualisation, and prediction, showcasing the versatility of machine learning across various domains.

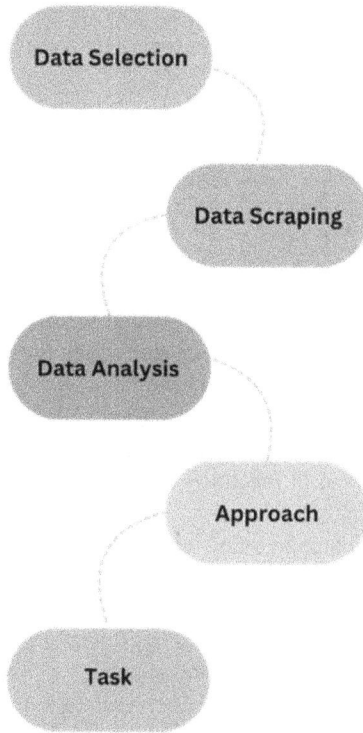

FIGURE 12.2 Procedure of sentiment analysis.

- **E-Commerce Website**: On an e-commerce website, customers can leave ratings and comments on a particular business or organisation. In this instance, a descriptive study was conducted on online stores that show product reviews or expert review websites with millions of reviews that are not review-specific websites.

DATA SCRAPING

It is also known as Feature Selection. It's important to remember that the first stage in developing a classification model is identifying relevant features in the dataset. As a result, during model training, a review may be translated into English and added to the feature vector. The term "Uni-gram" refers to a technique that considers a single word; "Bi-gram" refers to a technique that considers two words; and "Tri-gram" refers to a technique that considers three words. (Razon A et al., 2015). Characteristics that prioritise the use of language above a methodological basis are called pragmatic. It is the study of how perception and context are associated in linguistics and related disciplines. Investigating phenomena like as implicature, speech acts, relevance, and dialogues are all part of the study of pragmatics. Punctuation is employed, like exclamation marks, to draw attention to a statement's strength, whether it be positive or negative. Two other punctuation signs are the question mark and the apostrophe.

Sentiment analysis uses emojis, which are face expressions, to represent emotions. A vast range of human emotions is represented by various emoticons. Emoticons help to convey a writer's attitude or voice in a sentence, which makes sentiment analysis easier.

Expressions like lol and rofl. These are commonly employed to heighten the humour in a statement. It makes it acceptable to assume that an informal phrase in the text supports sentiment analysis, considering how opinion tweets are written.

DATA ANALYSIS

It is also known as Feature Extraction when we attempt to glean important information from the textual data. A crucial step in sentiment classification is feature extraction (Kumar R et al., 2024), which entails taking important information out of the text input and instantly impacts the model's functionality. The process involves extracting relevant information that encapsulates the main concepts in the text. Other characteristics were included in the study (Venugopalan M et al., 2015) because it could be challenging to extract features from text. After being lowered during the pre-processing stage, punctuations are frequently removed from text, but they can also be used to extract features.

- **Terms Frequency**: It's among the simplest ways to convey characteristics that are becoming more and more popular for information retrieval in many different NLP applications, like sentiment analysis. A single word (a unigram) or a group of two or three words (a bi-gram or a tri-gram) is considered, with the terms count denoting attributes. The existence of the word indicates a value of either 0 or 1. The number that indicates how frequently a phrase occurs in the provided content is called term frequency. To achieve better outcomes, the weighted TF-IDF (Term Frequency–Inverse Document Frequency) approach can be employed to assess the significance of each token.
- **Parts of Speech Tagging**: It is the technique of identifying a word in a text based on its definition and context is also known as grammatical tagging. The many types of tokens include nouns, verbs, determiners, adjectives, adverbs, and prepositions. For example, the phrase "What a beautiful weather it is" may have the following tags: what: Pronoun, a: Determiner, beautiful: Adjective, weather: Noun, it: Pronoun, is: Verb (Straka M et al., 2016). An adjective is more frequently employed in sentiment mining since it better captures the emotion of an opinion (Weerasooriya T et al., 2016). One of the easiest methods for extracting text characteristics is Bag of Words (BoW) (Qader et al., 2019). BoW will explain where words appear in a document. Each phrase's vector is constructed by using a word vocabulary represented by a bag. This paradigm's main flaw is that it disregards the grammatical meaning of the text. The BoW technique performs better in most circumstances when its performance is assessed using TF-IDF.

FEATURE SELECTION APPROACH

By assessing the feature selection methodology, a data feature is found. A trait could be unnecessary, important, or insignificant. Superfluous and redundant features are removed using a variety of feature selection techniques. The process of "feature selection" finds and removes unnecessary and irrelevant properties from the feature list (Joshi A, Tiwari H, 2023), improving the accuracy of sentiment categorisation. Lexicon-based and statistical approaches are used in sentiment analysis for feature selection in the work of Hailong and Wenyan (2014) and Duric et al. (2012). Features in lexicon-based methods are created by humans. To create a small feature set, the process usually starts with gathering words that evoke powerful emotions. These methods have the advantage of being effective since they take particular attention to each component. Selecting handmade characteristics is an involved and time-consuming procedure. Four general categories are used to group statistical strategies for feature selection, which are described in brief below:

- **Filter methodology** is a selection process that is most frequently employed. Without utilising any machine learning techniques, it picks the features by considering the general characteristics of the training set. A number of statistical criteria are used to grade the feature, and the characteristics with the best scores are then selected. They work effectively with datasets that have a large number of attributes and are inexpensive to compute. The terms "document frequency," "chi-square," "information gain," and "mutual information" are all used to describe basic filter methods.
- **Wrapper methodology** is a technique that is based on algorithms for machine learning and relies on the results of those algorithms (Joshi & Goyal, 2019). Due to this reliance, methods can find the best feature set for that particular modelling process, but they are often computationally expensive and iterative. Feature subsets created by forward or backward selection combined with different learning algorithms e.g., NB (Naive Bayes) &SVM are examples of wrapper techniques.
- **Embedded Approach** is an approach that integrates the process of feature selection with the modelling algorithm's execution. It makes use of feature selection integrated with categorisation techniques. As a result, it uses less computing power than the wrapper method. This method is algorithm-specific, though. Numerous decision tree algorithms, including LASSO (Least Absolute Shrinkage and Selection Operator)and CART (Classification and Regression Tree), as well as other methods (Hssina et al., 2014), are commonly the foundation of embedded approaches.
- **Hybrid methodology** is a tactic that blends filter and wrapper techniques; hybrid methods typically combine many techniques to provide the best feature subset. Hybrid strategies usually employ many ways to attain high performance and accuracy. There are now various hybrid feature selection algorithms available (Chiew et al., 2019).

TASK

It includes a variety of critical actions necessary for a thorough study and interpretation of textual material. Completing these assignments will help you comprehend and classify the feelings that are represented in the text without having to worry about plagiarism. Among them are:

SUBJECTIVITY CLASSIFICATION

This fundamental stage entails locating subjective signals, sentimental language, and subjective concepts in text. Subjectivity categorisation uses words and phrases that are suggestive of subjectivity, including "hard," "amazing," and "cheap," to differentiate between text components that are objective and subjective. To ensure an unbiased analysis, the purpose is to separate out objective data for additional processing.

- **Sentiment Classification**: Sentiment analysis has extensively studied the task of sentiment classification, which seeks to ascertain the sentiment expressed in every text passage. It entails classifying text based on predefined categories of sentiment, such as positive, negative, or neutral. Determining the polarity—positive or negative—is an important step. While there are systems that incorporate a neutral category, machine learning techniques are frequently used to effectively predict sentiment across different languages and areas.
- **Implicit Language Detection**: Implicit language detection focuses on recognising complex forms of language, such as sarcasm, irony, and comedy, which can considerably affect sentiment analysis. It can be difficult to identify implicit language as it frequently comprises unclear speech that might change the polarity and meaning of a statement. The use of punctuation, emoticons, and laughing emotions is an example of traditional methods for effectively identifying implicit language cues.
- **Aspect-Based Sentiment Analysis**: It relies heavily on aspect extraction, which is the process of locating particular aspects or characteristics that are stated in text. Aspect-based sentiment analysis differs from typical sentiment analysis in that it concentrates on specific textual parts.
- **Working of Sentiment Analysis**

The training and prediction phases are fundamental components of sentiment analysis, as shown in Figure 12.3, involving the preparation of models and the utilisation of those models to analyse text data. Below is a breakdown of each stage:

- **Training Phase and Prediction Phase**: In this phase, machine learning models are prepared using labelled training data. This data consists of text samples along with their corresponding sentiment labels. Pre-processing of the training data usually involves tokenisation (splitting the text into individual words or tokens), elimination of stop words (words that occur frequently, such as "and" and "the"), and maybe lemmatisation, or stemming (words reduced to their most fundamental form). To create

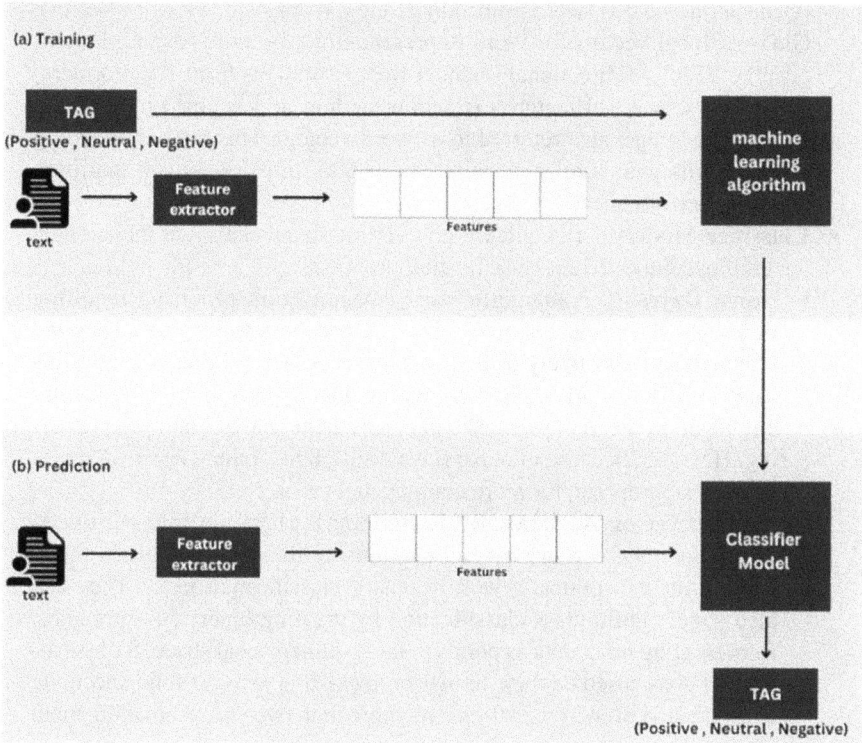

(a) Training

TAG
(Positive , Neutral , Negative)

text

Feature extractor

Features

machine learning algorithm

(b) Prediction

text

Feature extractor

Features

Classifier Model

TAG

(Positive , Neutral , Negative)

FIGURE 12.3 Training and prediction phase.

numerical or vector representations of the pre-processed text input that machine learning algorithms can comprehend. Once the model is trained and validated, it is ready for deployment to predict sentiments in unseen or new text data. The same preparation procedures (such as stop word removal and tokenisation) used in the training phase are applied to the fresh text data during the prediction phase. The same feature extraction methods that were employed during training are then applied to convert the pre-processed text input into numerical or vector representations. Subsequently, the trained machine learning model receives the translated text data, which predicts the sentiment label (positive, negative, or neutral). In order to understand the sentiment indicated in the text data, the predicted sentiment labels may finally be examined and evaluated. This makes a wide range of applications possible, including sentiment analysis of social media postings, product reviews, customer feedback, and more.

* **Feature Extraction**: Feature extraction is performed to transform the previously processed text input into vector or numerical representations that machine learning algorithms can comprehend. Machine learning text classification techniques will replace the traditional method of extracting text using a bag-of-words or bag-of-n-grams based on their frequency

(Qader et al., 2019), word embeddings e.g., Word2Vec (Word to Vector), GloVe (Global Vectors for Word Representation), or more advanced methods like BERT (Bidirectional Encoder Representations from Transformers) embeddings. A novel feature extraction method is developed by utilising word embeddings, also referred to as word vectors. This kind of encoding allows words with similar meanings to display similarly, which improves classifier performance.

- **Classifier Models**: Let's quickly go over the many statistical models that are employed in different classification processes:
  - **Naive Bayes**: For straightforward categorisation problems requiring little data and resources, naive Bayes algorithms work great. They are effective and less likely to overfit since they have strong bias and low variation. They work well with ongoing data updates and are frequently employed in text analysis tasks like sentiment analysis and spam filtering. However, because of naive Bayes' simplicity, other classifiers might be more appropriate for more complicated tasks.
  - **Support Vector Machines**: By determining the best hyperplane to divide data points into two groups and maximising the margin between them, it performs exceptionally well in binary classification tasks. They can also handle multi-class classification by creating binary sub-problems. Representing input data as points in multi-dimensional space, SVMs categorise texts based on their similarity to existing texts, enabling accurate classification even in scenarios with more than two classes, making them perfect for applications such as sentiment analysis.
  - **Logistic Regression**: It is a statistical method used for binary classification tasks, where the output is a probability score indicating the possibility of an observation falling into a specific class.
  - **Linear Regression**: This statistical technique models the relationship between a dependent variable and one or more independent variables by fitting a linear equation to observed data.

APPLICATION OF SENTIMENT ANALYSIS

Sentiment analysis, with its versatility and applicability, has become a cornerstone in various industries, offering insights and solutions to diverse business challenges. Across finance, retail, hospitality, technology, and beyond, sentiment analysis finds numerous applications, contributing to informed decision-making and enhanced customer experiences. Listed below are some of the most prevalent and impactful ways of application of sentiment analysis:

- **Finance**: In the world of finance, sentiment analysis has various advantages. It spreads over many parts of the sector with its diverse uses. Sentiment analysis is essential in the financial sector for interpreting investor sentiment, consumer confidence, and market sentiment. Financial organisations obtain crucial insights into prevalent market emotions by methodically analysing feelings presented through a variety of sources. Their profound comprehension empowers them to predict market patterns, evaluate investment hazards, and optimise trading tactics for maximum benefits. Furthermore, sentiment analysis is a powerful tool in the fight against fraud, as it makes it possible to spot unusual sentiments that can point to fraud as well as suspicious trends in financial transactions. Financial institutions may effectively reduce risks, streamline decision-making procedures, and maintain the integrity of the financial markets by utilising sentiment analysis in these roles.

- **Healthcare**: In the healthcare industry, sentiment analysis assists healthcare providers in understanding patient feedback, improving patient experiences, and enhancing healthcare outcomes. By analysing patient reviews, social media discussions, and healthcare surveys, healthcare organisations can identify areas for service improvement, address patient concerns, and personalise patient care. Sentiment analysis also enables healthcare providers to track patient sentiment towards treatments, medications, and healthcare providers, facilitating evidence-based decision-making and patient-centric care delivery. Jiménez-Zafra et al. (2019) brought to light the difficulties in applying sentiment analysis in the healthcare sector because of the specific and specialised language used in this domain. Twitter messages regarding the experiences of patients were incorporated into the public health analysis by Clark et al. (2018) using Twitter's Streaming API about 5 million tweets concerning breast cancer were produced over the course of a year. The tweets were classified using a CNN model and a standard LR (Logistic Regression) classifier after pre-processing. Raising public awareness, rallying support, and enjoying successful treatment outcomes were all connected. In a nutshell, sentiment analysis may be used to analyse social media content created by patients to gain a deeper understanding of their needs and perspectives.

- **Hospitality**: In the hospitality industry, sentiment analysis helps hotels, restaurants, and travel agencies monitor customer satisfaction and enhance guest experiences. Through the examination of social media mentions, online reviews, and customer feedback surveys, hospitality companies can pinpoint areas in need of development, immediately resolve guest complaints, and tailor services to suit individual tastes. Sentiment analysis also enables hospitality businesses to track sentiment trends, identify emerging travel preferences, and adapt their offerings accordingly. According to sentiment research, this is one of the most enticing industries. Hotels can make improvements by identifying the aspects that garner the most positive and negative comments by using sentiment analysis of reviews for their establishments. Because they might select the component that receives the greatest criticism should be improved, the service operators stand to benefit the most.

- **Stock Market**: One effective technique for predicting stock prices is sentiment analysis because it combines a thorough investigation of numerous news sources relevant to the stock market with the tracking of stock price variations. This multimodal technique comprises obtaining data from multiple avenues, including news articles, blogs, social media platforms like Twitter, and even financial information. Investors can obtain important insights into investor mood, market sentiment, and public opinion regarding individual companies or the overall market trends by utilising sentiment analysis methodologies. These messages may be subjected to sentence-level sentiment analysis, which would allow for the determination of the general polarity of the texts containing news about a certain company (Xing et al., 2018), used to ascertain if the trend will be increasing or declining. Negative news typically resulted in a downward trend, whereas positive news typically caused an upward trend. Digital currency like Bitcoin and others are connected to a cutting-edge technology called Blockchain.

- **Voice of Customer**: Sentiment analysis helps businesses capture the Voice of the Customer (VoC) by collecting and analysing user input from various sources like chats, emails, surveys, and the internet. This analysis reveals patterns, recurring issues, and emerging concerns, aiding in crafting a compelling value proposition and targeting the right consumer base. By staying abreast of consumer sentiments, businesses can remain agile, adapt to changing market demands, and sustain product relevance. Integrating sentiment analysis enables organisations to listen attentively to customer feedback, drive innovation, and foster customer-centric strategies for long-term success.

CHALLENGES OF SENTIMENT ANALYSIS

Sentiment analysis presents several challenges, such as the frequency of non-standard writing styles, language variances, and high computational costs. We examine the more common sentiment analysis problems for specific kinds of sentiment frameworks. One of the most difficult problems in NLP is sentiment analysis, since even humans have trouble accurately interpreting sentiments.

Furthermore, unstructured sentiment has a lot of challenges. It describes writing that is informal, unimpeded, and unrestricted by restrictions. This type of text often contains multiple sentences, each potentially expressing both positive and negative aspects. Unstructured reviews tend to give greater insight into opinions than formal ones (Levashina et al., 2014). Features mentioned explicitly in a review segment are termed explicit features, while those implied but not explicitly stated are called implicit features. This study explores the relationship between the structure of respondents' perspectives and issues in sentiment analysis, recognising the critical nature of sentiment analysis in understanding textual sentiment accurately. Let's examine a few of the primary difficulties with machine-based sentiment assessment in more detail:

- **Tone and Subjectivity**: Texts can be broadly categorised into subjective and objective categories. Objective texts typically convey factual information without expressing explicit sentiments, whereas subjective texts reflect personal opinions, emotions, or perspectives. Let's take an example where you want to evaluate the tone of these two texts:

"This movie is amazing!"

"This movie is 90 minutes long."

In the first example, the statement "This movie is amazing!" conveys a subjective opinion, expressing positive sentiment towards the movie. On the other hand, the second example, "This movie is 90 minutes long," provides an objective fact about the movie's duration without expressing any sentiment.

- **Sarcasm and Irony**: Humans often use positive language to convey negative feelings when using irony and sarcasm, which makes it challenging for robots to understand without a complete comprehension of the event's context.

  Let's consider a real-life scenario where someone asks their friend, *"How was your meeting?"* and gets the following responses:

  Friend A: *"Oh, it was amazing. Just what I needed on a Friday afternoon."*
  Friend B: *"Absolutely fantastic. Best meeting ever."*

  In Friend A's response, the phrase *"Oh, it was amazing"* could be taken at face value as a positive remark. However, the added comment *"Just what I needed on a Friday afternoon"* introduces a hint of sarcasm, implying that the meeting was actually inconvenient and unwelcome at that time.

  In Friend B's response, the phrase *"Absolutely fantastic. Best meeting ever"* sounds overtly positive, but the exaggerated enthusiasm can be a clear indication of sarcasm, suggesting the meeting was far from enjoyable.

- **Context and Polarity**: All claims are made at some point, by some person, in some location, and have a context when it is spoken. Sentiment analysis becomes quite difficult in an empty environment. However, robots cannot learn about a context if it is not explicitly given. One of the problems caused by context is polarity shifting. Take a look at the following example:

  Imagine you're asking friends for their opinions about a new restaurant they recently visited.

  (i) If you ask, *"What did you like about the restaurant?"* Friend A responds, *"Everything about it."* Friend B responds, *"Absolutely nothing!"*

     In this context, Friend A's response is likely positive, indicating that they enjoyed everything about the restaurant. Conversely, Friend B's response is negative, suggesting that they didn't like anything about it.

     Now, let's change the context:

  (ii) If you ask, *"What did you dislike about the restaurant?"* Friend A responds, *"Everything about it."*

     Friend B responds, *"Absolutely nothing!"*

In this scenario, the sentiment of the responses shifts due to the change in context. Friend A's response, *"Everything about it,"* now indicates dissatisfaction, while Friend B's response, "Absolutely nothing!" implies satisfaction, as they couldn't find anything to dislike.

This example shows how different attitudes can be expressed with the same words depending on the situation in which they are delivered. Since context affects how language and emotions are interpreted, it is crucial to comprehend it in order to perform effective sentiment analysis.

These examples illustrate how sentiment analysis can be challenging due to the nuanced meanings of words and the importance of context in understanding the true sentiment behind a statement.

CONCLUSION

In Conclusion, sentiment analysis, a fundamental component of NLP, offers priceless insights into how people feel about digital content. Understanding customer behaviour and public opinion on diverse digital channels, such as social media and online reviews, is crucial. Sentiment analysis helps individuals, governments, and corporations make strategic decisions and helps them negotiate the challenges of the digital age. This paper has explored the numerous aspects of sentiment analysis, such as aspect-based sentiment analysis, emotion detection, and graded sentiment analysis, which have been examined in this work, along with the intricate details of feature extraction and data selection. Moreover, it has highlighted the diverse applications of it in domains such as finance, healthcare, and hospitality, underscoring its versatility and relevance. Sentiment analysis is widely used; however, it still has limitations due to context sensitivity, tone ambiguity, and emoji interpretation. To address these problems, more investigation and creativity are required to enhance sentiment analysis effectiveness. In the end, sentiment analysis is crucial for understanding human emotions and behaviours, which helps with decision-making and promotes better knowledge in a variety of fields. Research and development activities must continue as we navigate the digital terrain in order to properly use sentiment analysis's potential, which will increase our world's empathy, connectedness, and insights.

BIBLIOGRAPHY

Ain QT, Ali M, Riaz A, Noureen A, Kamran M, Hayat B, Rehman A. (2017). Sentiment analysis using deep learning techniques: A review *Int J Adv Comput Sci Appl (IJACSA)*, 8(6). http://doi.org/10.14569/IJACSA.2017.080657

Alqaryouti O, Siyam N, Abdel Monem A, Shaalan K (2024). Aspect-based sentiment analysis using smart government review data, *Appl Comput Inform* 20(1/2): 142–161. https://doi.org/10.1016/j.aci.2019.11.003

Behdenna S, Barigou F, Belalem G (2018) Document level sentiment analysis: A survey. *EAI Endorsed Trans Context-aware Syst Appl* 4(13): e2.

Bhatia P, Ji Y, Eisenstein J (2015) Better document-level sentiment analysis from RST discourse parsing. arXiv preprint arXiv:150901599.

Chiew KL, Tan CL, Wong K, Yong KS, Tiong WK (2019) A new hybrid ensemble feature selection framework for machine learning-based phishing detection system. *Inf Sci* 484:153–166.

Clark EM, James T, Jones CA, Alapati A, Ukandu P, Danforth CM, Dodds PS (2018) A sentiment analysis of breast cancer treatment experiences and healthcare perceptions across twitter. arXiv preprint arXiv:180509959.

Duric A, Song F (2012) Feature selection for sentiment analysis based on content and syntax models. *Decis Support Syst* 53(4):704–711.

El-Din Mohamed Hussein DM (2018). A survey on sentiment analysis challenges. *J King Saud Univ - Eng Sci*, 30(4), 330–338. https://doi.org/10.1016/j.jksues.2016.04.002

Ferrari A, Esuli A (2019) An NLP approach for cross-domain ambiguity detection in requirements engineering. *Autom Softw Eng* 26(3):559–598.

Fredriksen-Goldsen KI, Kim HJ (2017) The science of conducting research with LGBT older adults-an introduction to aging with pride: National health, aging, and sexuality/gender study (NHAS).

Hailong Z, Wenyan G, Bo J. (2014) Machine learning and lexicon based methods for sentiment classification: a survey. In: *2014 11th web information system and application conference*. IEEE, pp 262–265.

Hssina B, Merbouha A, Ezzikouri H, Erritali M (2014) A comparative study of decision tree id3 and c4. 5. *Int J Adv Comput Sci Appl* 4(2):13–19.

Jiménez-Zafra SM, Martín-Valdivia MT, Molina-González MD, Ureña-López LA (2019) How do we talk about doctors and drugs? sentiment analysis in forums expressing opinions for medical domain. *Artif Intell Med* 93:50–57.

Joshi A, Goyal SB "Comparison of Various Round Robin Scheduling Algorithms," *2019 8th International Conference System Modeling and Advancement in Research Trends (SMART)*, Moradabad, India, 2019, pp. 18–21, doi: 10.1109/SMART46866.2019.9117345

Joshi A, Kumar V, Chauhan N, Kumar A, Singh RK (2024). The intersection of AI, ML, and industry: A review of emerging trends in real-world applications. In *2024 4th International Conference on Advancement in Electronics & Communication Engineering (AECE)* (pp. 769–773). IEEE. https://doi.org/10.1109/AECE62803.2024.10911386

Joshi A, Kumar V, Thakur G, Chauhan N, & Singh RK (2025). A primer for governance. In R Kumar, A Abdul Hamid, N Ya'akub, T Nyamasvisva, & R Tiwari (Eds.), *Leveraging Futuristic Machine Learning and Next-Generational Security for e-Governance* (pp. 45–86). IGI Global Scientific Publishing. https://doi.org/10.4018/979-8-3693-7883-0.ch003

Joshi A, Tiwari H (2023). An overview of python libraries for data science, *Journal of Engineering Technology and Applied Physics*, 5(2):85–90.

Kumar A, Akgec G, Gupta T, Bhatia A, Raj R (2023). Twitter data sentiment analysis forstock market prediction using machine learning. *Int J Eng Sci Technol* 2023: 86–90.

Kumar M, Ali Khan S, Bhatia A, Sharma V, Jain P "A Conceptual introduction of Machine Learning Algorithms," *2023 1st International Conference on Intelligent Computing and Research Trends (ICRT), Roorkee*, India, 2023, pp. 1–7, doi: 10.1109/ICRT57042.2023.10146676

Kumar R, Joshi A, Sharan HO, Peng SL, Dudhagara CR (Eds.). (2024). *The Ethical Frontier of AI and Data Analysis*. IGI Global.

Levashina J, Hartwell CJ, Morgeson FP, Campion MA (2014) The structured employment interview: narrative and quantitative review of the research literature. *Pers Psychol* 67(1):241–293.

Lu B, Ott M, Cardie C, Tsou BK (2011) Multi-aspect sentiment analysis with topic models. In: *2011 IEEE 11th international conference on data mining workshops*. IEEE, pp 81–88.

Pandya S, Mehta P (2020). *A Review on Sentiment Analysis Methodologies*, Practices and Applications.

Qader W, Ameen M, Musa, & Ahmed B. (2019). An overview of bag of words; importance, *Implement Appl Challeng.* 200–204. 10.1109/IEC47844.2019.8950616

Razon A, Barnden J (2015) A new approach to automated text readability classification based on concept indexing with integrated part-of-speech n-gram features. In: *Proceedings of the international conference recent advances in natural language processing,* pp. 521–528.

Saunders D (2021) Domain adaptation for neural machine translation. PhD thesis, University of Cambridge.

Schouten K, Frasincar F (2015) Survey on aspect-level sentiment analysis. *IEEE Trans Knowl Data Eng* 28(3):813–830.

Serrano-Guerrero J, Olivas JA, Romero FP, Herrera-Viedma E (2015). Sentiment analysis: A review and comparative analysis of web services. *Inform Sci,* 311:18–38. https://doi. org/10.1016/j.ins.2015.03.040

Singh BP, Joshi A (2024). Ethical Considerations in AI Development. In *The Ethical Frontier of AI and Data Analysis* (pp. 156–179). IGI Global.

Straka M, Hajic J, Straková J (2016) UDPipe: trainable pipeline for processing CoNLL-U files perform- ing tokenization, morphological analysis, pos tagging and parsing. In: *Proceedings of the tenth international conference on language resources and evaluation (LREC'16),* pp 4290–4297.

Venugopalan M, Gupta D (2015) Exploring sentiment analysis on twitter data. In: *2015 eighth international conference on contemporary computing (IC3).* IEEE, pp 241–247.

Verma P, Bhardwaj T, Bhatia A, Mursleen M (2023). Sentiment Analysis "Using SVM, KNN and SVM with PCA". In: Bhardwaj, T., Upadhyay, H., Sharma, T.K., Fernandes, S.L. (eds) *Artificial Intelligence in Cyber Security: Theories and Applications. Intelligent Systems Reference Library,* vol 240. Springer, Cham. https://doi. org/10.1007/978-3-031-28581-3_5.

Wankhade M, Rao ACS, Kulkarni C (2022). A survey on sentiment analysis methods, applications, and challenges. *Artif Intell Rev* 55, 5731–5780. https://doi.org/10.1007/ s10462-022-10144-1

Weerasooriya T, Perera N, Liyanage S (2016) A method to extract essential keywords from a tweet using NLP tools. In: *2016 sixteenth international conference on advances in ICT for emerging regions (ICTer).* IEEE, pp 29–34.

Xing FZ, Cambria E, Welsch RE (2018) Natural language based financial forecasting: a survey. *Artif Intell Rev* 50(1):49–73.

Yang B, Cardie C (2014) Context-aware learning for sentence-level sentiment analysis with posterior regularization. In: *Proceedings of the 52nd annual meeting of the association for computational linguistics* (Volume 1: Long Papers), pp 325–335.

13 A Comprehensive Survey of Early Kidney Disease Prediction Models Using Machine Learning Approach

Nita Dakhare and Chitra Dhawale

INTRODUCTION

Kidney Disease, as a quiet global epidemic, has silently affected the lives of millions of individuals. Kidney Disease has a prevalence rate of 10% among the Indian population. Destroying kidney function is the characteristic of Kidney Disease and presents a considerable public health challenge among the list of diseases. The disease, which targets renal function and gradually leads to chronic pathological factors, tends to be recognized at its later stages, when few treatment options are available and treatment is expensive. Not only does this condition lower the quality of life of patients at an early age, but increases the financial cost to the healthcare system for this disease worldwide. Kidney Disease, which deteriorates gradually in kidney function over an extended period. Kidney Disease can have a range of root causes, including renal disease, hypertension, genetically connected causes in other chronic diseases, and autoimmune conditions. The kidneys, which are essential for maintaining the equilibrium of inner tissue, suffer from a slow development in the damage caused by Kidney Disease, compromising the processes of filtration and regulation. However, during the first outbreak of symptoms, many Idiopathic or idiopathic nature; the signs of the disease are concealed. Kidney Dis-ease's wide prevalence required a thorough examination of its epidemiology, risk factors, and causal effects of genetic and environmental influences. Kidney Disease can be classified according to the glomerular filtration rate (GFR) into various stages. The above methods can enable a better design of progression. However, Kidney Disease has a significant correlation that shedding light on its various aspects of the consequences on the human body. Current diagnostic methods, as well as therapeutic innovation, will continue to redefine and understand how Kidney Disease should be approached; i.e. body symptom management or renal conservative management.

DOI: 10.1201/9781003516590-13

Kidney Disease can be categorized in terms of stages based on the kidney damage and reduction in kidney function severity. The most popular classification system of Kidney Disease comprises the division into stages using the GFR developed by the National Kidney Foundation (NKF). The system includes five stages and accurately describes the progressive nature of the diseases:

Stage 1:   Normal or High GFR Kidney Damage.
             The following traits apply to the type of Kidney Disease: GFR is elevated or normal. Although there might be some kidney damage such as protein in the urine or structural irregularities, the organs' ability to function is unaffected.
Stage 2:   Moderate GFR Decline.
             This category shares characteristics with Kidney Disease in its initial stages. GFR is rather lower. Signs of renal damage still exist.
Stage 3:   GFR Declines Moderately.
             There are two categories for the third stage:
Stage 3A: The GFR Ranges from 45 to 59 ml/min.
             GFR in Stage 3B is between 30 and 44 ml/min.
Stage 4:   A Substantial Decline in GFR.
             At this point, patients frequently have a variety of issues and require more extensive medical care.
Stage 5:   End-Stage Renal Disease, or Kidney Failure.
             This type of Kidney Disease is the most severe and calls for kidney replacement therapy, including a kidney transplant.

The patient's GFR indicates the severity of their Kidney Disease, whether kidney damage is present, and associated symptoms and complications. It is crucial to track the development of Kidney Disease so that medical professionals can adjust their care or interventions according to the severity of the condition. The earlier kidney illness is identified and treated, the more likely it is that complications will be avoided and the disease will not worsen. Clinical screening guidelines recommend that individuals at risk or those with Kidney Disease-related symptoms be screened regularly and consult a healthcare provider without further delay. The advent of machine learning has been the focal point of innovation in the healthcare industry in recent years. Thanks to this state-of-the-art technology, a great amount of medical data is now accessible, which creates new chances for the early diagnosis of illnesses like renal disease (Joshi & Goyal, 2019). With the use of machine learning and its immense capacity, this study sets out to address the problems associated with Kidney Disease and alter the predictive landscape.

MOTIVATION FOR EARLY KIDNEY DISEASE PREDICTION

Kidney Disease is a silent killer, often reaching advanced stages before causing noticeable symptoms. This latency makes early detection and intervention crucial for improving patient outcomes and reducing the disease's immense burden on healthcare systems. Here's why studying, analyzing, and developing Kidney Disease prediction using machine learning is a compelling research topic:

- **The Urgency of the Problem**: Global Health Threat: Kidney Disease affects millions worldwide, with its prevalence steadily increasing.
  - **Silent Progression**: Early stages often lack symptoms, leading to delayed diagnosis and worse outcomes.
  - **Significant Burden**: Kidney Disease is a major risk factor for cardio-vascular disease, diabetes, and other complications, straining healthcare resources.
- **The Promise of Machine Learning**
  - **Pattern Recognition**: Machine Learning algorithms can analyze vast amounts of clinical data to identify subtle patterns and relationships between risk factors and Kidney Disease development (Joshi & Goyal, 2019).
  - **Early Detection Potential**: Accurate prediction models could enable earlier diagnosis, allowing for timely intervention and improved prognosis.
  - **Personalized Medicine**: Machine Learning can help tailor treatment plans based on individual risk profiles, optimizing care and resource allocation.
- **Current Limitations and Research Gaps**
  - **Existing Diagnostic Methods**: Traditional methods like blood tests and urinalysis have limitations in sensitivity and specificity.
  - **Limited Understanding of Kidney Disease Progression**: Complex interplay of genetic, environmental, and lifestyle factors remains unclear.
  - **Need for Robust and Interpretable Models**: Developing Machine Learning models that healthcare professionals can trust and understand is crucial for clinical adoption.
- **Potential Impact of Research**: Develop a highly accurate and reliable Machine Learning model for Kidney Disease prediction. This could be a valuable tool for clinicians, enabling earlier diagnosis and improved patient care.
  - **Gain Deeper Insights into Kidney Disease Risk Factors**: Your research can contribute to a better understanding of the complex factors driving Kidney Disease development.
  - **Inform the Development of Personalized Prevention and Treatment Strategies**: Early and accurate prediction can pave the way for targeted interventions based on individual risk profiles.
  - **Advance the Field of AI in Healthcare**: Your work can contribute to the growing body of research demonstrating the potential of Machine Learning in improving clinical decision-making and patient outcomes.

In conclusion, researching Kidney Disease prediction using machine learning is a timely and impactful endeavor with the potential to revolutionize how we manage this critical disease. By leveraging the power of AI, we can unlock new possibilities for early detection, personalized care, and ultimately, saving lives.

NEED AND SCOPE OF EARLY KIDNEY DISEASE PREDICTION MODELS USING MACHINE LEARNING APPROACH

The imperative for early detection and prediction of Kidney Disease cannot be over-stated. Kidney Disease affects individuals of all ages and backgrounds, and its prevalence continues to rise. It is estimated that millions of people worldwide are affected by Kidney Disease, with a considerable number unaware of their condition until its advanced stages. This delay in diagnosis not only limits treatment options but also places a significant economic burden on healthcare systems.

The need for precise and timely Kidney Disease prediction models is evident. Such models have the potential to transform healthcare by enabling healthcare professionals to identify at-risk patients earlier, initiate interventions, and ultimately improve patient outcomes. Machine Learning, with its ability to analyze vast datasets and identify complex patterns, offers a promising avenue for Kidney Disease prediction.

This study seeks to contribute to the realm of healthcare by developing accurate predictive models for Kidney Disease using Machine Learning techniques. By leveraging a comprehensive dataset encompassing a range of patient variables, we aim to create a model capable of identifying individuals at risk of developing Kidney Disease at an early stage.

Identifying individuals at risk of developing Kidney Disease involves assessing various factors and markers that may indicate a higher likelihood of developing this condition. Kidney Disease is a progressive condition where the kidneys gradually lose their function over time. Early identification of individuals at risk is crucial for implementing preventive measures and timely intervention.

MODELS/METHODS FOR EARLY KIDNEY DISEASE PREDICTION USING MACHINE LEARNING

It is impossible to overstate the significance of early Kidney Disease detection and prediction. This is because Kidney Disease is non-discriminatory to age or background, and the condition is on the rise. Reportedly, millions of people across the globe have Kidney Disease, and a large proportion are unaware of the condition's existence until the advanced stage. Although the lack of knowledge among the majority of the populace will seek medical attention late, the situation imposes an economic burden on healthcare systems. Therefore, precise and timely early kidney prediction models are urgently needed to transform healthcare. Such models could enable physicians and other medical practitioners to identify at-risk patients early enough to start preventive interventions and achieve better patient outcomes. Due to its ability to handle large datasets and intricate pattern recognition, machine learning holds great promise for the early diagnosis of renal illness (Singh & Joshi, 2024). The following are the current machine learning models and techniques used to predict renal disease early on (Table 13.1)

TABLE 13.1
Early Kidney Disease Prediction Machine Learning Models

Model/method	Description	Features (examples)	Performance metrics	Advantages	Disadvantages
Logistic regression [1]	A linear model is suitable for binary classification tasks.	Age, blood pressure, glucose, BMI, serum creatinine, albumin, etc.	Confusion matrix, ROC-AUC, F1 score, accuracy, recall, and precision	• Simple and interpretable. • Capable of handling big datasets effectively. • Offers approximations of probability.	• Makes the assumption that the attributes and the log chances of the outcome have a linear connection. • If the target and the features being connected are nonlinear, it could not perform as well.
Decision trees [2]	Tree-like models that make decisions based on input features.	Serum creatinine, albumin, hemoglobin, eGFR, proteinuria, etc.	F1 score, accuracy, ROC-AUC, confusion matrix, sensitivity/specificity	• Easy to interpret and visualize. • Handles non-linearity and interactions well. • No need for feature scaling.	• Underfit when class differences are not large. • Overfitting is prone, especially with small datasets. • Sensitive to small data variations.
Random forest [3]	Ensemble decision trees that improve generalization and reduce overfitting.	eGFR, proteinuria, diabetes, hypertension, serum creatinine, etc.	Sensitivity, specificity, accuracy, ROC-AUC, F1 score	• Reduces overfitting by combining multiple trees. • Handles non-linearity and interactions well. • Robust to noise and outliers.	• Lack of robustness to noise. • Can be computationally expensive. • Do not have the interpretability of individual decision trees.
Support vector machines [4]	Locates the high-dimensional hyperplane that divides the most classes effectively.	Age, gender, smoking, cholesterol, serum creatinine, etc.	Confusion matrix, ROC-AUC, F1 score, accuracy, recall, and precision	• Functions well in spaces with several dimensions. • Flexible with many kernel functions. • Effective in capturing complex relationships.	• Memory may be expansive, particularly with datasets of high dimensions. • Assume performance of the vertical data model is dependent on the form of kernel and hyper-parameters.

(Continued)

TABLE 13.1 (Continued)

Model/method	Description	Features (examples)	Performance metrics	Advantages	Disadvantages
Neural networks [5]	Deep learning models with interconnected nodes that can capture complex patterns.	Serum urea, urine output, family history, serum creatinine, etc.	ROC–AUC, mean squared error, accuracy, precision, recall	• Can capture complex relationships in data. • Suitable for large datasets. • Can automatically learn relevant features.	• Be powerful engines as opposed to humans. • Computationally expansive, especially with detailed structure. • Might not suit relatively small volumes.
Gradient boosting [6]	Gradient boosting is an ensemble technique where errors from the previous iteration are corrected by successively increasing the number of trees.	Serum phosphorus, calcium, potassium, hemoglobin, etc.	Confusion matrix, accuracy, F1 score, ROC–AUC, Log loss	• It uses various weak learners • It can deal with non-linearity and interactions. • It is not influenced easily by outliers and noise.	• Can be sensitive to hyperparameter tuning. • Computationally more expensive than individual decision trees. • May require careful tuning to prevent overfitting.
K-Nearest Neighbors [7]	It predicts the most common class in k-nearest neighbors of a sample and classifies the sample as it is.	Serum sodium, C-reactive protein, hemoglobin, etc.	Precision–recall curve, ROC–AUC, accuracy, F1 score	• It is very simple and easy to interpret. • There is no need for training. • It is tough on outliers.	• It is computationally bound and delivers very inefficient results for large datasets. • It is sensitive to certain irrelevant or unnecessary variables. • Performance depends on the distance metric and the choice of k.

Model	Description	Features	Evaluation Metrics	Advantages	Disadvantages
Naïve Bayes [8]	Probabilistic model based on Bayes' theorem, suitable for text classification and simple tasks.	Age, blood pressure, glucose, BMI, serum creatinine, etc.	Confusion matrix, ROC-AUC, F1 score, accuracy, recall, and precision	• It is very easy to understand and very computationally effective • Can handle high-dimensional data well. • Is robust to irrelevant features	• Assumes independent features which is not the case in some problems • Does not make full use of correlated features
XGBoost [9]	It is an optimized gradient boosting library. It is optimized for efficiency and performance.	eGFR, proteinuria, serum creatinine, hypertension, etc.	AUC-ROC, Log loss, F1 score, accuracy, confusion matrix	• Faster and scalable • Regularized to prevent overfitting • Handles missing data well • Feature importance estimation is available	• Very sensitive to hyperparameters • It can be very computationally expensive • Less interpretable compared to simpler model is the best
LightGBM [10]	Gradient boosting framework designed for speed and efficiency	Serum creatinine, albumin, eGFR, hemoglobin, etc.	ROC-AUC, F1 score, accuracy, Log loss, confusion matrix	• Fast and efficient, especially with large datasets. • Supports categorical features without one-hot encoding. • Good scalability.	• Limited interpretability compared to simpler models. • May require tuning of parameters.
CatBoost [11]	It's a gradient boosting library that works well with categorical features and is very easy to set up. It requires much less data preprocessing.	Age, blood pressure, glucose, BMI, eGFR, etc.	Accuracy, AUC-ROC, Log loss, F1 score, confusion matrix	• Handles categorical features well. • Robust to noisy data. • Efficient training. • Automatic handling of missing values.	• May require tuning of hyperparameters. • Computationally more expensive than simpler models. • Limited interpretability.
SVM with RBF Kernel [12]	Support vector machines using radial basis function kernel for handling non-linear relationships.	Serum creatinine, albumin, eGFR, proteinuria, etc.	Confusion matrix, ROC-AUC, F1 score, accuracy, recall, and precision	• Functions well in spaces with several dimensions. • Flexible with many kernel functions. • Good at capturing intricate connections.	• Computational and memory issues with large datasets. • Performance depends upon hyperparameter tuning and kernel selection. • Limited interpretability.

PERFORMANCE MEASURES OF EARLY KIDNEY DISEASE PREDICTION MACHINE LEARNING MODELS

The exact set of these metrics varies depending on the dataset and methodology, and experimental setup used in the study. In most cases, these metrics are heavily dependent on the data and the task of this data. However, based on my general understanding of the algorithms and the research papers, here is a qualitative assessment of their performance. Actual numbers may vary significantly depending on the tasks and the data (Table 13.2).

RESEARCH GAPS IN EARLY KIDNEY DISEASE PREDICTION MODELS USING MACHINE LEARNING APPROACH

Despite promising advancements, research on Kidney Disease prediction using Machine Learning still faces several critical gaps:

- **Limited Data Availability**: Large, high-quality datasets encompassing diverse populations and comprehensive clinical factors are often scarce.
- **Generalizability**: Models trained on limited datasets may not perform well when applied to different populations or settings.
- **Hybrid Models**: Most early Kidney Disease Prediction Machine Learning Models are not Hybrid in nature. Hybrid models have potential for improving the prediction of Kidney Disease.

TABLE 13.2

Performance Measures of Early Kidney Disease Prediction Machine Learning Models

Model/method	Accuracy	Precision	Recall	F1 score	ROC-AUC
Logistic Regression [1]	Moderate	Moderate	Moderate	Moderate	Moderate
Decision Trees [2]	Moderate to High	Can be vary	Can be vary	Can be vary	Moderate to high
Random Forest [3]	High (Often)	Moderate to high	Moderate to high	Moderate to high	High
Support Vector Machines (SVM) [4]	High (Often)	Can be vary	Can be vary	Can be vary	High
Neural Networks [5]	High (Can be)	Can be vary	Can be vary	Can be vary	High (can be)
Gradient Boosting [6]	High (Often)	Can be vary	Can be vary	Can be vary	High
K-Nearest Neighbors (KNN) [7]	Moderate	Moderate	Moderate	Moderate	Moderate
Naive Bayes [8]	Moderate	Moderate	Moderate	Moderate	Moderate
XGBoost [9]	High (Often)	High	High	High	High
LightGBM [10]	High (Often)	High	High	High	High
CatBoost [11]	High (Often)	High	High	High	High
SVM with RBF Kernel [12]	High (Often)	Can be vary	Can be vary	Can be vary	High

---

RECOMMENDATIONS FOR FURTHER RESEARCH

This provides recommendations for further research and areas of exploration that stem from our study on Kidney Disease prediction using Machine Learning. These suggestions aim to advance the field, address existing gaps, and contribute to the continuous improvement of Kidney Disease diagnosis and management.

- **Robustness and Generalization**: Future research should focus on the external validation of Kidney Disease prediction models in diverse populations and healthcare settings. This will assess the models' generalization across different patient demographics and data sources.
- **Real-Time Data Integration**: Exploring the integration of real-time data streams, such as wearable device data or continuous monitoring data, into Kidney Disease prediction models is essential. This can provide more dynamic and up-to-date insights for healthcare decision-makers.
- **Model Explainability and Trust**: The development and implementation of more explainable Machine Learning models for Kidney Disease prediction should be a priority. Ensuring that models provide comprehensible explanations for their predictions is crucial for clinician trust and adoption.
- **Patient-Centered Interpretability**: Research should aim to improve patient-centered model interpretability. This involves developing user-friendly interfaces and educational materials that empower patients to understand and engage with predictive models in their healthcare decisions.
- **Data Quality and Integration**: Standardization of healthcare data formats and terminologies should be explored to enhance data quality and interoperability across different healthcare systems.
- **Longitudinal Data Analysis**: Longitudinal data analysis can provide insights into Kidney Disease progression and treatment response. Future research can investigate the use of Machine Learning for analyzing longitudinal data and predicting disease trajectories.
- **Ethical and Privacy Considerations**: Research should continue to address fairness and bias issues in Kidney Disease prediction models. Developing strategies to mitigate bias and ensure equitable predictions for all patient groups is essential.
- **Privacy-Preserving Methods**: Exploring privacy-preserving Machine Learning techniques, such as federated learning or secure multiparty computation, can enable collaborative model development while safeguarding patient privacy.
- **Multimodal Data Integration**: Investigating the fusion of multiple data sources, including genetic data, imaging data, and clinical notes, can provide a holistic view of Kidney Disease prediction and enhance model accuracy.

CONCLUSION

All things considered, this review offers a thorough analysis of the range of machine-learning algorithms used for early Kidney Disease prediction. The research examines the variety of predictive analytics and their possible use in the context of healthcare by taking into account ensemble methods, logistic regression (LR), decision trees (DT), neural networks (NN), etc. The examination of features, performance metrics, as well as strengths and limitations of each model promotes a more in-depth understanding of their respective applications and foundations in Kidney Disease early prediction. Even though the survey diversifies the application of machine learning models, they all converge on one crucial point: early detection and intervention are the best tools to manage Kidney Disease. While each model has unique advantages and considerations, the choice of each should be closely tailored to the particular characteristics of the dataset, clinical needs, and computational resources. Moreover, this survey not only contributes to the existing knowledge but also indicates new directions and trends in early Kidney Disease prediction research. Given that the availability of health care data continues to expand, while machine-learning techniques evolve, it is possible to anticipate the growing accuracy and efficiency of the Kidney Disease prediction model. In terms of practical implications, the findings of this survey could guide the decision-makers in using a particular model for predicting Kidney Disease at early stages. Therefore, this chapter helps promote evidence-based decisions in this field and provides some recommendations on how to achieve better outcomes and treat kidney-related issues.

BIBLIOGRAPHY

Alsekait, D. M., Saleh, H., Gabralla, L. A., Alnowaiser, K., El-Sappagh, S., Sahal, R., & El-Rashidy, N. "Toward comprehensive chronic Kidney Disease prediction based on ensemble deep learning models," *Applied Sciences*, vol. 13, p. 3937, 2023.

Chen, T., & Guestrin, C. "XGBoost: A Scalable Tree Boosting System," in *Proceedings of the 22nd ACM SIGKDD International Conference on Knowledge Discovery and Data Mining*, 2016a, pp. 785–794.

Chen, X., & Guestrin, C. "XGBoost: A scalable tree boosting system," in *Proceedings of the 22nd ACM SIGKDD International Conference on Knowledge Discovery and Data Mining*, 2016b, pp. 785–794.

Chittora, P. et al., "Prediction of chronic kidney disease - A machine learning perspective," *IEEE Access*, vol. 9, pp. 17312–17334, 2021.

Debal, D. A., & Sitote, T. M. "Chronic kidney disease prediction using machine learning techniques," *The Journal of Big Data*, vol. 9, p. 109, 2022.

Dritsas, E., & Trigka, M. "Machine learning techniques for chronic kidney disease risk prediction," *Big Data and Cognitive Computing*, vol. 6, p. 98, 2022.

Gulati, V., & Raheja, N. "Comparative analysis of machine learning techniques based on chronic kidney disease dataset," in *IOP Conference Series: Materials Science and Engineering*, 1131, 012010.

Hassan, M. M., Hassan, M. M., Mollick, S. et al. A comparative study, prediction and development of chronic kidney disease using machine learning on patients clinical records. *Human-Centric Intelligent Systems*, vol. 3, pp. 92–104, 2023.

Hastie, T., Tibshirani, R., & Friedman, J. *The Elements of Statistical Learning: Data Mining, Inference, and Prediction*, Springer, 2009.

Ifraz, G. M., Rashid, M. H., Tazin, T., Bourouis, S., Khan, M. M. "Comparative analysis for prediction of kidney disease using intelligent machine learning methods", *Computational and Mathematical Methods in Medicine*, vol. 2021, 10 p, 2021. Article ID 6141470.

Iftikhar, H., Khan, M., Khan, Z., Khan, F., Alshanbari, H. M., Ahmad, Z. A comparative analysis of machine learning models: A case study in predicting chronic kidney disease. *Sustainability*, vol. 15, p. 2754, 2023.

Ilyas, H., Ali, S., Ponum, M., Hasan, O., Mahmood, M. T., Iftikhar, M., & Malik, M. H. Chronic kidney disease diagnosis using decision tree algorithms. *BMC Nephrology*, vol. 22(1), p. 273, 2021.

Islam, M. A., Majumder, M. Z. H., & Hussein, Md. A. "Chronic kidney disease prediction based on machine learning algorithms," *Journal of Pathology Informatics*, vol. 14, 100189, 2023. ISSN 2153-3539.

Jain, S., Patel, M., & Jain, K. "A comparative analysis of ML Stratagems to estimate chronic kidney disease predictions and progression by employing electronic health records," in *Emerging Trends in Data-Driven Computing and Communications: Proceedings of DDCIoT 2021*. Springer Singapore, 2021.

Joshi, A., & Goyal, S. B. "Comparison of Various Round Robin Scheduling Algorithms," in *2019 8th International Conference System Modeling and Advancement in Research Trends (SMART), Moradabad, India*, 2019, pp. 18–21, doi: 10.1109/SMART46866. 2019.9117345.

Kaur, C., Kumar, M. S., Anjum, A., Binda, M. B., Mallu, M. R., & Al Ansari, M. S. "Chronic kidney disease prediction using machine learning," *Journal of Advances in Information Technology*, vol. 14, no. 2, pp. 1798–2340, 2023 (Online).

Ke, G. et al., "LightGBM: A highly efficient gradient boosting decision tree," *Advances in Neural Information Processing Systems*, vol. 2017, pp. 3146–3154, 2017.

Khalid, H., Khan, A., Khan, M. Z., Mehmood, G., Qureshi, M. S., "Machine learning hybrid model for the prediction of chronic kidney disease", *Computational Intelligence and Neuroscience*, vol. 2023, 14 p, 2023. Article ID 9266889.

Kumar, R., Joshi, A., Sharan, H. O., Peng, S. L., & Dudhagara, C. R. (Eds.). (2024). *The Ethical Frontier of AI and Data Analysis*. IGI Global.

Lapi, F., Nuti, L., Marconi, E., Medea, G., Cricelli, I., Papi, M., Gorini, M., Fiorani, M., Piccinocchi, G.-N., & Cricelli, C. "To predict the risk of chronic kidney disease (CKD) using Generalized Additive2 Models (GA2M)," *Journal of the American Medical Informatics Association*, vol. 30, no. 9, pp. 1494–1502, 2023.

Lederer, J., & Pan, R. "Understanding Gradient Boosting Machines," arXiv preprint arXiv:1902.07558, 2019.

Liu, Y., Yu, J., & Yuan, C. "An effective stock index forecasting framework based on support vector machine" *IEEE Access*, vol. 7, pp. 105918–105929, 2019.

Prokhorenkova, L., Gusev, G., Vorobev, A., Dorogush, A. V., & Gulin, A. "CatBoost: unbiased boosting with categorical features," in *Advances in Neural Information Processing Systems*, 2018, pp. 6638–6648.

Rady, E.-H. A., & Anwar, A. S. "Prediction of kidney disease stages using data mining algorithms," *Informatics in Medicine Unlocked*, vol. 15, 100178, 2019, ISSN 2352-9148.

Ramana, C. V., Kumar, J. V., Sravani, N., Virajitha, M., & Vivek, V. "Performance analysis of machine learning classifier for predicting chronic kidney disease," *IJIRT*, vol. 8, no. 4, 2021, ISSN: 2349-6002.

Reshma, S., Shaji, S., Ajina, S. R., Vishnu Priya, S. R., & Janisha, A. "Chronic kidney disease prediction using machine learning," *International Journal of Engineering Research & Technology (IJERT)*, vol. 9, no. 7, 2020.

Ribeiro, M. T., Singh, S., & Guestrin, C. "'Why should I trust you?': Explaining the predictions of any classifier," in *Proceedings of the 22nd ACM SIGKDD International Conference on Knowledge Discovery and Data Mining*, 2018, pp. 1135–1144.

Singh, B. P., & Joshi, A. (2024). Ethical considerations in AI development. In R. Kumar, A. Joshi, H. Sharan, S. Peng, & C. Dudhagara (Eds.), *The ethical frontier of AI and data analysis* (pp. 156–179). IGI Global Scientific Publishing. https://doi.org/10.4018/979-8-3693-2964-1.ch010.

Tekale, S., et al. "Prediction of chronic kidney disease using a machine learning algorithm." *International Journal of Advanced Research in Computer and Communication Engineering*, vol. 7, no. 10, pp. 92–96, 2018.

Zhang, X., Huang, Y., Shi, W., & Dai, W. "High-dimensional data regression analysis based on ensemble learning algorithms," *Neuro-computing*, vol. 381, pp. 242–253, 2020.

Zhang, Y., & Yang, Q. "A survey on multi-view learning," arXiv preprint arXiv:1802.05365, 2018.

Zhao, J., Zhang, Y., Qiu, J. et al. "An early prediction model for chronic kidney disease." *Scientific Reports*, vol. 12, p. 2765, 2022.

Zhou, Z. H., Wu, J., & Tang, W. "Exploring deep learning and transfer learning for k-nearest neighbor," *Neurocomputing*, vol. 309, pp. 124–135, 2018.

14 Navigating Healthcare Security Challenges in the Era of 6G Connectivity

A Futuristic Perspective

Sai Satya Navya Sri Vasamsetti, Gisala Venkatesh, and Manas Kumar Yogi

INTRODUCTION

The internet has become an integral part of our lives in the 21st century, providing access to social networking, online shopping, data storage, gaming, online study, and online jobs. However, the internet's widespread use has led to the development of cybercrime, as it has become a significant issue in various spheres of life due to its relative benefits. Hence, security has unequivocally been a crucial aspect in present and future wireless communication networks, including 5G and 6G (Raja & Asghar, 2020). In recent years, advancements in wireless communication technologies have been driving significant changes across various sectors, and healthcare is no exception. The emergence of 6G technology, with its promise of ultra-fast data transmission, ultra-low latency, and massive connectivity, is poised to revolutionize healthcare delivery. This chapter explores the opportunities that 6G technologies bring to the healthcare industry, focusing on how they can enhance telemedicine, remote patient monitoring, and medical education, thereby enabling real-time collaboration and data-driven decision-making.

THE PROMISE OF 6G IN HEALTHCARE

6G technology offers unprecedented benefits for healthcare professionals. It enables real-time, high-quality video consultations, facilitating telemedicine and ensuring that patients receive timely and accurate diagnoses and treatments regardless of their location. Remote patient monitoring becomes more efficient with the ability to transmit large volumes of data instantaneously, allowing for continuous monitoring and timely interventions.

DOI: 10.1201/9781003516590-14

Furthermore, 6G can transform medical education by enabling virtual reality (VR) and augmented reality (AR) applications, providing immersive learning experiences for medical students and professionals (Agee & Gates, 2013).

REVOLUTIONIZING HEALTHCARE WITH 6G

- **Telemedicine**: High-definition video consultations and real-time data sharing between patients and healthcare providers improve the quality of remote care.
- **Remote Patient Monitoring**: Continuous monitoring of vital signs through wearable devices and sensors ensures proactive health management (Rahman & Rahman, 2022) and early detection of health issues.
- **Medical Education**: VR and AR applications offer immersive training experiences, allowing medical professionals to practice complex procedures in a simulated environment.

LITERATURE REVIEW

Recent research highlights significant advancements in integrating 6G technologies into healthcare systems, promising enhanced telemedicine, advanced IoT devices for real-time monitoring, and AI-driven diagnostics, as shown in Table 14.1. Key developments include AI-based network management for optimized resource allocation, predictive analytics for early disease detection, secure patient data sharing via blockchain technology, real-time haptic feedback for remote surgeries enabled by ultra-low latency, and comprehensive Internet of Medical Things (IoMT) ecosystems for seamless device interoperability. These innovations aim to improve patient outcomes, increase healthcare accessibility, and reduce costs.

NAVIGATING SECURITY CHALLENGES IN THE 6G ERA: SAFEGUARDING HEALTHCARE DATA AND NETWORKS

While the benefits of 6G in healthcare are substantial, they come with significant security challenges. The increased data transmission rates and extensive connectivity in 6G networks heighten their vulnerability to cyber-attacks. The massive volumes of sensitive patient data being transmitted and stored pose serious privacy concerns (Gupta et al., 2024).

Key Security Challenges

- **Increased Exposure to Cyber Threats**: The extensive infrastructure of 6G networks, spanning across various devices and communication nodes, poses a heightened risk of cyber-attacks due to the multitude of potential entry points. Robust cybersecurity strategies must continuously evolve to address these diverse attack surfaces effectively.

TABLE 14.1

Current Research Work Summarizing Recent Research Work on the Integration of 6G Technology in Healthcare Systems

Research work	Advancements	Challenges	Merits
Pyone et al., 2017	• Enhanced telemedicine with ultra-low latency - Advanced IoT devices for real-time monitoring - AI (Artificial Intelligence) and ML integration for diagnostics	• Data privacy and security concerns High infrastructure costs • Interoperability issues	• Improved patient outcomes through timely interventions • Increased accessibility to healthcare services
Surekha and Rahman, 2022	• AI-driven network management • Predictive analytics for patient care • Seamless connectivity for remote areas	• High computational requirements • Algorithmic bias and fairness • Regulatory compliance	• Proactive healthcare management • Reduced healthcare costs • Enhanced patient monitoring
Sfar et al., 2022	• Secure patient data sharing with blockchain • Decentralized data storage • Enhanced data integrity and transparency	• Scalability of blockchain solutions • Energy consumption of blockchain • User acceptance	• Enhanced data security • Improved patient trust • Reduced fraud and errors
Nguyen et al., 2022	• Real-time haptic feedback • High precision remote surgery • Reduced latency for critical applications	• Reliability of haptic feedback • Network robustness • Ethical concerns regarding remote surgery	• Improved surgical outcomes • Access to specialized surgeries • Training and simulation opportunities
Rahman et al., 2023	• Comprehensive IoMT ecosystems - Enhanced sensor data fusion - Real-time health analytics	• Battery life of IoMT devices • Data standardization <Network congestion	• Continuous patient monitoring • Early detection of health issues • Personalized healthcare

- **Protection of Confidential Health Data**: Ensuring the privacy of vast volumes of sensitive patient information transmitted over 6G networks requires not only strong encryption protocols but also comprehensive data access controls and monitoring mechanisms. Compliance with global privacy regulations is essential to maintain patient trust and legal adherence.

- **Complex Integration Demands**: Integrating disparate healthcare devices and systems within unified 6G infrastructures necessitates meticulous planning to bridge interoperability gaps and mitigate security vulnerabilities. Effective collaboration between healthcare providers and technology vendors is crucial to ensure seamless data exchange without compromising system integrity.
- **Adapting Security Measures at Scale**: As 6G networks expand exponentially, scalable security frameworks must anticipate and respond to evolving threats swiftly. Proactive measures such as threat intelligence sharing and continuous security audits are essential to fortify network defences and safeguard against emerging cybersecurity risks.

PROPOSED SOLUTIONS

To address the security challenges inherent in 6G networks, a hybrid mechanism combining game theory and federated learning (FL) offers robust solutions. This approach leverages game theory to design incentive structures that motivate secure data sharing and resource allocation among healthcare providers and patients. Simultaneously, FL ensures that sensitive patient data remains decentralized and protected, utilizing collaborative model training across distributed devices. By integrating these methodologies, the hybrid approach not only enhances data security but also optimizes the efficiency and reliability of healthcare services within the advanced framework of 6G networks (Ali et al., 2022).

GAME THEORY FOR SECURITY

Game theory can be applied to design incentive mechanisms that encourage cooperation and discourage malicious behaviour within the smart healthcare system (Patel et al., 2022). For example, incentive-compatible mechanisms can be created to incentivize patients to securely share their health data with healthcare providers while protecting their privacy. This approach ensures that all stakeholders act in the best interest of the system's overall security.

APPLICATION OF GAME THEORY IN HEALTHCARE NETWORKS

1. **Formulating Incentives**: Design strategies that encourage secure and transparent data exchange while discouraging unauthorized activities. This involves creating systems that incentivize proactive engagement and impose penalties for actions that compromise data integrity or confidentiality.
2. **Engaging Participants**: Educate all stakeholders within the healthcare ecosystem about the benefits of collaboration and the potential consequences of non-participation (Sharma & Guleria, 2023). By fostering a shared understanding of mutual advantages and responsibilities, stakeholders are motivated to actively contribute to the collective success of the network.

3. **Continuous Monitoring**: Apply game theory models to consistently monitor network dynamics and adapt incentives accordingly. This dynamic
   approach ensures that incentives are aligned with evolving circumstances
   and effectively address emerging challenges or threats to data security and
   system efficiency (Mohammed et al., 2023).

GAME THEORY WITH STACKELBERG SECURITY EQUILIBRIUM APPROACH IN WBAN (GTSSE)

The main objective of the proposed work is to maintain healthcare (i.e., medical
information) at a high-security level without any threats. The maintenance is also
designed to ensure minimal energy consumption and response time. Wearable body
sensors are used to identify and monitor the patient's health records, which are maintained in personal systems. Wireless Body Area Networks (WBAN) have exclusive
architectures to adapt to medical data applications. At each stage of the WBAN, the
system is designed with a high flexibility rate to accommodate different patient information platforms (Figure 14.1).

These sensors provide real-time health monitoring of patients from multiple locations. The network setup involving body sensors is designed for scalability and efficient collection of patient data. Biosensors are integrated into the network to monitor
health metrics across several patients simultaneously (Subramanian et al., 2022). A
local personal computer (PC) is linked to the network for analysing medical data
stored on the server (Figure 14.2).

Security is upheld within the Game-Theoretic Secure Sensing Environment
(GTSSE) methodology through relay points and employing mathematical
formulations to determine authoritative power positions. The GTSSE approach has
engineered the system to operate at a heightened level of security, facilitating efficient

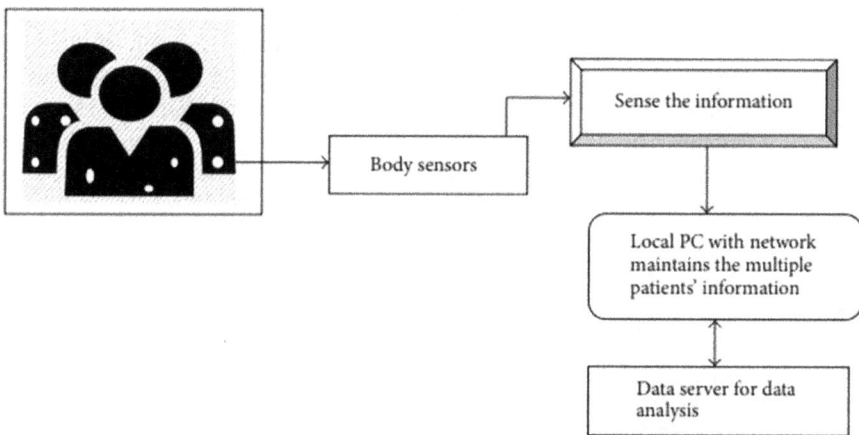

FIGURE 14.1   Architecture diagram of GTSSE approach (Yaqoob et.al., 2022).

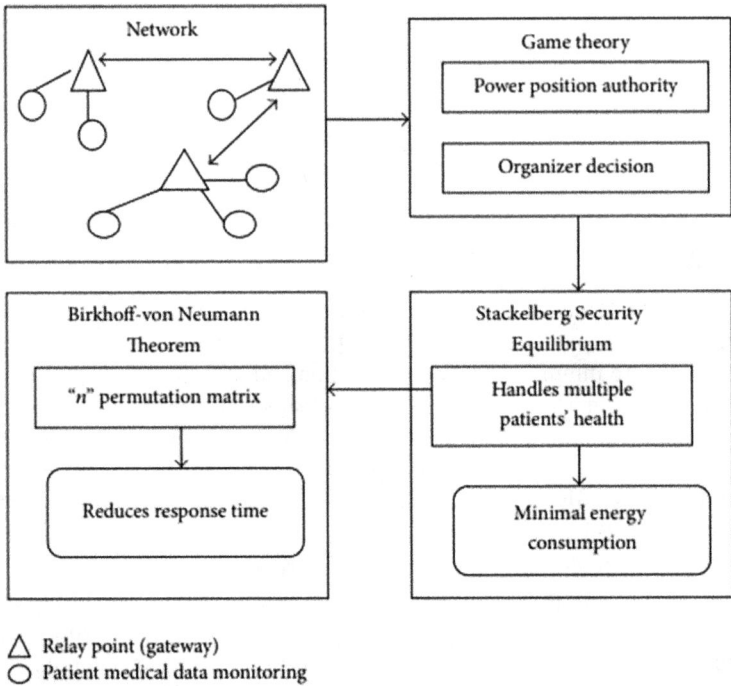

FIGURE 14.2   Steps of monitoring patients' information.

allocation of limited resources for patient information storage (Batista et al., 2023). The GTSSE framework is designed to prevent jamming and attacks while utilizing body sensor networks.

In the context of game theory, a participant within the WBAN system plays a crucial role in making informed and strategic decisions. Within the realm of body sensor health monitoring, game theory provides a detailed depiction of strategic interactions among multiple entities. The GTSSE approach offers a robust solution to game theory applications, enabling the implementation of optimal strategies with effective outcomes. This approach leverages the principles of game theory to design mechanisms that ensure secure and efficient data transmission and resource allocation within WBANs, enhancing the overall performance and reliability of health monitoring systems. A game player's strategy encompasses a comprehensive plan for actions across all potential scenarios, ensuring the secure management of patient disease levels within a resilient framework. Game theory provides a mathematical framework for effectively analysing information from multiple patients using Stackelberg Security Equilibrium. This equilibrium ensures strategic planning, where a leader entity establishes policies first, followed by responses from other entities, thereby optimizing decision-making in healthcare scenarios involving sensitive patient data.

GAME THEORY IN INTRUSION DETECTION SYSTEMS (IDS)

Game theory is a field that studies strategic interactions among rational players, focusing on optimizing their benefits. It offers efficient and robust distributed algorithms, making it useful in wireless networks for modelling, analysing, and designing distributed schemes. Hence, in this aspect, game theory is utilized to study and forecast the future behaviour of the complicated attacks in present and future networks. Furthermore, it aids in the characterization of the intricate nature of these attacks and facilitates the prediction of their future patterns, hence enhancing the ability to assess and prepare for effective responses. The wireless network components commonly seen in contemporary settings encompass vehicle ad hoc networks (VANETS), drone networks, and high-speed trains (HST). These components consist of a combination of mobile and stationary nodes, each equipped with a range of communication technologies and infrastructure (Janay & Sarkara, 2023). Intrusion detection systems (IDS) are used to safeguard networks from both internal and external cyber threats. The IDS employs anomaly detection policies to identify malicious activities perpetrated by attackers. Cooperative games are those where players cooperate to optimize a common goal, while non-cooperative games are those where players don't cooperate. Furthermore, the use of a distributed architecture that incorporates prediction and detection algorithms allows for the optimization of processes by using both mobile nodes and centralized infrastructure to enhance efficiency and effectiveness.

IDS employ anomaly detection to protect networks from cyber threats. Cooperative games optimize shared goals, while non-cooperative games involve independent decision-making. Distributed architectures with prediction and detection algorithms enhance network security by leveraging mobile nodes and centralized infrastructure efficiently (Figure 14.3).

Game theory is commonly recognized as a mathematical framework that can be employed to analyse the dynamics of conflict between a defender (IDS) and attackers, with the aim of determining the optimal strategy for the defence in accurately identifying a suspicious target as malevolent. Therefore, to safeguard the integrity of the prevailing intelligent network against significant and perhaps fatal cyber threats, a number of cyber games have been developed. These games predominantly employ non-cooperative game theory as a means to address issues pertaining to prediction and decision-making. In the context of such a particular game, participants strive to optimize their own payoffs while simultaneously decreasing the payoffs of their adversaries (Kharche & Kharche, 2023). The primary aim of a non-cooperative game is to establish a state of Nash Equilibrium (NE) between the attacker and the IDS. In this condition, the attacker deploys malicious software targeting networking and IoT nodes, while the IDS employs its detection mechanism to safeguard legitimate users.

This chapter, therefore, proposes utilizing the intruder attack pattern through channel modelling to facilitate the analysis of intrusions into host networks by employing game theory and devising counter-protection strategies. The proposed intrusion detection scenario further aims to identify and combat security challenges in the IoT framework by focusing on perception, network, middleware, and application layers. It therefore suggests integrating network slicing, machine learning techniques, and a game theory approach to effectively address these challenges.

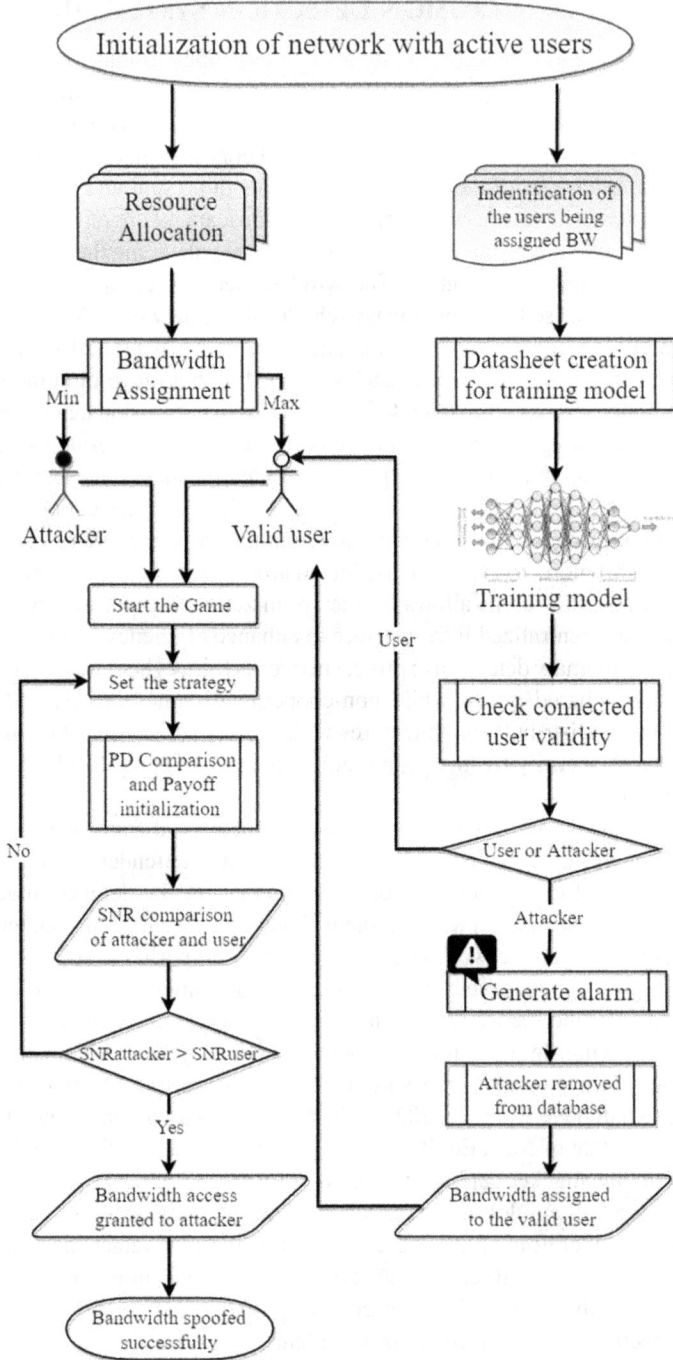

FIGURE 14.3   Flow process of Intrusion Detection Systems (IDS).

TYPES OF GAMES IN IDS

- **Cooperative Game**: Nodes collaboratively monitor and report intrusions to enhance detection accuracy.
- **Non-cooperative Game**: Nodes independently decide on intrusion detection based on individual strategies and payoffs.
- **Zero-Sum Game**: Gain of one node is a loss for another, modelling adversarial interactions between attackers and defenders.
- **Bayesian Game**: Nodes use probabilistic reasoning to make decisions under uncertainty, considering potential attacker strategies.

FEDERATED LEARNING IN HEALTHCARE: ENHANCING DATA PRIVACY AND EFFICIENT RESOURCE ALLOCATION

FL revolutionizes collaborative model training across distributed healthcare devices, such as wearables and medical sensors, by preserving patient privacy through localized data processing (Ahmad & Harjula, 2024). This approach ensures data security by avoiding direct sharing of raw data, thus mitigating risks related to data breaches and unauthorized access.

FEDERATED LEARNING PROCESS

- **Local Model Training**: Healthcare devices independently train machine learning models using their local data sets, ensuring that sensitive patient information remains decentralized and secure.
- **Model Aggregation**: Locally trained models are aggregated centrally without transmitting raw data. This aggregation process consolidates insights from diverse data sources while maintaining individual data privacy.
- **Global Model Update**: The centrally aggregated model is updated and redistributed to devices for further training iterations. This iterative process enhances model accuracy over time without compromising data confidentiality.

CLIENT SELECTION

To reduce communication costs in FL, a practical approach involves limiting the number of participating clients or selecting only a subset of parameters for updates during each training round. This selection process can be randomized or strategically targeted. Specifically, parameters that are farthest from their local optima, indicated by larger gradients, can be prioritized.

The central server plays a crucial role in managing the resources of diverse clients. It evaluates the state of each client's resources, including wireless channel conditions, computational power, and the volume of relevant data. Based on this analysis, the server determines which clients should participate in the current training task.

In making decisions, the server optimizes data, energy, and CPU (Central Processing Unit) resources to minimize energy consumption, training latency, and

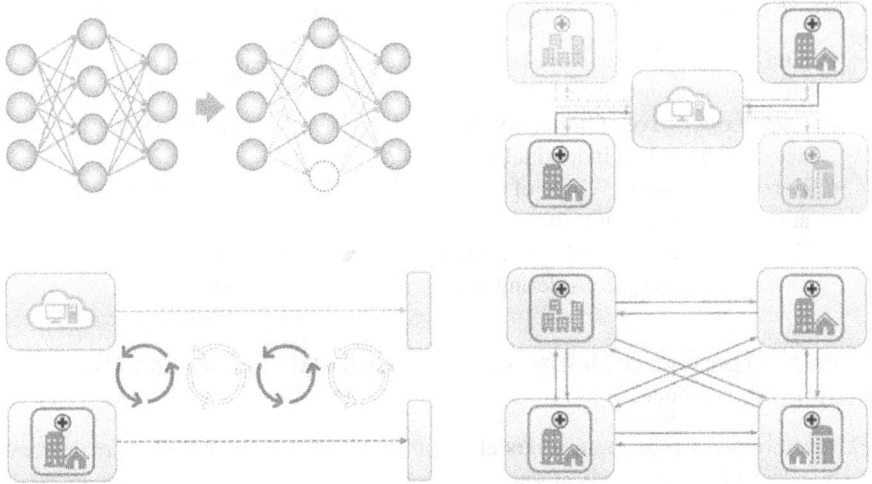

FIGURE 14.4   Communication-efficient federated learning mechanism.

bandwidth costs. This technique enables dynamic optimization of data and energy management in mobile devices participating in FL, without prior knowledge of network dynamics. It ensures efficient resource allocation, enhancing the performance and sustainability of the FL process (Figure 14.4).

GAME THEORY FOR FEDERATED LEARNING SECURITY

Game theory plays a pivotal role in governing interactions between the server and edge devices within FL (Ning et al. 2020). It facilitates the design of incentive mechanisms that motivate participants to share their data and computational resources while ensuring the system's security and efficiency (Quy et al., 2023). Game theory effectively balances the trade-offs between training rewards and costs, thereby maximizing utility for each participating node.

MECHANISM AND APPROACH

1. **Incentive Mechanism**: The server implements an incentive structure tailored to each node's contributions. By offering rewards based on individual participation, nodes are encouraged to share their data securely, promoting overall system efficiency and collaboration.
2. **Dynamic Contribution Measurement and Incentive Mechanism**: A dynamic approach is employed to continuously assess each node's contributions. This adaptive mechanism adjusts incentives based on real-time performance, ensuring sustained participation and data contribution throughout the FL process.

3. **Secure Aggregation**: To safeguard data privacy during model aggregation, secure aggregation techniques are employed. These methods ensure that even if an unauthorized entity gains access to the aggregated data, they cannot discern the specific data points contributed by individual nodes, thereby preserving confidentiality and preventing data leakage.

Below, the mathematical models for each of the mechanisms and approaches described above are outlined:

1. **Incentive Mechanism**
   Objective: The objective is to incentivize nodes based on their contributions to the FL process.
   Mathematical Model:
   Let R_i denote the reward given to node i.
   Assumption: Rewards are proportional to the contribution of each node.

   $$R\_i = f\left(\{\text{Contribution}\}\_i\right)$$

   Where f is a function that computes the reward based on the contribution metric $\{\text{Contribution}\}\_i$

   Implementation:

   $\{\text{Contribution}\}\_i$ can be quantified based on factors such as the amount of data contributed, computational resources used, or the quality of contributed models.
   The exact form of f could vary (linear, logarithmic, etc.) depending on the desired incentive structure.

2. **Dynamic Contribution Measurement and Incentive Mechanism**
   Objective: To dynamically adjust incentives based on the real-time performance of nodes.
   Mathematical Model:

   Let $\{\text{Contribution}\}\_i(t)$ denote the contribution of node i at time t
   Dynamic Adjustment:

   $$R\_i(t) = g\left(\{\text{Contribution}\}\_i(t)\right)$$

   Where g is a function that adjusts R_i based on $\{\text{Contribution}\}\_i(t)$
   Adaptation:
   $\{\text{Contribution}\}\_i(t)$ is continuously updated based on the node's performance metrics, which could include metrics like accuracy improvement, latency, or resource utilization.
   The function g dynamically adjusts incentives to maintain optimal participation and fairness among nodes.

3. Secure Aggregation

Objective: To aggregate model updates securely without compromising individual node data privacy.

Secure Aggregation Technique:

The Federated Averaging algorithm with differential privacy mechanisms can be used to achieve secure aggregation.

Suppose $\{w_i(t)\}$ are the model updates from each node i at iteration t

Each node i adds noise $\{N\}\_i$ to its update to achieve differential privacy.

The server aggregates the perturbed updates to obtain the global update $\mathbf{w}_{\text{global}}(t)$

$$\mathbf{w}\text{global}(t) = \sum_{i=1}^{n}(wi(t) + Ni)$$

Privacy Preservation:

The noise Ni ensures that even if an attacker gains access to the aggregated update $\mathbf{w}\text{global}(t)$ they cannot deduce the exact contributions $w_i(t)$ from individual nodes.

Differential privacy parameters (e.g., noise variance) are chosen to balance privacy and utility.

These models encapsulate the core mechanisms and approaches described in the context of FL, each addressing specific aspects such as incentive structure, dynamic adaptation, and data privacy.

RESULTS AND DISCUSSIONS

Federated Learning with Game Theory: The integration of game theory into FL creates a dynamic and secure environment for healthcare data processing. The proposed algorithm leverages the concepts of contributions and incentives to ensure effective participation and collaboration among nodes in the network. Below is the detailed description of the algorithm:

ALGORITHM: FL GAME THEORY

INPUT:

- num_nodes: Integer – number of nodes participating
- contributions: List of Floats – contributions of each node
- incentives: List of Floats – incentives offered by the server

---

OUTPUT:

- Generates a plot

STEPS:

1. Plotting Initialization:
   - Initialize a plotting canvas for bar charts.
2. Loop through Each Node:
   - For each `node_id` from `0` to `num_nodes - 1` do:
     - Plot a bar at position `node_id` for `contributions [node_id]` with the label 'Contributions'.
     - Plot a bar at position `node_id` for `incentives [node_id]` with the label 'Incentives'.
3. Labelling:
   - Label the x-axis as 'Node ID'.
   - Label the y-axis as 'Value'.
   - Title the plot as 'Federated Learning with Game Theory'.
   - Include a legend to distinguish between 'Contributions' and 'Incentives'.
4. Display the Plot:
   - Render the plot to visualize the contributions and incentives for each node (Figure 14.5).

This algorithm visualizes the contributions and incentives of each node participating in the FL process. By plotting these values, it is possible to analyse the effectiveness of the incentive mechanisms in promoting data sharing and collaboration.

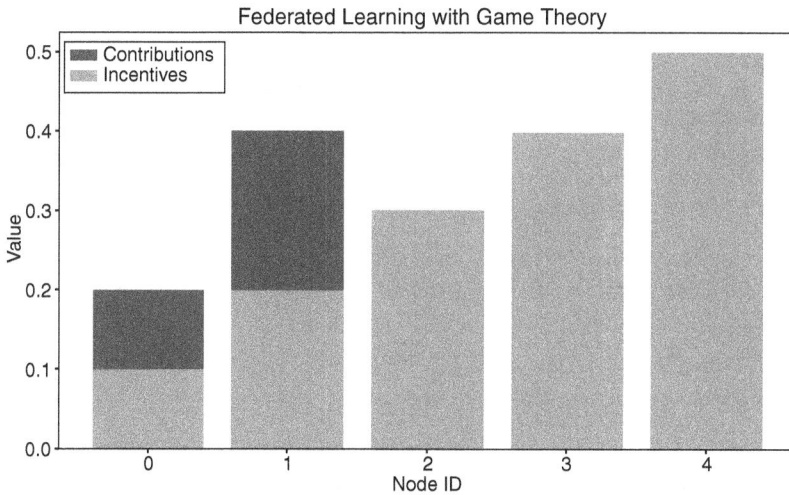

FIGURE 14.5 Plot of contributions, incentives with proposed hybrid method.

RESULTS

The application of the FL Game Theory algorithm resulted in a bar chart that visually represents the contributions and incentives of each node. The chart clearly illustrates how the incentive mechanisms reward nodes based on their contributions, encouraging higher participation and collaboration in the FL process.

GAME THEORY-BASED INCENTIVE CALCULATION FOR FEDERATED LEARNING

The incentive mechanism based on game theory principles plays a crucial role in motivating nodes to participate and share data in the FL process. The following algorithm outlines the calculation of incentives for each node based on their performance relative to the global model.

ALGORITHM: CALCULATE INCENTIVE

INPUT:

- client_accuracy: Float – Accuracy of the local model (client)
- global_accuracy: Float – Accuracy of the global model
- alpha: Float – Incentive parameter
- beta: Float – Penalty parameter

OUTPUT:

- incentive: Float – Calculated incentive based on game theory principles

INCENTIVE CALCULATION:

```
Set incentive = alpha * client_accuracy + beta * (client_
  accuracy - global_accuracy)
// optionally ensure non-negative incentives
If incentive < 0 then:
Set incentive = 0
```

RETURN INCENTIVE

This algorithm calculates the incentive for each node based on its local model's accuracy and the global model's accuracy. The incentive is computed using the formula:

$$\text{Incentive} = \alpha \times \text{client\_accuracy} + \beta \times \left(\text{client\_accuracy} - \text{global\_accuracy} \right)$$

The incentive parameters (α and β) allow for fine-tuning the reward and penalty applied to the nodes based on their performance. By ensuring that incentives are non-negative, the algorithm maintains motivation for nodes to improve their contributions (Figure 14.6).

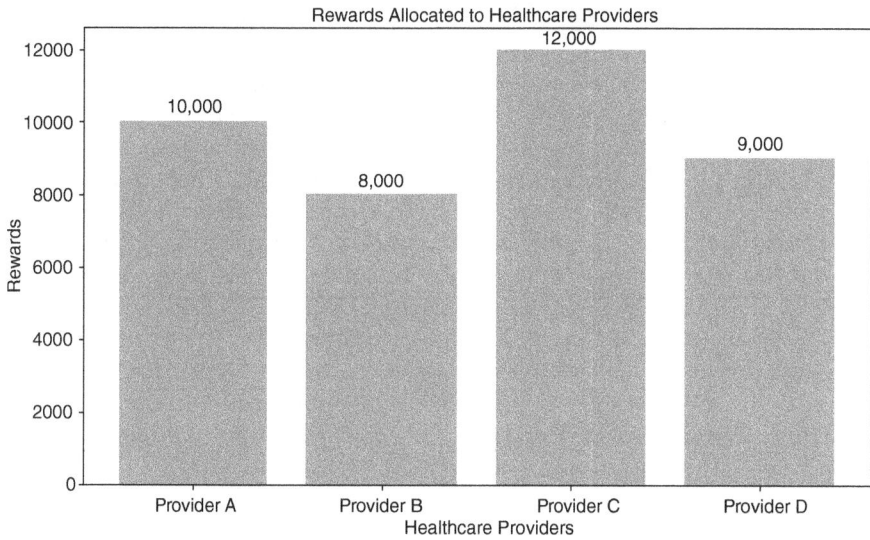

FIGURE 14.6   Rewards allocated to healthcare providers.

The bar chart depicting rewards allocated to different healthcare providers in a FL process holds significant importance in several dimensions of healthcare and technology integration:

- **Incentivizing Data Contribution**: The rewards allocated reflect how healthcare providers are incentivized based on their contributions to FL. Providers with higher rewards typically contribute more valuable gradients or model updates, fostering a collaborative environment where participants are motivated to share their resources effectively. This approach is critical as it encourages broader participation and ensures a diverse dataset, which is essential for training robust and generalized machine learning models in healthcare applications.
- **Quality Assessment and Improvement**: The varying heights of the bars reflect differences in the quality or quantity of contributions from different providers. This can serve as a quality assessment metric, helping stakeholders identify which providers are consistently contributing high-quality data or models. It also enables continuous improvement efforts by highlighting areas where additional support or resources may be needed to enhance contributions from underperforming providers.
- **Transparency and Accountability**: By visualizing rewards publicly, the chart promotes transparency in how rewards are distributed among healthcare providers. This transparency fosters trust among participants and stakeholders by demonstrating fairness and accountability in the allocation process. It also encourages providers to uphold standards of data integrity and security, knowing that their contributions are valued and rewarded fairly.

- **Decision-Making Support**: The graph aids decision-making processes within FL initiatives by providing a clear overview of resource allocation. Stakeholders can utilize this information to strategically allocate resources, prioritize support for top-performing providers, and identify opportunities for collaboration or intervention as needed. This data-driven approach enhances the efficiency and effectiveness of FL projects in healthcare by facilitating informed decision-making based on quantitative insights.
- **Promoting Collaboration and Innovation**: Ultimately, the graph promotes collaboration and innovation in healthcare by illustrating the collective impact of FL efforts. It encourages providers to collaborate on shared goals, leverage each other's strengths, and collectively advance healthcare research and technology. By showcasing the benefits of participation, the graph inspires continuous innovation and improvement in leveraging data for healthcare advancements.

In practical applications, these algorithms can be tailored to specific healthcare scenarios, such as telemedicine and remote patient monitoring. By adjusting the incentive parameters, healthcare providers can optimize the balance between data privacy and the benefits of collaborative learning. The integration of game theory and FL thus offers a robust framework for enhancing healthcare security and efficiency in the era of 6G connectivity (Figure 14.7).

The line plot illustrating the evolution of the contribution metric over time for a healthcare provider in FL can have several impactful implications for researchers in the field:

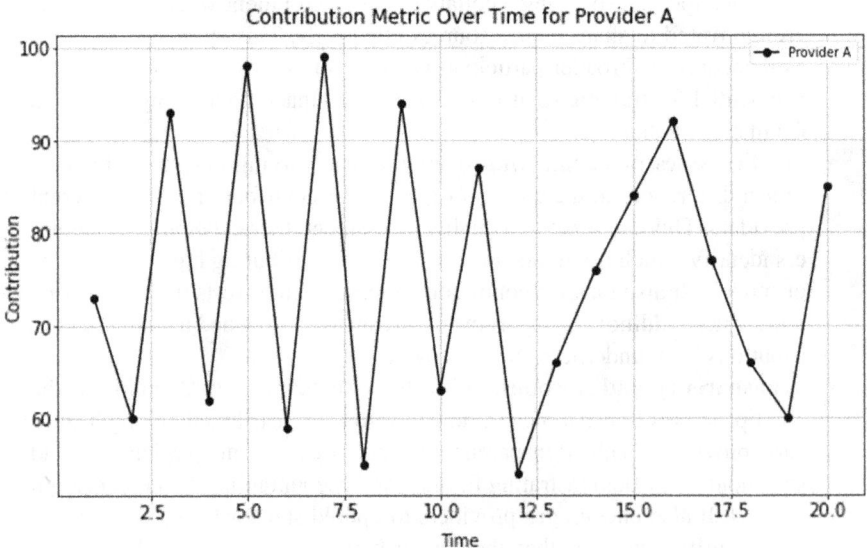

FIGURE 14.7   Plot of contribution metric wrt time for Healthcare provider A.

- **Temporal Analysis of Participation**: Researchers can analyse the fluctuation patterns in contribution metrics over time. This provides insights into how engaged healthcare providers are in the FL process across different time periods. Understanding these patterns helps in assessing the sustainability of participation and identifying factors influencing provider involvement.

- **Identifying Trends and Anomalies**: The graph enables researchers to identify trends, such as increasing or decreasing participation rates over time. Sudden spikes or dips in contribution metrics can indicate specific events or interventions impacting provider behaviour. Detecting anomalies prompts further investigation into underlying causes, which may range from technological issues to shifts in policy or participant motivation.

- **Assessing Impact of Interventions**: Researchers can use the line plot to evaluate the effectiveness of interventions aimed at increasing contributions over time. For instance, implementing incentives, educational programs, or performance feedback mechanisms can be tracked through changes in contribution metrics. This data-driven approach helps in refining strategies to optimize participant engagement and data sharing.

- **Benchmarking and Comparison**: The plot facilitates benchmarking efforts by comparing contribution metrics across different healthcare providers or within the same provider over time. Researchers can identify top-performing providers and study their practices to derive best practices that can be shared across the FL network. It also enables fair comparisons by normalizing metrics against time-related variations.

- **Supporting Policy and Decision-Making**: The visual representation of contribution evolution aids in policy formulation and strategic decision-making. Researchers can utilize insights from the plot to advocate for supportive policies that sustain participation and foster collaboration among healthcare providers. Decision-makers can leverage this information to allocate resources effectively and prioritize initiatives that drive long-term engagement and success.

- **Longitudinal Insights into Collaboration Dynamics**: By observing how contribution metrics evolve longitudinally, researchers gain a deeper understanding of the collaborative dynamics within FL ecosystems. This includes studying patterns of data sharing, model updates, and the evolution of collaborative relationships among providers. Such insights are crucial for designing future research collaborations and improving the overall efficiency of FL approaches (Figure 14.8).

The above graph, which compares model updates before and after secure aggregation with differential privacy, holds significant importance for security and privacy designers in the following ways:

- **Visualizing Privacy Enhancements**
  - **Illustration of Differential Privacy**: The graph visually demonstrates how differential privacy techniques add noise to model updates after aggregation. This is crucial for designers as it shows how individual

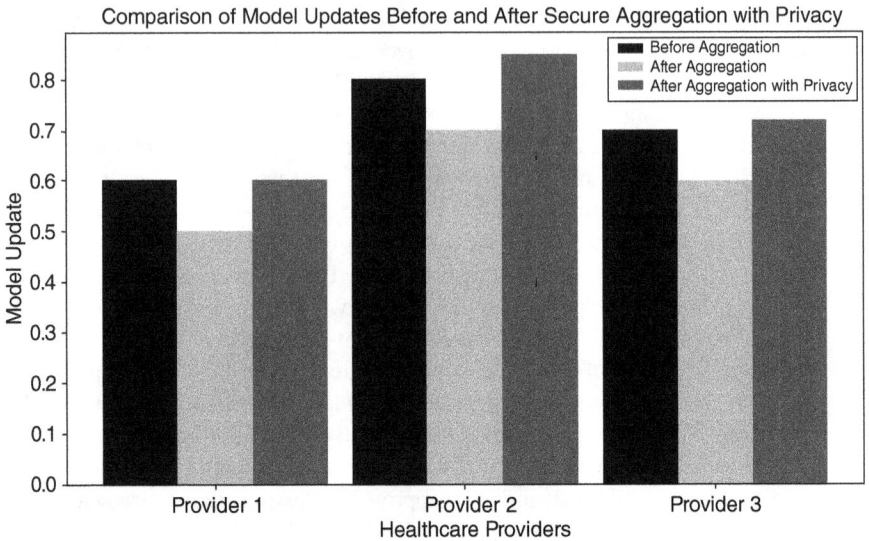

FIGURE 14.8 Privacy-based model updates by various healthcare providers.

contributions are obfuscated while still allowing meaningful aggregation for model improvement.

- **Understanding Privacy Guarantees**: Designers can use this graph to showcase to stakeholders and decision-makers how differential privacy provides strong privacy guarantees by preventing malicious actors from deducing specific contributions from individual healthcare providers.
- **Assessing Privacy vs. Utility Trade-Offs**
  - **Balancing Privacy and Model Accuracy**: The comparison between model updates before and after differential privacy allows designers to evaluate the trade-offs between privacy protection and model accuracy. They can adjust the level of noise (as shown in the graph) to find an optimal balance that meets both privacy requirements and performance goals.
- **Communication with Stakeholders**
  - **Effective Communication Tool**: Graphical representations serve as powerful tools for conveying complex concepts such as differential privacy to non-technical stakeholders. Designers can utilize this graph to clearly explain how secure aggregation with differential privacy safeguards sensitive healthcare data while maintaining the effectiveness of FL models.
- **Decision Support**
  - **Supporting Decision-Making**: By visually presenting the impact of differential privacy on model updates, the graph helps security and privacy designers make informed decisions about the implementation of privacy-preserving techniques. They can use the insights gained from the graph to refine their strategies and ensure compliance with regulatory requirements.

- **Promoting Adoption of Privacy Technologies**
  - **Encouraging Adoption**: Demonstrating the effectiveness of differential privacy through graphical representation can encourage healthcare organizations and providers to adopt FL technologies. By illustrating how secure aggregation techniques preserve data privacy while facilitating collaborative model training, stakeholders gain confidence in the technical feasibility and benefits of leveraging sensitive patient data for improved healthcare outcomes. This approach highlights integrating privacy-preserving technologies in FL initiatives.

The scatter plot in Figure 14.9 depicting the trade-off between privacy (differential privacy noise level) and utility (model accuracy or convergence rate) in FL provides valuable insights into the intricate dynamics researchers encounter when balancing data privacy with model performance. Below is a detailed analysis of the graph:

The plot typically shows a curve where increasing the differential privacy noise level enhances privacy protection might degrade model accuracy or slow down convergence rates. Researchers use this visual representation to find an optimal balance, ensuring that privacy measures do not excessively compromise the utility of FL models. By analysing this trade-off, stakeholders can make informed decisions on setting appropriate privacy parameters.

- **Understanding Differential Privacy and Utility**
  - **Differential Privacy**: Differential privacy is a crucial concept in FL to protect individual data privacy while aggregating insights across distributed data sources. Higher differential privacy noise levels indicate stronger privacy protections but potentially lower utility due to added noise in the aggregated model.

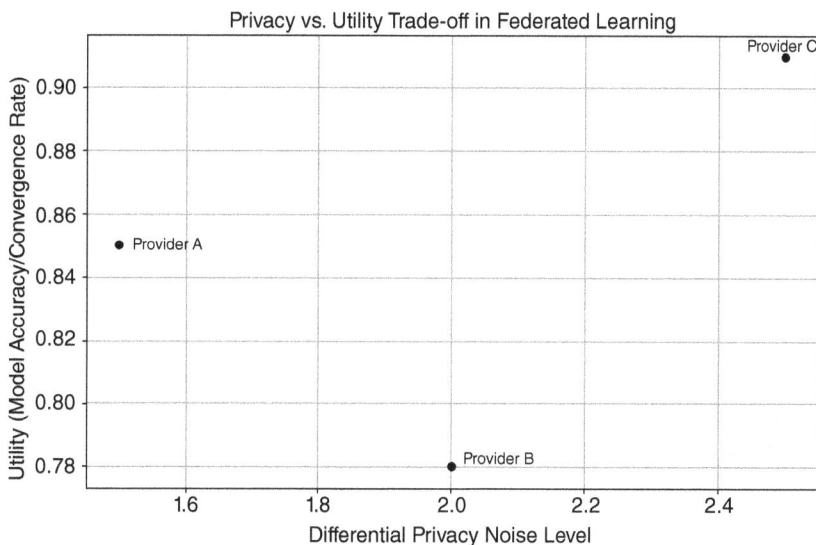

FIGURE 14.9 Trade-off between privacy and utility.

- **Utility (Model Accuracy/Convergence Rate)**: Utility measures how well the FL model performs its intended task, such as predicting outcomes or improving model convergence rates. Higher utility scores indicate better model performance, often correlated with lower privacy protections.

ANALYSIS OF THE SCATTER PLOT

- **Privacy vs. Utility Trade-Off**: The scatter plot illustrates an inverse relationship between differential privacy noise levels and utility scores. As differential privacy noise levels increase (indicating stronger privacy protections), there is typically a decrease in utility scores, reflecting potential compromises in model accuracy or convergence rates. This trade-off underscores the challenge of balancing data privacy with maintaining optimal performance in FL applications.
- **Provider-Specific Insights**: Each point on the plot represents a healthcare provider, offering insights into how different providers manage the trade-off between privacy and utility. Providers with lower differential privacy noise levels often achieve higher utility scores, suggesting less noisy data aggregation and potentially more accurate models. Conversely, providers opting for higher privacy levels sacrifice some utility for enhanced privacy protections.
- **Optimization Considerations**: Researchers can utilize this plot to optimize differential privacy parameters based on their specific use case and regulatory requirements. It serves as a visual guide to finding a balance that meets acceptable privacy standards while maximizing model utility. For instance, in scenarios where stringent privacy regulations are mandated, providers may need to accept a trade-off of slightly reduced utility to ensure compliance with privacy regulations. This approach facilitates informed decision-making in FL implementations, aligning technical optimizations with regulatory and operational constraints.
- **Impact of Privacy Enhancements**: Observing outliers or clusters in the plot can indicate instances where certain providers excel in maintaining high utility despite stringent privacy protections. These cases highlight potential best practices or technological innovations that mitigate the traditional privacy-utility trade-off, such as advanced privacy-preserving techniques like differential privacy with tailored noise mechanisms or efficient data pre-processing methods. These insights encourage the adoption of effective privacy enhancements while maintaining robust model utility in FL settings.
- **Policy and Research Implications**: Policymakers and researchers can use this analysis to inform policy decisions and research directions in FL. It underscores the importance of developing scalable privacy-preserving solutions that minimize data exposure while maximizing the utility of collaborative machine learning models. Moreover, it encourages further exploration into hybrid approaches that blend differential privacy with other privacy-enhancing technologies to achieve optimal trade-offs (Figure 14.10).

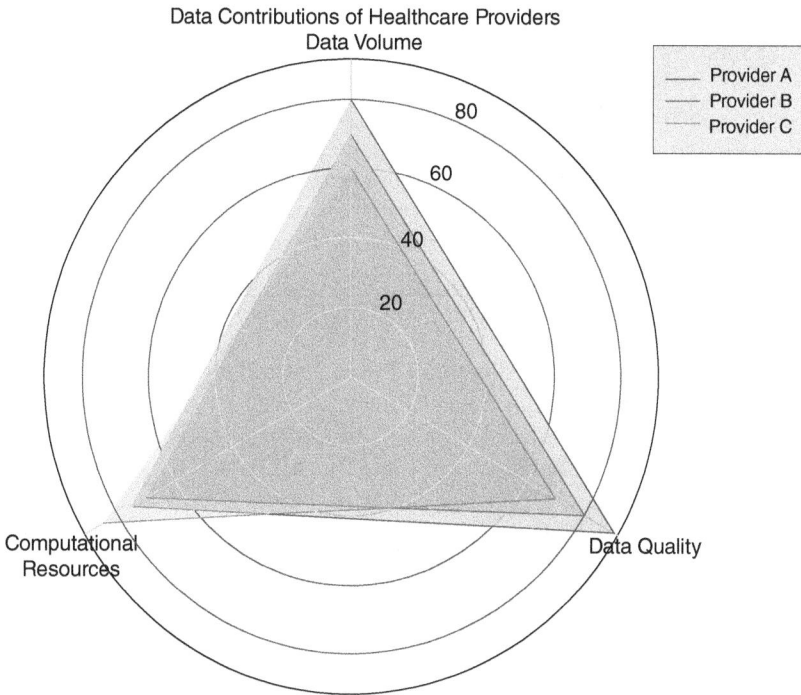

FIGURE 14.10 Degree of data contribution during federated learning by various health providers.

The radar graph depicting data contributions from various healthcare providers holds profound significance within healthcare systems, particularly in the context of data-driven decision-making and collaborative model development through FL. Below, a comprehensive exploration of its importance is provided:

- **Enhancing Collaborative Healthcare**: The radar graph serves as a visual tool to showcase the diverse contributions of healthcare providers in terms of data volume, quality, and computational resources. In FL, where data privacy is paramount, each provider retains control over their data while contributing collectively to the development of robust machine learning models. This collaborative approach enables healthcare systems to leverage a broader and more representative dataset without compromising individual data privacy, thereby enhancing the accuracy, reliability, and generalizability of predictive models.
- **Optimizing Resource Allocation**: By illustrating each provider's strengths across multiple dimensions, such as their data volume, quality, and computational capabilities, the radar graph aids in optimizing resource allocation. Healthcare organizations can strategically allocate resources based on providers' contributions, focusing investments on areas where additional support or infrastructure is needed to enhance data collection, processing efficiency, or data quality assurance.

- **Promoting Accountability and Transparency**: The radar graph promotes accountability and transparency among healthcare providers by clearly depicting their contributions. It encourages providers to uphold data quality standards and actively participate in collaborative initiatives aimed at improving healthcare outcomes. This transparency fosters trust among stakeholders and regulatory bodies, reinforcing compliance with data protection regulations and ethical standards governing healthcare data usage. This approach ensures that all stakeholders are informed about the contributions and responsibilities of each participant in FL initiatives, thereby enhancing overall accountability and promoting ethical practices in healthcare data management.
- **Facilitating Decision-Making and Prioritization**: In healthcare systems, informed decision-making relies heavily on accurate data insights. The radar graph facilitates decision-making by offering a comparative analysis of each provider's capabilities and contributions. Healthcare administrators and data scientists can prioritize initiatives based on providers' strengths and weaknesses identified in the radar chart, ensuring targeted interventions to address specific healthcare challenges effectively.

The radar graph serves as a pivotal visual representation in healthcare systems, empowering stakeholders to leverage collective data contributions effectively, optimize resource utilization, uphold privacy standards, and drive impactful advancements in healthcare delivery and research. Its role in fostering collaboration and informed decision-making underscores its critical importance in shaping the future of healthcare through data-driven innovation and patient-centric care.

These algorithms and their results underscore the importance of interdisciplinary collaboration and the need for standardized security protocols to address the unique challenges posed by 6G technology in healthcare. As the healthcare industry continues to evolve with advancements in wireless communication, the integration of innovative solutions like game theory and FL will be crucial for ensuring secure and efficient healthcare delivery.

CASE STUDIES

CASE STUDY 1: ENHANCING TELEMEDICINE WITH 6G CONNECTIVITY IN RURAL AREAS

Background: In a rural region with limited access to medical facilities, a healthcare provider implements 6G-enabled telemedicine services. The goal is to overcome the geographical and infrastructural barriers that hinder access to quality healthcare. The high-speed and low-latency capabilities of 6G ensure that patients can have real-time consultations with specialists who may be located hundreds of miles away.

Implementation: Using 6G technology, the healthcare provider offers high-definition video consultations, enabling doctors to examine patients remotely as effectively as in person (Quy et al., 2023). Advanced sensors and diagnostic tools connected through the 6G network allow for comprehensive remote examinations, including vital signs monitoring and imaging diagnostics.

Game Theory Application: Providers apply game theory to design incentive mechanisms that encourage patients to securely share their health data. By offering benefits such as reduced consultation fees, access to exclusive health programs, and personalized health tips, patients are incentivized to actively participate. These strategies are carefully crafted to demonstrate the value of data sharing while ensuring patients retain control over their privacy and personal information.

Federated Learning Application: To protect patient privacy, FL employs on-device training of diagnostic models. Each patient's data remains locally on their device and contributes through locally computed model updates. These updates, which are transmitted to a central server periodically, are encrypted and aggregated rather than raw data, following stringent privacy protocols (Chataut et al., 2024). This approach ensures that sensitive health data stays secure throughout the process, leveraging collective intelligence to enhance the accuracy and effectiveness of telemedicine services.

Outcomes:

- **Improved Access to Care**: FL facilitates on-device training of medical models, enabling patients in remote areas to access timely medical consultations without extensive data transmission to central servers, thereby reducing latency and supporting real-time decision-making.
- **Enhanced Data Privacy**: Utilizing techniques like differential privacy and secure aggregation, FL ensures patient data remains encrypted and anonymized throughout model training.
- **Patient Engagement**: Incentive mechanisms, designed using game theory, encourage active patient participation in securely sharing health data.

This approach highlights how FL optimizes healthcare accessibility, preserves data privacy, and enhances patient engagement through efficient and secure data management practices.

CASE STUDY 2: ADVANCING REMOTE PATIENT MONITORING WITH 6G TECHNOLOGY

Background: A metropolitan hospital integrates 6G technology into its remote patient monitoring system. This integration aims to provide continuous and accurate tracking of patient health metrics, especially for chronic disease management and post-operative care.

Implementation: Wearable devices connected via 6G continuously monitor vital signs such as heart rate, blood pressure, and glucose levels. These devices transmit data in real-time to healthcare providers, enabling immediate intervention when necessary. The ultra-low latency of 6G ensures that data is updated instantaneously, allowing for timely responses to any abnormalities.

Game Theory Application: To enhance data accuracy and timeliness, the hospital implements a reward system based on game theory principles. Patients are incentivized to maintain regular data uploads through rewards such as health credits, access to premium healthcare services, and participation in wellness programs. This system not only motivates patients to adhere to their monitoring schedules but also helps in maintaining a steady flow of accurate health data.

Federated Learning Application: FL ensures that sensitive patient data remains on local devices, where wearable devices perform local computations to update monitoring models. Only encrypted and aggregated model updates are shared with the central server, which integrates these updates to refine the monitoring system. This method enables continuous improvement of monitoring algorithms while maintaining stringent patient privacy protections.

Outcomes:

- **Proactive Health Management**: Continuous monitoring facilitated by FL enables early detection of potential health issues, facilitating proactive interventions to improve patient outcomes.
- **Data Privacy and Security**: FL ensures robust patient data privacy by keeping sensitive information on local devices and only transmitting encrypted model updates to a central server.
- **Patient Compliance**: Incentive mechanisms based on game theory enhance patient adherence to monitoring protocols.

CASE STUDY 3: TRANSFORMING MEDICAL EDUCATION AND TRAINING WITH 6G TECHNOLOGY

Background: A leading medical school adopts 6G technology to enhance its educational offerings. The school introduces VR- and AR-based training programs to provide immersive learning experiences for medical students and professionals.

Implementation: The medical school develops a 6G-enabled platform that offers VR simulations of surgical procedures, AR-assisted anatomy classes, and interactive case studies. These advanced training modules allow students to practice and refine their skills in a controlled, virtual environment that mimics real-life scenarios.

Game Theory Application: To boost engagement and collaborative learning, the platform incorporates game theory to incentivize participation. Students earn points and rewards for participating in collaborative sessions, completing simulations, and achieving high performance in assessments. This competitive yet collaborative environment fosters a deeper engagement with the training material and encourages peer learning.

Federated Learning Application: FL is employed to iteratively enhance training models using feedback from student interactions. As students engage with VR and AR modules, their performance data and feedback update the training algorithms locally. These updates are aggregated to improve the overall quality and accuracy of training content, ensuring its relevance and effectiveness over time.

Outcomes:

- **Enhanced Learning Experiences**: VR and AR technologies offer realistic and immersive training environments, enhancing skill acquisition and retention through interactive simulations and scenarios.
- **Continuous Improvement**: FL facilitates the continuous evolution of training content by integrating real-time feedback from student interactions.
- **Student Engagement**: Incentive mechanisms, guided by game theory principles, foster active student participation and collaboration.

Integrating VR, AR, FL, and game theory-based incentives optimizes learning environments by enhancing engagement, improving content relevance, and promoting continuous skill development in medical education and training.

CASE STUDY 4: PERSONALIZED MENTAL HEALTH SUPPORT USING 6G TECHNOLOGY

Background: A mental health organization aims to revolutionize personalized mental health support through the integration of 6G technology. Harnessing the high-speed and low-latency capabilities of 6G networks, the organization seeks to deliver tailored therapy and counselling services with unprecedented efficiency and responsiveness. By leveraging these advanced telecommunications capabilities, individuals can access seamless interactions and real-time support, enhancing the accessibility and effectiveness of mental health interventions. This approach promises to transform how mental health services are delivered, offering immediate assistance and personalized care irrespective of geographical location or time constraints.

Implementation: The organization develops a mobile application that connects patients with mental health professionals through video calls, chat, and AI-driven support. The app also includes self-help tools, such as mood tracking, meditation exercises, and cognitive behavioural therapy (CBT) modules, which are enhanced by the fast and reliable connectivity of 6G.

Game Theory Application: To encourage continuous engagement and participation, the organization uses game theory to design a reward system. Patients earn points and badges for completing therapy sessions, regularly using self-help tools, and achieving personal mental health goals. These rewards can be redeemed for additional therapy sessions, wellness products, or exclusive content, motivating patients to stay active in their mental health journey.

Federated Learning Application: Implementing FL in mental health support systems is indeed a promising approach. It strikes a balance between personalization and privacy, which are crucial in such sensitive domains. By keeping machine learning models local to each patient's device and only sharing aggregated updates with the central server, you minimize the risk of exposing sensitive data while still benefiting from collective insights. This method not only enhances data security but also improves the effectiveness of therapy recommendations by tailoring them to individual usage patterns and feedback. It's a great example of leveraging technology to improve healthcare without compromising patient privacy.

Outcomes:

- **Personalized Support**: Patients receive customized therapy and self-help tools tailored to their unique needs and progress.
- **Enhanced Privacy**: FL ensures that sensitive mental health data is not exposed, maintaining high standards of privacy and confidentiality.
- **Increased Engagement**: Game theory-based incentives encourage consistent participation and engagement, leading to better mental health outcomes.
- **Continuous Improvement**: The FL approach allows the mental health support system to continuously evolve based on real-time feedback and usage data, ensuring that the content remains relevant and effective.

By implementing 6G technology and innovative security mechanisms, these case studies illustrate how healthcare providers can enhance service delivery, improve patient outcomes, and ensure data privacy. The strategic use of game theory and FL provides a robust framework for overcoming the unique challenges posed by 6G in healthcare, paving the way for a secure and efficient future.

Future Directions for Strengthening Healthcare Security in the 6G Era

Looking ahead, it is essential to explore new technologies and methodologies to strengthen healthcare security in the 6G era. Future directions include:

- **Smart Computers and Special Databases**: Enhance the security and efficiency of 6G networks with advanced encryption and data management capabilities. These technologies ensure that patient data remains secure and accessible only to authorized personnel, leveraging robust encryption methods such as homomorphic encryption and blockchain-based storage to protect sensitive healthcare information effectively.
- **Interdisciplinary Collaboration**: Crucial for developing robust security solutions tailored for 6G networks, especially in healthcare contexts. By bringing together experts from healthcare, cybersecurity, and telecommunications, we can effectively address technical vulnerabilities and regulatory requirements. This approach ensures that healthcare systems leveraging 6G networks remain resilient against evolving cyber threats. Integrating

expertise from these diverse fields allows for comprehensive security strategies that protect patient data and maintain system integrity, thereby fostering trust and reliability in healthcare services. This collaboration is essential for advancing both technology and safety standards in the healthcare sector.

- **Standardized Security Protocols**: Establish robust protocols for data encryption, access control, and incident response across 6G healthcare networks. By defining standardized practices, such as adopting ISO (International Organization for Standardization)/IEC (International Electrotechnical Commission) 27001 for information security management and NIST (National Institute of Standards and Technology) Cybersecurity Framework for risk management, organizations can ensure consistency and interoperability in safeguarding patient data and mitigating security risks effectively.

- **Regulatory Compliance**: Adhere rigorously to regulatory frameworks and compliance requirements such as GDPR (General Data Protection Regulation), HIPAA (Health Insurance Portability and Accountability Act), and other relevant regulations in the 6G era. Compliance ensures that healthcare providers maintain the highest standards of patient data security and privacy, fostering trust among patients and stakeholders while mitigating legal and reputational risks associated with data breaches or non-compliance.

CONCLUSION

The advent of 6G technology holds immense promise for revolutionizing healthcare through advancements in remote patient monitoring, telemedicine, and data-driven decision-making. However, with these advancements come significant security challenges that must be effectively addressed to protect the privacy and integrity of sensitive healthcare data.

As 6G networks integrate technologies like AI, VR, and blockchain, the attack surface for malicious actors expands dramatically. Securing the network of connected medical devices, digital twins, and real-time data streams demands a multifaceted approach. This includes implementing advanced encryption, robust access controls, and proactive threat detection mechanisms.

Moreover, the introduction of quantum computing capabilities in 6G necessitates the development of quantum-resistant cryptographic algorithms to safeguard against emerging threats. Collaboration between healthcare providers, technology firms, and regulatory bodies is essential to navigate these challenges. Establishing comprehensive data governance frameworks, rigorous cybersecurity protocols, and promoting a culture of security awareness among healthcare professionals are crucial steps.

Additionally, decentralized security solutions such as blockchain-based data management and distributed ledger technologies can enhance the resilience of 6G-enabled healthcare systems against cyber threats. By prioritizing security and privacy as foundational elements of the 6G revolution in healthcare, organizations can fully harness its transformative potential.

This approach not only improves patient outcomes and operational efficiency but also ensures the confidentiality and trustworthiness of medical data in an increasingly interconnected world.

REFERENCES

Agee, M. D., & Gates, Z. (2013). Lessons from game theory about healthcare system price inflation: evidence from a community-level case study. *Applied Health Economics and Health Policy*, 11, 45–51.

Ahmad, I., & Harjula, E. (2024, May). Adaptive Security in 6G for Sustainable Healthcare. In *Nordic Conference on Digital Health and Wireless Solutions* (pp. 38–47). Cham: Springer Nature Switzerland.

Ali, M., Naeem, F., Tariq, M., & Kaddoum, G. (2022). Federated learning for privacy preservation in smart healthcare systems: A comprehensive survey. *IEEE Journal of Biomedical and Health Informatics*, 27(2), 778–789.

Batista, E., Lopez-Aguilar, P., & Solanas, A. (2023). Smart health in the 6G era: bringing security to future smart health services. *IEEE Communications Magazine*.

Chataut, R., Nankya, M., & Akl, R. (2024). 6G networks and the AI revolution—Exploring technologies, applications, and emerging challenges. *Sensors*, 24(6), 1888.

Gupta, M., Sharma, P., & Kalra, R. (2024). Federated Learning and Artificial Intelligence in E-Healthcare. In *Federated Learning and AI for Healthcare 5.0* (pp. 104–118). IGI Global.

Janay, P., & Sarkara, A. (2023). Secure data transmission in the era of 6G: Challenges and solutions. *Algorithm Asynchronous*, 1(1), 8–15.

Kharche, S., & Kharche, J. (2023). 6G intelligent healthcare framework: A review on role of technologies, challenges and future directions. *Journal of Mobile Multimedia*, 19(3), 603–644.

Mohammed, M. A., Lakhan, A., Abdulkareem, K. H., Zebari, D. A., Nedoma, J., Martinek, R., ... Garcia-Zapirain, B. (2023). Energy-efficient distributed federated learning offloading and scheduling healthcare system in blockchain based networks. *Internet of Things*, 22, 100815.

Nguyen, D. C., Pham, Q. V., Pathirana, P. N., Ding, M., Seneviratne, A., Lin, Z., ... Hwang, W. J. (2022). Federated learning for smart healthcare: A survey. *ACM Computing Surveys (Csur)*, 55(3), 1–37.

Ning, Z., Dong, P., Wang, X., Hu, X., Guo, L., Hu, B., ... Kwok, R. Y. (2020). Mobile edge computing enabled 5G health monitoring for Internet of medical things: A decentralized game theoretic approach. IEEE *Journal on Selected Areas in Communications*, 39(2), 463–478.

Patel, V. A., Bhattacharya, P., Tanwar, S., Gupta, R., Sharma, G., Bokoro, P. N., & Sharma, R. (2022). Adoption of federated learning for healthcare informatics: Emerging applications and future directions. *IEEE Access*, 10, 90792–90826.

Pyone, T., Smith, H., & van den Broek, N. (2017). Frameworks to assess health systems governance: a systematic review. *Health Policy and Planning*, 32(5), 710–722.

Quy, V. K., Chehri, A., Quy, N. M., Han, N. D., & Ban, N. T. (2023). Innovative trends in the 6G era: A comprehensive survey of architecture, applications, technologies, and challenges. *IEEE Access*, 11, 39824–39844.

Rahman, A., Hossain, M. S., Muhammad, G., Kundu, D., Debnath, T., Rahman, M., & Band, S. S. (2023). Federated learning-based AI approaches in smart healthcare: concepts, taxonomies, challenges and open issues. *Cluster Computing*, 26(4), 2271–2311.

Rahman, S., & Rahman, M. Z. U. (2022). Blockchain framework for cognitive sensor network using non-cooperative game theory. *IEEE Access*, 10, 60114–60127.

Raja, B. S., & Asghar, S. (2020). Disease classification in health care systems with game theory approach. *IEEE Access*, 8, 83298–83311.

Sfar, A. R., Natalizio, E., Mazlout, S., Challal, Y., & Chtourou, Z. (2022). Privacy preservation using game theory in e-health application. *Journal of Information Security and Applications*, 66, 103158.

Sharma, S., & Guleria, K. (2023). A comprehensive review on federated learning based models for healthcare applications. *Artificial Intelligence in Medicine*, 146, 102691.

Subramanian, M., Rajasekar, V., Ve, S., Shanmugavadivel, K., & Nandhini, P. S. (2022). Effectiveness of decentralized federated learning algorithms in healthcare: a case study on cancer classification. *Electronics*, 11(24), 4117.

Surekha, S., & Rahman, M. Z. U. (2022). Blockchain framework for cognitive sensor network using non-cooperative game theory. *IEEE Access*, 10, 60114–60127.

Yaqoob, M. M., Nazir, M., Yousafzai, A., Khan, M. A., Shaikh, A. A., Algarni, A. D., & Elmannai, H. (2022). Modified artificial bee colony based feature optimized federated learning for heart disease diagnosis in healthcare. *Applied Sciences*, 12(23), 12080.

15 Practical Application
Case Studies in 6G Healthcare

Devansh Singhal, Ananya Singhal, Shikha Agarwal, Anil Chauhan, and Aarti Chaudhary

INTRODUCTION

Following the COVID-19 epidemic, healthcare has emerged as one of individuals' most crucial necessities. People are increasingly concerned about their health, leading to a greater reliance on the healthcare system. The healthcare business, like the rest of the world, must improve to keep up with the rapid rate of change and development. It needs to be more precise, rapid, and efficient. For years, the Internet of Things (IoT) has played an important role in reducing the burden on medical practitioners (Baker *et al.*, 2017), boosting the use of preventative care and therapy at home rather than relying on traditional reactive and facility-based techniques (Zhao *et al.*, 2017). As the population ages and the incidence of illnesses and outbreaks, such as COVID-19, increases, along with a growing number of people with long-term health concerns, the need for IoT in the medical field has significantly risen. However, this increasing demand raises the question of whether present technology can meet these demands. The most recent phase of cellular networks and related technologies may be key to resolving this challenge (Mucchi *et al.*, 2020).

We predict more automation as 6G technology progresses in the coming decade. Although 5G technology has not been fully established, certain issues have already surfaced. Consequently, relying on 6G is recommended. Technological innovation will continue to rise, and healthcare should be at the forefront of this revolution. 6G will enhance the usage of e-healthcare gadgets and technology that allow doctors to acquire real-time patient reports more precisely and quickly. 6G communication technology for healthcare demands high data speeds (≥ 1 Tbps), high operating frequencies (≥ 1 THz), low end-to-end latency (≤ 1 ms), high dependability (10-9), high mobility (≥ 1000 km/h), and a wavelength of less than 300 μm [5]. Reviewing current statistics, a report from Juniper Research found that the growth of AI-driven chatbots in healthcare will average 320% per annum. Statista predicts that the global healthcare AI market will approach a trillion dollars by 2030, with an average annual growth of three-quarters from 2022 to 2030 (Bhat & Alqahtani, 2021).

The usage of 6G technology has substantially benefited the biomedical and healthcare engineering fields. This technology is expected to revolutionise the industry efficiently, from remote activity surveillance to remote robotic surgery

DOI: 10.1201/9781003516590-15

(Nova et al., 2021). E-healthcare developed from a desire to enhance healthcare delivery. Its quick expansion has been fuelled by rising demand for improved services, perceived ease of use and usefulness, widespread availability of computing and telecommunications equipment, and rapid advancements in mobile networks.

E-healthcare services, which are accessed via cell phones, laptops, and other mobile devices, rely heavily on the communication network. As these services become more popular, the demand for fast and dependable networks will increase. This book chapter discusses numerous application cases for how 6G technology is helping to improve the healthcare industry. It also includes case studies that demonstrate the advantages of 6G technology in healthcare, such as Intelligent Wearable Devices (IWD), Telesurgery, and the use of Augmented Reality (AR) and Virtual Reality (VR) for Training. Additionally, it explores the potential of 6G technology to transform patient monitoring systems, allowing for continuous and more accurate tracking of vital signs and health metrics (S. Chen *et al.*, 2020).

These developments will allow healthcare providers to make more informed judgments and deliver better patient care. The use of 6G in healthcare is predicted to result in considerable improvements in treatment results, patient happiness, and overall efficiency. As we look to the future, 6G technology has the potential to completely transform the healthcare business, providing solutions to some of the most critical issues confronting both healthcare practitioners and patients.

LITERATURE SURVEY

This literature review delves into the wide-ranging potential applications and future developments of 6G technology, with a particular emphasis on its transformative effects in healthcare. The study "6G Technology Use Cases and Future Prospects" addresses the shortcomings of 5G and suggests improvements for applications such as VR, AR, unmanned mobility, Industry 4.0, and pervasive connectivity. Furthermore, "Practical Applications of 6G in Unmanned Mobility" explores how 6G can enhance transportation by improving the safety and efficiency of autonomous vehicles and drones (Table 15.1).

The study "Advanced Communication Techniques and Network Architectures for 6G" investigates how combining artificial intelligence (AI) and 6G may enhance network management and allow real-time decision-making, which is crucial for applications requiring high accuracy and low latency. Similarly, "6G Wireless Systems: Vision and Requirements" emphasises the need for faster data rates and reduced latency to allow multimodal extended reality (XR), connected robotics and autonomous systems (CRAS), and wireless brain–computer interfaces (BCI).

AI and machine learning (ML) are poised to revolutionise disease detection, diagnosis, and treatment within the healthcare sector. These technologies promise significant advancements (Joshi & Tiwari, 2023), enhancing patient care as outlined in discussions on AI and ML applications in healthcare.

The integration of federated learning (FL) and edge computing introduces innovative methods for privacy-preserving data processing and real-time applications such as telesurgery. These advancements are detailed in studies focusing on Federated Learning and Edge Computing.

TABLE 15.1

Literature Survey

Title of paper	Findings	Use cases
6G Technology Use Cases and Future Prospects	Provides an overview of potential uses and future advances in 6G technology. It examines the limitations of current 5G networks and proposes enhancements to meet future requirements.	Virtual Reality (VR), Augmented Reality (AR), Unmanned Mobility, Industry 4.0, Pervasive Connectivity
Practical Applications of 6G in Unmanned Mobility	The research focuses on the practical application of 6G technology in unmanned mobility. It gives detailed insights into how 6G can revolutionise the transportation industry by enhancing the safety and efficiency of autonomous vehicles and drones.	Unmanned mobility
Advanced Communication Techniques and Network Architectures for 6G	The research discusses the integration of AI for improved network management and real-time decision-making.	Communication techniques, Artificial Intelligence (AI)
6G Wireless Systems: Vision and Requirements	The implementation of 5G networks has demonstrated its limitations. These restrictions have prompted efforts to define the next-generation 6G wireless system. 6G is intended to incorporate applications such as autonomous systems and extended reality (XR). It will explore more high-frequency bands and converge with upcoming technological trends. Each use case discussed will need better performance metrics than 5G has greater data throughput and decreased latency. To provide immersive experiences, XR will require ultra-reliable low-latency communication (URLLC) and improved mobile broadband (eMBB). CRAS will necessitate low latency and high-quality (HD) map broadcasts.	Multisensory extended reality (XR), connected robotics and autonomous systems (CRAS), and wireless brain–computer interfaces (BCI).
AI and Machine Learning in Healthcare	AI and ML enhance the ability to detect, diagnose, and treat diseases with more accurate results. AI-driven chatbots are increasing in number helping in assisting patients and healthcare providers.	Artificial Intelligence (AI), Machine Learning (ML)
Federated Learning and Edge Computing	Federated learning (FL) and edge computing will transform healthcare. FL enables training machine learning models across decentralised devices while protecting data privacy, which is critical in healthcare. Edge computing brings data processing closer to where it is required, lowering latency and bandwidth use. This is critical for applications such as telesurgery, which need real-time data processing.	Edge Computing, Telesurgery

Title	Description	Keywords
6G-Enabled Internet of Things: Vision, Techniques, and Challenges (Shubham Gargrish et al., 2019)	The research provides an extensive overview of how 6G technology is expected to transform the Internet of Things (IoT). It focuses on the vision for 6G, the enabling techniques, and the challenges that need to be addressed.	Internet of Things (IoT)
DOCOMO 6G White Paper	The paper presents an in-depth exploration of 6G technology. It focuses on its envisioned use cases, technological advancements, and the potential benefits for society and various industries.	
A Comprehensive Survey on 6G Wireless Networks: Vision, Research Activities, Challenges, and the Road Ahead	This survey paper provides a detailed examination of the current state of 6G. It identifies key areas of focus, ongoing activities, and the challenges that lie ahead.	
Detecting Dangers in Medical Imaging Data Using 6G Wireless Sensor Networks and AI Technology	This study emphasises the significance of enhancing security standards in systems that analyse medical pictures, especially when used on 6G mobile networks. By highlighting FUZET's capability to eliminate security (Singh & Joshi, 2024) risks and safeguard essential healthcare information, It makes an important contribution to the continuing efforts to improve the security and dependability of medical imaging systems in the healthcare industry.	URLLC, Fuzzy Analytic Hierarchy Process (FAHP), and TOPSIS (Technique for Order Preference Based on Similarity to the Ideal Solution).
Remote Cardiac System Monitoring Using 6G IoT Communication and Deep Learning (Banga et al., 2024)	This study proposes a framework for remote cardiac monitoring by integrating 6G-IoT communication technology with deep learning algorithms. The ultra-reliable, low-latency capabilities of 6G-IoT facilitate the real-time transmission of high-fidelity cardiac data from wearable sensors to healthcare providers (Banga et al., 2024).	Internet of Things (IoT), Deep Learning (DL), Cardiac System Monitoring, URLLC
Smart Healthcare System Wi-Fi and a 6G fog network enable communication	This paper presents an innovative approach to privacy-preserving healthcare applications by integrating 6G and IoT devices with deep learning and fog computing technologies. The use of quantum federated regressive Bayes neural networks enhances data security and privacy, while the fog computing module ensures low-latency, real-time data processing.	Fog computing technologies, Internet of Things (IoT), Deep Learning (DL), Neural networks

Additionally, 6G technology holds promise in transforming the Internet of Things (IoT) landscape within healthcare. It is expected to enable real-time monitoring and management of patient data, enhancing the efficiency and effectiveness of healthcare services as highlighted in discussions on 6G-enabled IoT.

These technological innovations represent pivotal steps toward improving healthcare delivery, ensuring privacy, and advancing real-time medical applications in diverse healthcare settings.

Research such as "Detecting Dangers in Medical Imaging Data Using 6G Wireless Sensor Networks and AI Technology" and "Remote Cardiac System Monitoring Using 6G IoT Communication and Deep Learning" outlines frameworks for secure, real-time medical data transmission [28]. "Smart Healthcare System Wi-Fi and a 6G Fog Network Enable Communication" discusses the integration of 6G, IoT, deep learning, and fog computing for privacy-preserving healthcare applications, emphasising enhanced data security and low-latency processing. Overall, this review highlights the significant advancements that 6G technology will bring to healthcare and other fields, paving the way for more efficient, secure, and real-time applications.

CASE STUDIES

The case study highlights the diverse potential applications of 6G technology within the healthcare sector, emphasising its central role and various impactful areas. Intelligent Wearable Device (IWD) is a notable advancement, leveraging 6G for real-time health monitoring and data analysis, thereby enhancing patient care with continuous and accurate tracking of vital signs. Telesurgery represents another crucial application, with 6G's ultra-low latency and high reliability enabling remote surgeries, allowing surgeons to operate on patients from different locations with minimal delay and high precision.

AR and VR in healthcare are expected to gain significantly from 6G, providing high-resolution, immersive experiences for medical training, patient education, and rehabilitation. The advancement of unmanned mobility via 6G will increase the safety and efficiency of autonomous vehicles and drones, revolutionising healthcare logistics by assuring the speedy and dependable transportation of medical supplies. High Altitude Platform Stations (HAPS) will play an important role in delivering dependable connectivity to remote places, guaranteeing ongoing access to healthcare services and real-time data sharing.

6G-enabled Internet of Things (IoT) will enhance anomaly detection, allowing advanced networks to monitor health data and provide early warnings for potential health issues. Enhanced security protocols, such as fuzzy encryption, will protect sensitive health data, ensuring privacy and defence against cyber threats. The concept of Hospital-to-Home Service will see significant improvements with 6G, facilitating seamless transitions from hospital to home (H2H) care through connected health devices that enable continuous patient monitoring and support.

Using Deep Learning and Fog Computing with 6G technology will bring data processing closer to the source, reduce latency and enhance real-time decision-making capabilities. Additionally, enhanced remote monitoring systems supported by 6G will allow healthcare providers to track patient health more effectively and intervene

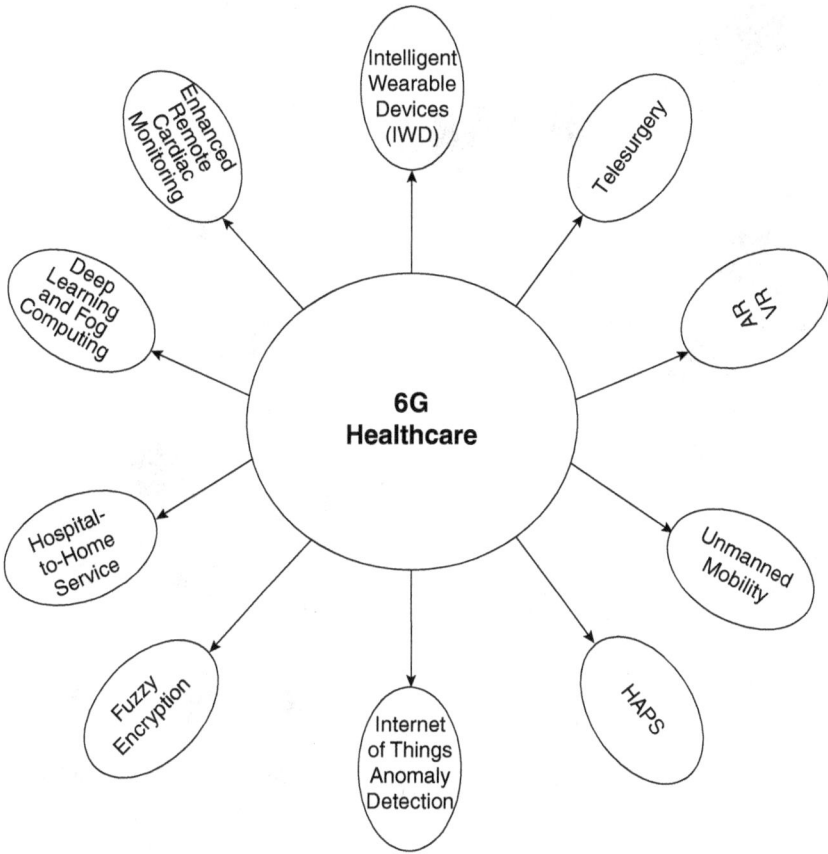

FIGURE 15.1 Case studies under healthcare.

promptly when necessary. In summary, this case study illustrates how 6G technology can revolutionise various aspects of healthcare, enhancing patient monitoring, remote care, data security, and connectivity in underserved regions (Figure 15.1).

INTELLIGENT WEARABLE DEVICES (IWD)

6G technology is set to revolutionise the healthcare sector by offering integrated smart health services. IWD equipped with advanced sensors and AI capabilities play a pivotal role. These devices continuously monitor vital signs and provide real-time data to healthcare providers. For instance, smart bandages can monitor wound healing progress and alert providers to infections. With 6G, these devices will transmit data instantly and reliably, enhancing the prediction of potential health issues or disease progression.

The implementation of 6G technology promises improved communication reliability, facilitates big data analytics, and strengthens the management of epidemics and pandemics in healthcare settings.

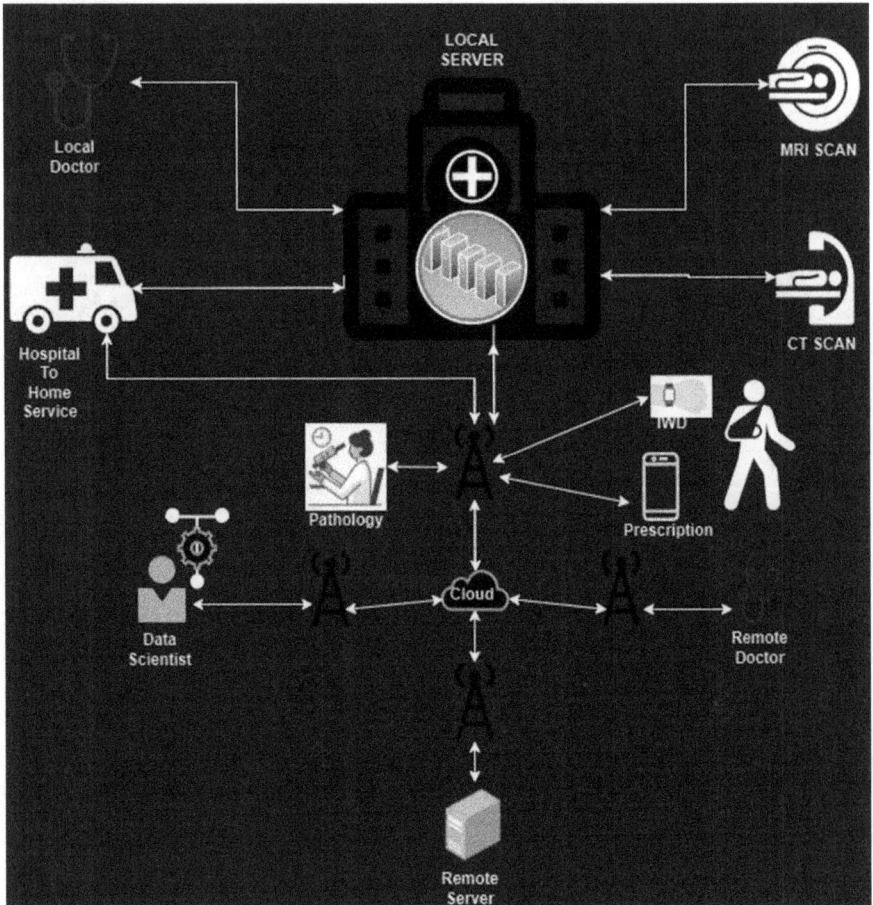

FIGURE 15.2   Data collection by wearable devices.

The technology works by integrating tangible items, detectors, and other components into a single network. Networked devices can communicate with one another to get critical information, explore data, and complete tasks (Chiuchisan et al., 2014; Chauhan et al., 2021). Cyber-physical IoT applications will benefit from using several devices to detect, control, and process models (Figure 15.2).

TELESURGERY

Telesurgery allows remote surgical procedures using robotic systems. 5G has made strides here, but limitations remain. 6G promises ultra-low latency and reliable connections. This will make telesurgery safer and more feasible. It will benefit rural and underserved areas by providing access to specialised surgical care. Surgeons can perform complex procedures remotely.

VIRTUAL REALITY (VR) AND AUGMENTED REALITY (AR) FOR TRAINING

The technology combines tangible items, detectors, and other components into a single system. AR makes actual items look more digital. It also has different sensory abilities, including hearing, seeing, touching, and feeling. AR combines real-time interaction with detailed 3D representations of both digital and physical objects. VR is a computer-created environment that does not exist. High data rates are required for high-quality services like streaming high-resolution movies.

While 5G triggered early adoption for AR/VR, these applications require a system capacity above 1 Tbps and per-user data rates in Gbps. The latency must be extremely low to enable real-time user interaction in the immersive environment (Zorzi *et al.*, 2020). This is fulfilled by 6G. AR and VR with 6G will transform healthcare training. They create immersive, realistic training environments. Medical students and surgeons can simulate complex procedures. This reduces surgical errors and improves healthcare quality. 6G will ensure smooth data transmission for uninterrupted training experiences.

The introduction of 6G technology will allow specialists to watch over those needing it via satellite. Holographic communication and AR can aid with diagnostic accuracy. Doctors may simulate surgery in VR without using persons who are real. It will be beneficial in dangerous, sophisticated operations or surgeries. All of these smart gadgets will have a 6G internet connection. AR and VR can be quite valuable in the healthcare field and have various benefits. This technique is used in MR for neurosurgery, oral and maxillofacial surgery, spine surgery, and other applications. AR and VR have the potential to significantly improve healthcare.

UNMANNED MOBILITY

Advanced capabilities are essential for intelligent automobiles to process information swiftly and make autonomous decisions. The emergence of 6G technology represents a transformative leap for autonomous driving systems, offering high data rates, ultra-low latency (below 1 ms), and exceptional reliability (above 99.99999%). These features are critical for ensuring the safe and efficient operation of autonomous vehicles.

6G's ability to support massive machine-type communications (mMTC) is particularly advantageous (Y. Taniguchi *et al.*, 2022), facilitating seamless communication among numerous sensors and devices within vehicles and infrastructure. This robust connectivity is vital for maintaining consistent performance, preventing accidents, and ensuring passenger safety in autonomous driving scenarios.

Furthermore, the high data rates provided by 6G will not only enhance safety protocols but also optimise traffic management and enrich infotainment systems. These technological advancements broaden the scope for applications such as faster emergency response times, thereby enhancing the overall efficiency and dependability of autonomous vehicle operations.

In conclusion, 6G technology is set to significantly enhance the capabilities of intelligent automobiles, ushering in an era of safer, more efficient, and interconnected autonomous driving experiences.

HIGH ALTITUDE PLATFORM SERVICE (HAPS)

HAPS, known as High Altitude Pseudo-Satellites, are unmanned aerial vehicles positioned in the stratosphere at an altitude of around 20 km. They are specifically designed to provide extensive coverage for communication networks. These platforms can cover wide areas, with a cell radius exceeding 50 km, and they also function as backhaul support for portable base stations.

A significant advantage of HAPS lies in its ability to extend communication services to remote and challenging terrains, including mountainous regions, oceans, and potentially even outer space in the future. The deployment of portable base stations that can seamlessly connect to HAPS enables the provision of timely communication solutions for temporary networks, whether in industrial settings or during large-scale events.

The integration of HAPS technology is crucial for facilitating immediate communication support during emergencies, thereby enhancing overall recovery efforts and emergency response capabilities. This capability ensures the maintenance of critical communication links, even in remote or inaccessible areas, significantly bolstering the resilience and effectiveness of communication networks across diverse operational scenarios.

INTERNET OF THINGS ANOMALY DETECTION

Virtual worlds, wearable technologies, and networked systems provide massive amounts of data for the health and fitness sectors. This surge is largely due to the rapid expansion of the metaverse. In this evolving landscape, it is crucial to protect the security and integrity of healthcare and fitness data. Uniqueness recognition serves as an essential tool for identifying variations from ordinary examples, ensuring security while enhancing the quality of care and execution (Zhu *et al.*, 2024).

The use of data fusion techniques allows for the integration of various data streams from different IoT devices and virtual environments. This integration offers a full view of information that is required for accurate identification of anomalies. Blockchain technology protects documents by keeping a visible and immutable record of all data transactions that occur. The implementation of Improved Isolation Forest (IIF) algorithms, optimised with Particle Swarm Optimization, enables real-time detection of anomalies. This is crucial for identifying and responding to abnormal patterns quickly, thereby maintaining the integrity and performance of the healthcare and fitness systems (Zhu *et al.*, 2024).

FUZZY ENCRYPTION FOR MEDICAL IMAGE DATA

A weak encryption method was developed to address security vulnerabilities associated with 6G wireless technology in healthcare image communications. This approach combines homomorphic encryption, the fuzzy analytical hierarchy process (FAHP), and the TOPSIS framework to assess solutions based on their closeness to an ideal solution. This integrated technique considerably enhances the security evaluation of 6G web-based systems that analyse medical picture data, protecting sensitive patient information while maintaining data integrity during transmission. The methodology enhances overall system resilience against potential cyber threats in the evolving digital healthcare landscape.

Fuzzy encryption is a combination of encryption and decision-making frameworks that ensures that the data remains encrypted during processing, thus maintaining confidentiality and integrity. The FAHP and TOPSIS framework improves security assessment by providing a structured decision-making approach to evaluate and prioritise any security risks.

The AI-assisted security risk identification using the XG boost algorithm utilises machine learning techniques to enhance the mitigation and identification of potential security risks. The same approach tested with AI assistance further improves the accuracy and efficiency of the security risk identification process.

The fuzzy analytical hierarchy process (FAHP) builds upon the analytical hierarchy process (AHP) by incorporating fuzzy logic. This allows FAHP to handle the inherent ambiguity and subjectivity that come with human decision-making. Instead of requiring precise numerical values, FAHP empowers decision-makers to utilise linguistic terms like "high," "medium," or "low." These terms are then translated into fuzzy numbers for analysis, enabling a more nuanced representation of human judgement.

TOPSIS is a multi-criteria decision-making method. This ideal solution embodies the best possible scenario across all considered criteria. By evaluating the distance of each alternative from this ideal, TOPSIS provides a systematic approach to ranking options in complex decision-making scenarios.

HOSPITAL-TO-HOME SERVICE

Ambulances are crucial in transporting individuals, ensuring oxygen supply, and maintaining road safety standards. However, current ambulance systems often lack advanced capabilities for efficient emergency response. There is an increasing demand for next-generation ambulances equipped with rapid response capabilities and AI-driven technology to evolve into intelligent vehicles of the future.

Emerging concepts like H2H (Hospital to Home) envision these intelligent vehicles as mobile hospitals. Utilising advanced AI and self-driving technology, H2H aims to reduce reliance on traditional healthcare services such as doctors and nurses. This concept operates similarly to ambulances but offers enhanced capabilities to deliver immediate medical care at accident scenes or during emergencies, potentially saving lives by providing critical treatment before patients reach hospitals.

The integration of 6G connectivity is crucial for H2H services, especially beneficial for elderly populations. This advanced communication technology facilitates seamless transmission of medical data, real-time diagnostics, and remote consultations, thereby improving the efficiency and effectiveness of mobile healthcare solutions.

In summary, the evolution towards AI-driven ambulances and mobile hospitals represents a significant advancement in emergency medical services. These innovations promise to expedite emergency responses and enhance healthcare outcomes, catering to critical situations more effectively.

ENHANCED REMOTE CARDIAC MONITORING

The emergence of 6G-IoT technology presents next-generation communication infrastructure that boasts URLLC data transmission, a critical feature for capturing real-time cardiac data. In life-threatening situations, it can help in immediate data transfer which can highly impact the patient's life (Banga *et al.*, 2024).

This technology uses 6G-IoT to transfer information from cutting-edge wearable sensors directly to medical care vendors. These sensors are specifically designed to capture high-fidelity cardiac signals, providing a detailed picture of a patient's heart function (Banga *et al.*, 2024).

Once received, the data undergoes analysis by a meticulously designed deep learning model. This model comprises a densely connected neural network optimised with a swish activation function (Banga *et al.*, 2024). Through extensive training on vast datasets, the model becomes adept at identifying patterns indicative of potential cardiac anomalies. This real-time analysis allows for immediate intervention when necessary, significantly improving upon traditional monitoring methods.

Furthermore, the integration of 6G-IoT communication guarantees the system's scalability and adaptability. This ensures seamless integration with future advancements in technology, fostering a robust solution for long-term remote cardiac monitoring.

ANOMALY DETECTION IN METAVERSE HEALTHCARE AND FITNESS DATA ANALYTICS

The rapid growth of the metaverse is generating a substantial volume of healthcare and fitness data, encompassing virtual environments, networked systems, and wearable technologies. Ensuring the security and integrity of this "big data" is critical for protecting patient privacy, increasing medical quality, and improving performance metrics. This paper presents a unique approach for detecting anomalies in metaverse healthcare and fitness data analytics using 6G IoT.

6G's ultra-low latency and high bandwidth facilitate real-time transmission and analysis of large datasets from diverse IoT devices integrated into virtual and fitness environments. This capability enables immediate identification of potential issues, promoting proactive healthcare and fitness management.

Effective anomaly detection relies on comprehensive, accurate datasets achieved through data fusion techniques. Integrating data streams from IoT devices provides a holistic view of patient health and fitness, enhancing the detection of anomalies that might otherwise be missed.

Given the sensitive nature of healthcare and fitness data, robust security measures are crucial. Blockchain technology ensures data integrity and traceability within the metaverse healthcare and fitness ecosystem, safeguarding against tampering and fostering trust.

This anomaly detection system is built around an optimised version of the Isolation Forest algorithm, bolstered by particle swarm optimization (PSO). This approach enables real-time anomaly detection in data streams, identifying deviations from normal patterns to flag potential health issues for early intervention and improved outcomes.

DEEP LEARNING AND FOG COMPUTING FOR PRIVACY-PRESERVING HEALTHCARE

The healthcare landscape is undergoing a transformative shift toward patient-centric care models dismantling any reliance on centralised hospital systems with the help of 6G networks. This evolution has made the healthcare network more robust and capable of managing the Instantaneous gathering and interpreting of huge amounts of patient information. A system proposed for the same leverages the synergistic capabilities of 6G communication infrastructure, Internet of Things (IoT) devices, and fog computing.

The system proposes body sensors designed for continuous health data monitoring. These seamlessly integrated IoT devices transmit the collected data to a geographically proximate fog computing unit. This approach minimises latency and communication overhead by processing the data at the network's edge and thus significantly reduces the amount of information requiring transmission to centralised servers.

The system incorporates a deep learning model for anomaly detection within healthcare data streams. This model is constructed upon the principles of quantum federated regressive Bayes neural networks, offering a robust framework for data security and privacy preservation. The federated learning approach ensures that patient data remains distributed across the network, mitigating the risk of unauthorised access. Additionally, the implementation of Bayesian neural networks empowers the model with the ability to continuously learn and adapt, enhancing its accuracy in anomaly detection over time.

HOSPITAL METAVERSE INTEGRATION (AHMAD *ET AL.*, 2024)

The integration of 6G technology to form a Hospital Metaverse will be the next big thing for the healthcare industry. This innovative approach envisions 6G supporting the entire patient care journey, from the initial emergency response through to rehabilitation.

6G enables us to eliminate time and space barriers within the hospital setting. Healthcare workflows will be optimised through improved communication, while massive connectivity empowers real-time data analytics, leading to better-informed decisions. Furthermore, 6G enhances mobility throughout hospitals. During emergencies and remote patient monitoring scenarios, seamless data transmission and situational awareness are ensured through the interconnectedness of patients, doctors, nurses, and medical equipment.

6G paves the way for large-scale metaverse implementation in healthcare. This technology facilitates the merging of the virtual and real worlds, creating a digital realm where patients and healthcare providers may communicate with computer-generated surroundings and other people in real time. This integration holds immense potential to address the challenges faced in remote healthcare settings where the physical presence of a healthcare professional might be limited.

The implementation of 6G in healthcare promises numerous benefits. Hospital processes are expected to become more streamlined, leading to improved quality of care and reduced costs. Additionally, 6G's focus on energy-efficient solutions aligns with the growing emphasis on sustainable practices within the healthcare sector. Given the sensitive nature of medical information, 6G networks are designed to ensure data stability and safety. Maintaining patient privacy and data security remains a critical aspect of any healthcare environment. Integrating stakeholder needs and existing healthcare regulations early in the research and development process is essential to prevent future roadblocks and ensure the successful implementation of 6G technology in healthcare.

THREATS AND ATTACKS IN 6G NETWORK

While 6G is still under development, it is vital to monitor for threats and assaults that might interrupt network operations. The following are some possible threats to the 6G network (Bakkiam David & Al-Turjman, 2022; Fischer, 2009). Malware, DDoS attacks, IoT botnets, spoofing attacks, rogue base stations, spoofing attacks, eaves-dropping, physical assaults, and man-in-the-middle (MITM) attacks are among the dangers. Malware, DDoS attacks, IoT botnets, spoofing attacks, rogue base stations, spoofing attacks, eavesdropping, physical assaults, and Man-in-the-Middle (MITM) attacks are among the dangers.

- **Malware**: Malware is expected to represent a significant threat to 6G networks, just as it does to existing mobile networks. Malware can acquire private information, interfere with network functionality, and cause network infrastructure damage.
- **DDoS Assaults**: DDoS assaults are a popular approach for disrupting network functionality. These assaults include several devices flooding a network with traffic, making normal traffic difficult, if not impossible, to get through.
- **Internet of Things (IoT) Networks**: The upcoming 6G networks are expected to handle a large number of IoT devices, which might be exposed to cyber assaults. These IoT gadgets could be utilised to form botnets that can execute Distributed Denial of Service (DDoS) attacks and various other types of attacks.

CONCLUSION AND FUTURE SCOPE

In today's rapidly changing world, people place a high value on their time. People want to save time by doing things swiftly. 6G is necessary to complete the assignment with precision and speed. The growth of 6G wireless technology favours the healthcare industry. This book chapter discusses case studies of 6G in the healthcare business, where we may utilise 6G to assist individuals improve their tasks and do them with more precision.

The case studies which are included in this book chapter are Intelligent Wearable Devices (IWD), Telesurgery, AR and VR for training, Unmanned Mobility, HAPS, Internet of thing Anomaly Detection, Hospital to Home service, and many other studies which can be enhanced under the development of 6G in healthcare.

The future for the 6G in healthcare is to build a strong and reliable network that provides more security (Kumar *et al.*, 2024) and gives better results. The future of 6G technology is brighter as the enhancing technology in the healthcare industry makes a huge impact on the health of the people. 6G technology can transform the medical sector by delivering ultra-fast dependable, and near-instant connectivity. Upcoming applications will range from high-precision remote procedures to cutting-edge tele-health sessions that combine real-life, virtual, and augmented worlds, as well as the deployment of AI-driven diagnostics and personalised treatment plans. Furthermore, 6G will accelerate the Internet of Medical Things (IoMT), allowing for continuous monitoring and real-time insights from devices worn or incorporated in the body. These advances will improve patient outcomes, promote preventive health habits, and increase access to high-quality medical treatment, particularly in distant and underserved areas.

BIBLIOGRAPHY

Ahmad, I., Ahmad, I., & Harjula, E. (2024). Adaptive security in 6G for sustainable health-care. In: Särestöniemi, M., et al. *Digital Health and Wireless Solutions. NCDHWS 2024. Communications in Computer and Information Science*, vol 2083. Springer, Cham. https://doi.org/10.1007/978-3-031-59080-1_3

Alawadhi, A., Almogahed, A., Mohammed, F., Ba-Quttayyan, B., & Hussein, A. (2024). Improving performance metrics in WBANs with a dynamic next beacon interval and superframe duration scheme. *Heliyon*, 10, 5, e26468.

Baker, S. B., Xiang, W., & Atkinson, I. (2017). Internet of things for smart healthcare: Technologies, challenges, and opportunities. *IEEE Access* 5, 26521–26544.

Bakkiam David, D., & Al-Turjman, F. (2022). Synonym-based multi-keyword ranked search with secure k-NN in 6G network. *IET Networks* 2022, 1–12.

Banga, A. S., Alenazi, M. M., Innab, N., Alohali, M., Alhomayani, F. M., Algarni, M. H., & Saidani, T. (2024). Remote cardiac system monitoring using 6G-IoT communication and deep learning. *Wireless Personal Communications*, 1–20.

Bhat, J. R., & Alqahtani, S. A. (2021). 6G ecosystem: Current status and 697 future perspec-tive, *IEEE Access*, 9, 43134–43167, doi: 10.1109/ACCESS.2021.3054833

Chauhan, S., Arora, R., & Arora, N. Researcher issues and future directions in healthcare using IoT and machine learning. In *Smart healthcare monitoring using IoT with 5G*, Ist., G. C. Meenu Gupta and V. H. C. de Albuquerque, Eds. Boca Raton, London, New York: CRC Press, Taylor and Francis Group, 2021, pp. 177–196.

Chen, S., Liang, Y., Sun, S., Kang, S., Cheng, W., & Peng, M. Vision, requirements, and tech-nology trend of 6g: How to tackle the challenges of system coverage, capacity, user data-rate and movement speed. *IEEE Wireless Communications*, 2020, 1–11.

Chen, Z., Ma, X., Zhang, B., Zhang, Y., Niu, Z., Kuang, N., et al. (2019). A survey on terahertz communications. *China Communications*, 16(2), 1–35.

Chiuchisan, I., Costin, H., & Geman O. (2014) Adopting the Internet of things technologies in healthcare systems. In: *2014 International Conference and exposition on Electrical and power engineering (EPE)*, pp 532–535.

Fischer, E. A. (2009). *Creating a National Framework for Cybersecurity: An Analysis of Issues and Options*; Nova Science Publishers: Hauppauge, NY.

Gargrish, S., Chauhan, S., Gupta, M., & Obaid, A. J. (2019). *6G Enabled IoT Wearable Devices for Elderly Healthcare.*

Hosseinzadeh, M., Hemmati, A., & Rahmani, A. M. 2022. *6G-Enabled Internet of Things: Vision, Techniques, and Open Issues.*

Joshi, A., & Tiwari, H. (2023). An overview of python libraries for data science. *Journal of Engineering Technology and Applied Physics*, 5(2), 85–90. https://doi.org/10.33093/jetap.2023.5.2.10

Kharche, S., & Kharche, J. (2023). 6G intelligent healthcare framework: A review on role of technologies, challenges and future directions, *Journal of Mobile Multimedia* 19(3), 603–644.

Kumar, R., Joshi, A., Sharan, H. O., Peng, S. L., & Dudhagara, C. R. (Eds.). (2024). *The Ethical Frontier of AI and Data Analysis*. IGI Global.

Li, C., Zhang, Z., & Xiao, H. (2024). Medical Image Data Security Risk Identification Based on 6G Wireless Sensor Networks and AI-Assisted Technology. Wireless Personal Communications, 1–19.

Li, J., & Li, J. (2024). Wireless Communication Based Smart Healthcare System Through 6G Fog Network. Wireless Personal Communication.

Mucchi, L. Jayousi, S. Caputo, S. Paoletti, E. Zoppi, P.; Geli, S.; Dioniso, P. How 6G Technology Can Change the Future Wireless Healthcare. In *Proceedings of the 2020 2nd 6G Wireless Summit (6G SUMMIT)*, Levi, Finland, 17–20 March 2020; pp. 1–6.

Nayak, S., & Patgiri, R. (2021). 6G communication technology: A vision on intelligent healthcare. In *Health informatics: A computational perspective in healthcare* (pp. 1–18). Singapore: Springer Singapore.

Nova, S. N., Rahman, M. S., & Chakraborty, C. (2021). "Patient's health surveil- 779 lance model using IoT and 6G technology," in *Green Technological 780 Innovation for Sustainable Smart Societies*, C. Chakraborty, Ed. Springer: Cham, Switzerland, pp. 191–209.

Porambage, P., Gur, G., Osorio, D. P. M., Liyanage, Madhusanka, Ylianttila, Mika, 6G Security Challenges and Potential Solutions, The 2021 Joint EuCNC & 6G Summit, Porto, Portugal (held online due to Coronavirus outbreak), 8–11 June 2021.

Saeed, M. M., Saeed, R. A., Abdelhaq, M., Alsaqour, R., Hasan, M. K., & Mokhtar, R. A. (2023). Anomaly detection in 6G networks using machine learning methods. *Electronics* 12(15), 3300.

Singh, B. P., & Joshi, A. (2024). Ethical considerations in AI development. In *The Ethical Frontier of AI and Data Analysis* 156–179. IGI Global.

Taha, B. B. A., Samson, R., Steponenaite, A., Ansari, S., Langdon, P. M., Wassell, I. J., Abbasi, Q. H., Imran, M. A., & Keates, S. (2021). 6G opportunities arising from the internet of things use cases: A review paper. *Future Internet* 13(6), 159.

Taniguchi, Y., Ikegami, Y., Fujikawa, H., Pathare, Y., Kutics, A., Massimo, B. et al. (2022). Counseling (ro)bot as a use case for 5G/6G, Complex & Intelligent Systems.

Zhao, W., Luo, X., & Qiu, T. (2017). Smart healthcare. *Applied Sciences* 7, 3–7.

Zhu, K. T., Wu, Y., Yang, R., & Yuan, Q. (2024). Anomaly detection in metaverse healthcare and fitness: Bigdata analytics using 6G-enabled internets of things. *Wireless Personal Communications*, 1–20.

Zorzi, Giordani, Polese, M., Mezzavilla, M., & Rangan, S. M. (2020, March). Toward 6G networks: Use cases and technologies. *IEEE Communications Magazine* 58(3), 55–61.

16 Proximal Femur Fracture Detection Using Deep Learning

Ruhi Gedam, Tarun Bhardwaj, Vibha Bora, Sushil Mankar, Vijay Surve, and Sharda Chhabria

INTRODUCTION

Femoral fractures, particularly among the elderly, present substantial challenges in clinical diagnosis and treatment. Accurate detection and classification of these fractures are pivotal for effective patient management and outcome optimization (Wang Shuai, et al. 2019). With the advancements in artificial intelligence (AI) and medical imaging technologies, there arises a significant opportunity to improve the diagnostic process through automated systems. In this context, this research endeavours to develop a sophisticated approach utilizing AI techniques, specifically employing the YOLOv8 model, for the detection and classification of femoral fractures.

The You Only Look Once version 8 (YOLOv8) model has garnered attention for its remarkable capabilities in object detection tasks. By adapting this model to femoral fracture detection, this study aims to enhance the accuracy, efficiency, and reliability of fracture identification in radiographic images. Leveraging the YOLOv8 model's architecture, which enables real-time inference with high accuracy, holds promise for transforming the diagnostic workflow in orthopaedic radiology.

However, manual interpretation of radiographic images for fracture detection is time-consuming and can be prone to human error. With the advent of artificial intelligence (AI) and its integration with medical imaging technologies, there exists a promising opportunity to revolutionize the diagnostic process through automated systems.

Through this research, we aim to address the pressing need for more robust and automated fracture detection systems in clinical practice. By harnessing AI technology, we anticipate significant advancements in the timely diagnosis and classification of femoral fractures, ultimately leading to improved patient care and outcomes. This chapter outlines the methodology, experimental setup, and expected contributions of utilizing the YOLOv8 model in femoral fracture detection and classification.

The primary challenge in diagnosing hip fractures lies in the variability of radiographic presentations and the potential for human error. Inexperienced clinicians may overlook subtle fractures, leading to delayed treatment and poorer patient

DOI: 10.1201/9781003516590-16

267

outcomes. Given the high incidence and severe consequences of missed hip fractures, there is an urgent need for solutions that enhance diagnostic accuracy and reliability.

In collaboration with N. K. P. Salve Institute of Medical Sciences & Research Centre and Lata Mangeshkar Hospital, Nagpur, this research aims to develop a sophisticated AI-based approach for the detection and classification of proximal femoral fractures using X-ray images. The research methodology involves the utilization of the You Only Look Once version 8 (YOLOv8) algorithm, renowned for its exceptional capabilities in object detection tasks. The YOLOv8 model will be adapted and trained on a dataset comprising X-ray images of patients with confirmed proximal femoral fractures, ensuring robust performance in fracture identification (Table 16.1).

The difference between fractured and healthy femur is shown in Figure 16.1.

DATA IMPLEMENTATION

- **Data Acquisition**: The dataset employed in this study was sourced from N. K. P. Salve Institute of Medical Sciences & Research Centre and Lata Mangeshkar Hospital, located on Hingna Road, Nagpur. This comprehensive collection comprises both normal and femoral fracture X-rays, making it a robust resource for training and validating AI models designed for fracture detection. Specifically, the dataset includes a total of 203 X-ray images, of which 130 depict femoral fractures and 73 are normal images without fractures.

  The balanced representation of normal and fractured femoral X-rays within this dataset is pivotal for developing a reliable AI diagnostic tool. The presence of both types of images ensures that the AI model can learn to distinguish between healthy and pathological conditions, enhancing its diagnostic accuracy and generalization capabilities.
- **Data Annotation**: The acquired dataset was annotated using the Roboflow platform, where each X-ray image was meticulously labelled using the polygon tool to delineate the regions corresponding to femoral fractures (Figure 16.2).

Before initiating the model training phase, a comprehensive data pre-processing pipeline was implemented to enhance the quality and suitability of the X-ray images for subsequent analysis (Figure 16.3). The pre-processing steps were meticulously designed to address common issues in medical imaging data, such as variability in image orientation, size, and contrast. These steps are crucial to ensure that the AI models receive consistent and high-quality input data, thereby improving their performance and reliability.

STEPS IN DATA PRE-PROCESSING

- **Automatic Orientation Correction**: X-ray images often come with varying orientations due to differences in how they are captured. Automatic orientation correction algorithms were applied to standardize the orientation of all images. This ensures that anatomical structures are consistently positioned, facilitating more effective feature extraction by AI models.

TABLE 16.1
Literature Review

Paper name	Model (algorithm) used	Dataset	Findings	Accuracy
"Artificial Intelligence (AI) vs. Human in hip fracture detection," "Helion.2022.e11366, Thailand (2022)"	YOLOv4	1000 Images	Through comparative studies against human experts, we observed that AI algorithms can match or even surpass human performance in detecting these fractures. Moreover, AI systems provide consistent accuracy in their diagnoses, eliminating variability caused by factors like fatigue or varying levels of experience among human practitioners. AI models may struggle with generalization, as they may not perform optimally across different patient populations or clinical settings.	95%
"Validation and Algorithmic audit of a deep learning system for the detection of proximal femoral fractures in patients in the emergency department: a diagnostic accuracy study," Lancet Digital Health 2022; 4:e351–58, Australia (2022)	Deep Learning	200 Images	In our investigation, we discovered that the deep learning system shows remarkable accuracy in detecting proximal femoral fractures among patients arriving at the emergency department, indicating its potential as a valuable diagnostic aid. The deep learning system offers swift and automated interpretation of medical images, potentially streamlining the fracture detection process compared to manual assessment by radiologists. Human oversight and validation are essential to ensure the reliability, safety, and clinical relevance of the deep learning system's diagnostic results, emphasizing the need for ongoing monitoring and evaluation.	

(Continued)

TABLE 13.1 (Continued)

Paper name	Model (algorithm) used	Dataset	Findings	Accuracy
"Artificial Intelligence for Hip Fracture Detection and Outcome Prediction: A Systematic Review and Meta-analysis." JAMA Network Open 2023; 6(3):e233391 (2023)	DenseNet-121 Architecture	627 images	By summarizing findings from various studies, the aim is to provide a clear picture of AI's diagnostic accuracy in identifying hip fractures and its ability to predict patient outcomes like mortality, morbidity, or functional recovery. This review approach allows us to compile evidence from multiple studies, giving clinicians, researchers, and policymakers a thorough understanding of AI's potential in hip fracture management. Despite its strengths, our meta-analysis may face challenges due to variations in study quality and design, which could affect the reliability and applicability of our findings.	85%
"Deep Learning for image-based detection of femoral fracture." International Journal of Computer Assisted Radiology and Surgery 14.9 (2019)	CNN, ResNet-18 with CBRAM	4189 images	The study delves into the use of advanced deep learning techniques for automatically detecting femoral fractures from medical imaging data, such as X-rays or CT scans. The anticipated findings are those that evaluate the algorithm's diagnostic accuracy, sensitivity, specificity, and its performance compared to traditional diagnostic methods or assessments made by human experts. By harnessing deep learning algorithms, we anticipate improvements in fracture detection sensitivity and specificity compared to conventional methods, potentially leading to more precise diagnoses and reduced instances of missed fractures. There are some concerns about generalization to real-world clinical settings arise due to the lack of external validation or testing on independent datasets, highlighting the need to ensure algorithm robustness and reliability across different clinical environments	92%

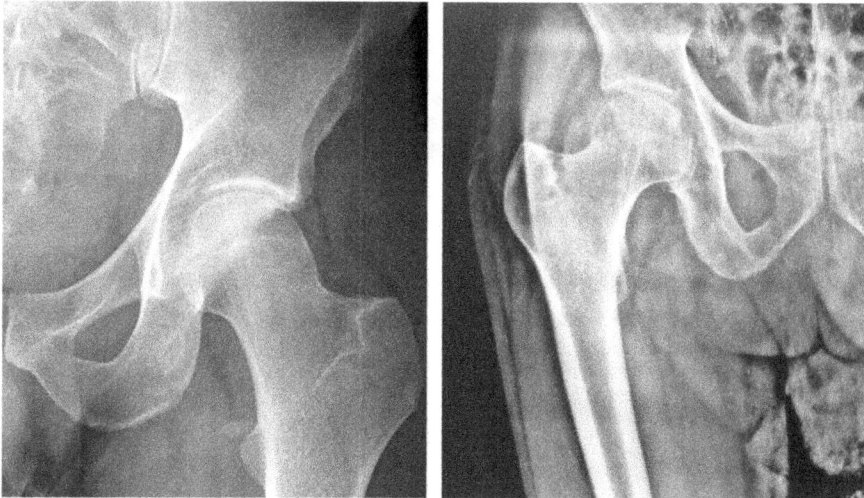

FIGURE 16.1   X-ray image of femur: (L) normal; (R) fractured.

Courtesy: N.K.P. Salve Institute of Medical Sciences & Research Centre and Lata Mangeshkar Hospital.

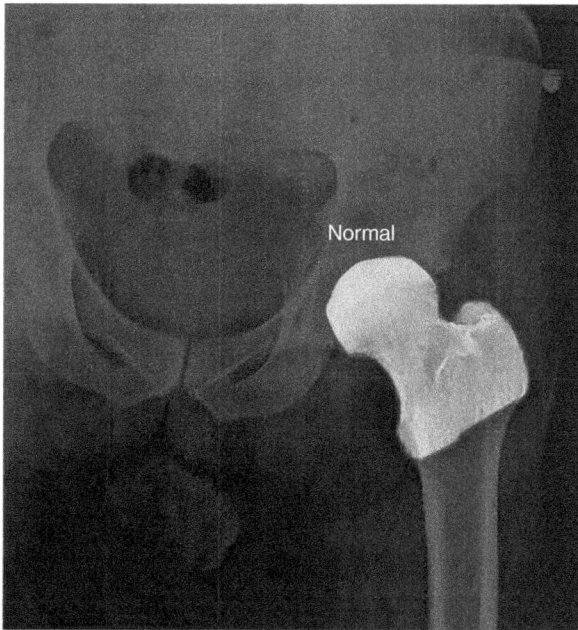

FIGURE 16.2   Example of annotated femur X-ray image (normal).

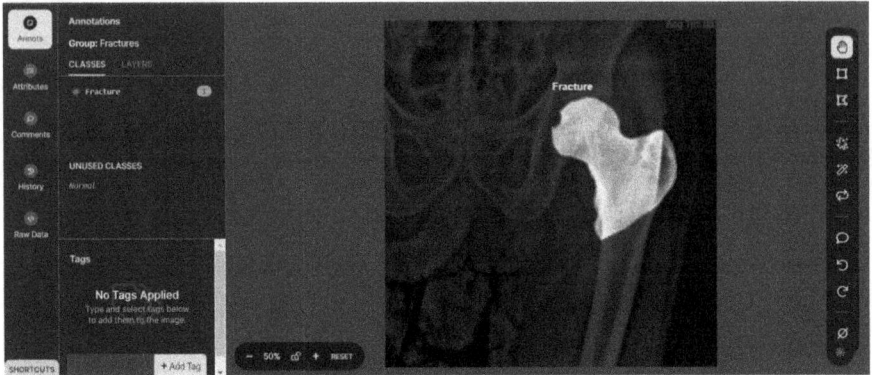

FIGURE 16.3 Example of annotated femur X-ray image (fracture).

- **Resizing to Standardized Resolution**: To ensure uniformity across the dataset, all images were resized to a standardized resolution of 640 × 640 pixels. This step involved stretching the images to fit this resolution, which balances the trade-off between maintaining detail and ensuring manageable computational load. Standardized image size is critical for batch processing and ensures that the input dimensions to the AI models remain consistent.
- **Contrast Adjustments Using Histogram Equalization Method**: Histogram Equalization was employed to automatically adjust the contrast of the images. This technique redistributes the intensity values of the pixels to enhance the overall contrast of the image. By doing so, it makes subtle features more visible and improves image clarity. This adjustment is particularly important in medical imaging where the visibility of fine details can significantly impact diagnostic accuracy.

Data Augmentation

To enhance the dataset and improve the generalization capabilities of the AI model, data augmentation techniques were systematically applied. Data augmentation involves creating modified versions of the original images to simulate a broader range of imaging conditions and anatomical orientations. This process helps to prevent over fitting, where the model performs well on the training data but poorly on unseen data.

The following augmentation methods were employed:

- **Cropping**: Cropping was performed with a minimum zoom level of 0% and a maximum zoom level of 20%. This means that up to 20% of the image's edges could be cropped, creating variations that help the model learn to recognize femoral fractures from partial views or different zoom levels.

- **Rotation**: Images were rotated randomly within a range of $-11°$ to $+11°$. This small rotation range was chosen to reflect realistic variations that could occur in clinical practice without excessively distorting the anatomical structures.

METHODOLOGY

MODEL SELECTION

Deep Learning model identified hip fractures with more accuracy For femoral fracture detection in medical imaging, the YOLOv8 model was chosen for its efficiency, accuracy, customization options, community support, and clinical relevance. Its single-stage architecture, computational efficiency, and high precision make it ideal for real-time detection tasks, crucial for timely diagnosis and clinical decision-making.

Before considering YOLOv8, the model was trained on YOLOv4. However, we found that:

- YOLOv4 is a more complex model compared to YOLOv8, which can lead to increased computational requirements during training and inference.
- YOLOv8 may offer enhanced speed and efficiency compared to YOLOv4, particularly in real-time object detection scenarios.
- YOLOv8 may have lower resource requirements, including memory and computational power, compared to YOLOv4. This can be advantageous in scenarios where hardware resources are limited or where efficient utilization of resources is a priority.

MODEL SPECIFICATION

In this study, we employed the YOLOv8 model to train a femoral fracture detection system using a dataset augmented to 767 images from an initial 203 images. We create training, validation and test sets The augmented dataset was then divided as 92% training, 5% validation, and 3% training to ensure robust model evaluation (Table 16.2).

TABLE 16.2
Dataset Specifications

Measure	Value
Actual no. of femoral X-ray images	203
No. of fractured femur images	130
No. of normal femur images	73
No. of images after augmentation	767
No. of images used in training	705
No. of images used in validation	36
No. of images used in testing	26

To facilitate model training in a cloud-based environment, notably Google Colab, installation of essential packages including Roboflow and Ultralytics was done. Subsequently, a new directory named 'dataset' was created in the home directory, where the augmented and pre-processed dataset was exported as a code snippet. This snippet facilitated seamless access to the dataset during model training.

- For the training phase, YOLOv8 was employed with the specified task='detect' and mode='train'. The model was trained for 250 epochs, and an image size of 640 was selected to ensure optimal detection performance.
- During validation, the model's performance was assessed using the task='detect' and mode='val'. The best weights obtained from the trained model were utilized to evaluate its accuracy and robustness.
- Finally, for prediction tasks, the trained model was deployed with the task='detect' and mode='predict'. The best weights obtained from model training were employed to make predictions on new unseen data.

IMPLEMENTATION

MODEL TRAINING

The training phase employed the YOLOv8 model, specifically tailored for the task of detecting femoral fractures. The following steps outline the training process in detail:

- **Task**: The task parameter was set to 'detect', indicating that the objective was object detection.
- **Mode**: The mode parameter was set to 'train', initiating the training phase.
- **Epochs**: The model was trained for 250 epochs, allowing ample time for the model to learn from the dataset and optimize its detection capabilities.
- **Image Size**: An image size of 640 pixels was chosen. This resolution was selected to balance the need for detailed feature detection and computational efficiency.

During the training phase, the model learned to identify and classify femoral fractures from the X-ray images. The training process involved optimizing the model's weights through back propagation and gradient descent, iterating over the dataset multiple times (epochs) to minimize the detection error.

PROCEDURE

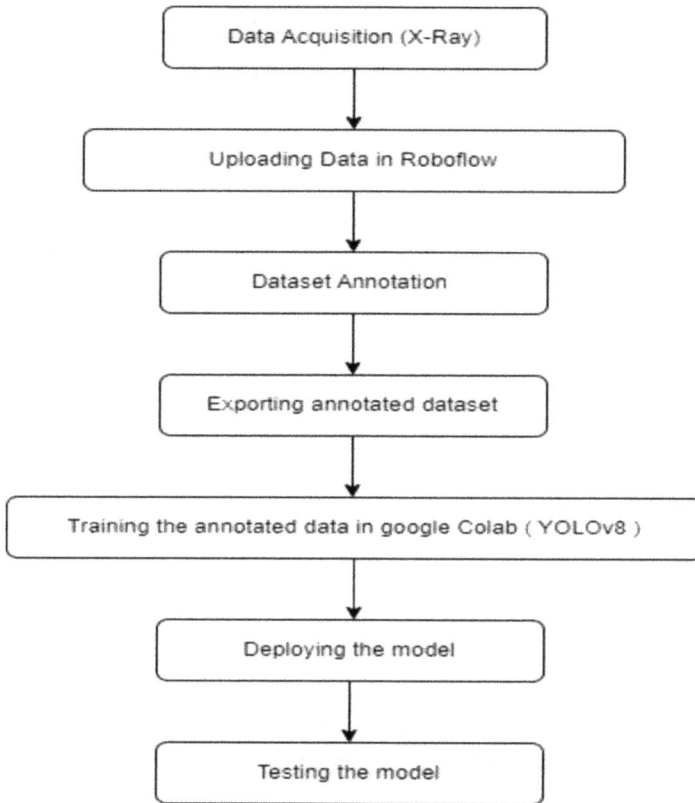

FIGURE 16.4   Flowchart of the work done.

MODEL DEPLOYMENT

Following the completion of the training phase, the femoral fracture detection model was seamlessly deployed onto the Roboflow platform. Roboflow provides a robust and accessible framework that facilitates the integration, testing, and evaluation of AI models in real-world scenarios.

Platform Integration

- The deployment process involved uploading the trained model to Roboflow, a platform known for its ease of use and comprehensive tools for computer vision projects.
- The deployment was streamlined through Roboflow's user-friendly interface, which supports various machine learning frameworks and models, including those trained using YOLOv8.

Model Hosting

- Roboflow offers cloud-based hosting for AI models, ensuring that the femoral fracture detection model is readily accessible for testing and inference. This cloud hosting eliminates the need for local infrastructure, reducing maintenance overhead and facilitating scalable deployment.

TESTING AND EVALUATION

Post-deployment, the model's performance was rigorously tested and evaluated using new X-ray images. This step is crucial for validating the model's efficacy and reliability in clinical settings.

Real-World Data Testing

- The deployed model was tested on a diverse set of new X-ray images to simulate real-world conditions. These images were not part of the original training or validation datasets, ensuring an unbiased assessment of the model's performance.
- The testing process involved running the model on these images and evaluating its ability to accurately detect femoral fractures.

Performance Metrics

- The model's efficacy was evaluated using key performance metrics, including accuracy, precision, recall, and F1 score. These metrics provide a comprehensive understanding of the model's detection capabilities and robustness.
- Precision measures the proportion of true positive detections among all positive detections made by the model, while recall assesses the proportion of true positives detected out of all actual positive cases. The F1 score, a harmonic mean of precision and recall, provides a balanced measure of the model's performance.

Evaluation Tools

- For evaluating model performance, offering visualizations and detailed reports that help in understanding the model's strengths and weaknesses.

CONCLUSION

Following the completion of the training phase, the deployed femoral fracture detection model underwent comprehensive testing on X-ray images that were distinct from those included in the training dataset. This testing phase aimed to assess the model's performance in identifying femoral fractures in real-world scenarios. A total of 15 unique X-ray images were carefully selected for this evaluation, ensuring a diverse representation of clinical cases and imaging conditions commonly encountered in medical practice.

TABLE 16.3
Model Analysis

Measure	Value (%)
mAP	92.3
Precision rate	83.6
Recall rate	86.6

During the testing process, the model exhibited remarkable accuracy, successfully detecting femoral fractures in 14 out of the 15 evaluated images. This high success rate underscores the robustness and effectiveness of the trained model in accurately identifying fractures from X-ray imagery. Notably, the sole misidentification observed was attributed to subtle differences in contrast and brightness levels present within one of the images, highlighting the model's sensitivity to variations in imaging parameters.

Quantitative analysis of the model's performance yielded noteworthy metrics, further affirming its efficacy in femoral fracture detection (Table 16.3).

These results underscore the potential clinical utility of the deployed model, suggesting its viability as a valuable tool for aiding orthopaedic diagnosis and treatment planning in medical practice (Figure 16.5).

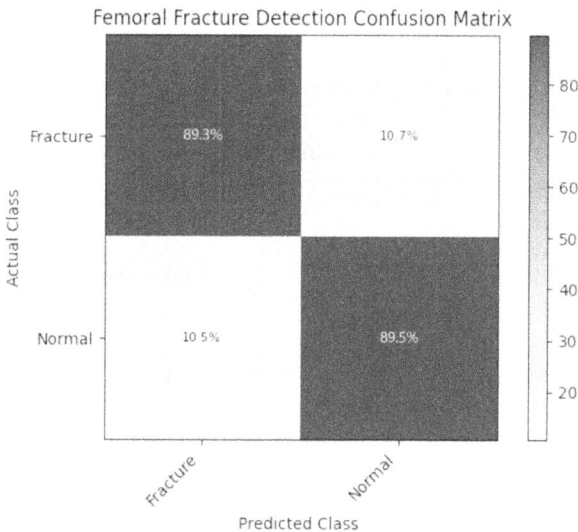

FIGURE 16.5 Confusion matrix of the deployed YOLOv8 model for proximal femur fracture detection.

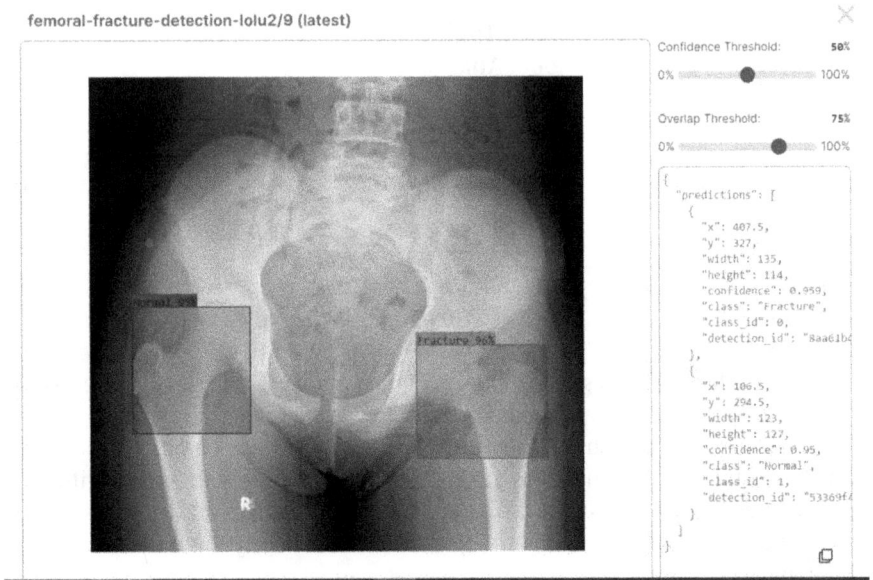

femoral-fracture-detection-Iolu2/9 (latest)

Confidence Threshold: 50%

0% ▬▬▬▬●▬▬▬▬ 100%

Overlap Threshold: 75%

0% ▬▬▬▬▬▬●▬▬ 100%

```
{
  "predictions": [
    {
      "x": 407.5,
      "y": 327,
      "width": 135,
      "height": 114,
      "confidence": 0.959,
      "class": "Fracture",
      "class_id": 0,
      "detection_id": "8aa61b6
    },
    {
      "x": 106.5,
      "y": 294.5,
      "width": 123,
      "height": 127,
      "confidence": 0.95,
      "class": "Normal",
      "class_id": 1,
      "detection_id": "53369f6
    }
  ]
}
```

FIGURE 16.6   Example 1 of an X-ray image being tested in the trained deployed model.

FINDINGS

Despite its impressive performance, the deployed femoral fracture detection model showed sensitivity to slight variations in contrast and brightness levels within X-ray images, hindering prediction accuracy. This limitation highlights the need for enhanced robustness and adaptability in medical imaging AI systems, especially in real-world clinical settings.

While the model exhibited high overall accuracy, occasional misidentifications underscore the necessity for further refinement to improve resilience to imaging variations. Additionally, external factors such as imaging equipment and patient demographics may influence model performance, necessitating ongoing optimization efforts for maximized clinical utility (Figures 16.6 and 16.7).

FUTURE SCOPE

After the successful identification of proximal femoral fractures with the YOLOv8 algorithm, the next step is to make the process even more refined. We want to teach our AI model to not just spot fractures, but to also categorize them into two important types: neck fractures and intertrochanteric fractures. This categorization is crucial because it helps doctors plan treatments tailored to each fracture type, ensuring the best possible care for patients. Our upcoming research will focus on fine-tuning the AI model's ability to tell these fractures apart using advanced techniques and a diverse range of X-ray images. The only challenge of utilizing AI in medicine is that physicians are reluctant to trust something they do not fully understand (Smith et al. 2022).

femoral-fracture-detection-lolu2/11 (latest)

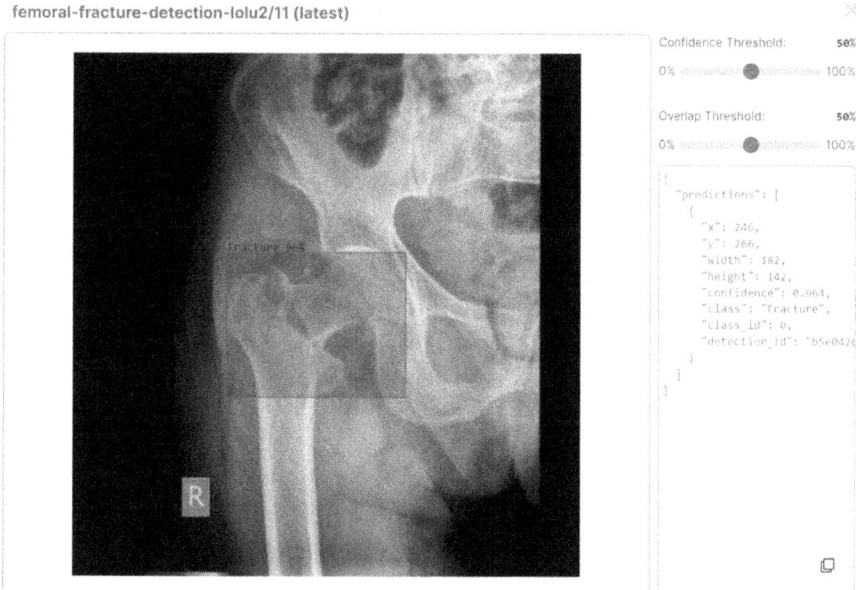

FIGURE 16.7 Example 2 of an X-ray image being tested in the trained deployed model.

Then, the model will go through intensive training sessions, tweaking its algorithms to become even better at recognizing the unique characteristics of each fracture type. After training, we'll rigorously test the model's accuracy using various X-ray images, seeking feedback from orthopaedic experts to ensure its practical usefulness in real-world medical settings. Ultimately, our goal is to develop an AI system that not only detects fractures but also helps doctors make more informed decisions, leading to improved care and outcomes for patients.

BIBLIOGRAPHY

Krogue, JD, Cheng, KV, Hwang, KM, Toogood, P, Meinberg, EG, Geiger, EJ, Zaid, M, McGill, KC, Patel, R, Sohn, JH, Wright, A, Darger, BF, Padrez, KA, Ozhinsky, E, Majumdar, S, Pedoia, V. (2020). Automatic hip fracture identification and functional subclassification with deep learning. *Radiology. Artificial Intelligence*, 2(2), e190023. https://doi.org/10.1148/ryai.2020190023

Lex JR, Michele JD, Koucheki R, Pincus D, Whyne C, Ravi B. (2023). Artificial intelligence for hip fracture detection and outcome prediction: A systematic review and meta-analysis. *JAMA Network Open* 6(3):e233391.

Oakden-Rayner L, Dunnmon J, Carneiro G, Ré C. (2020). Hidden stratification causes clinically meaningful failures in machine learning for medical imaging. *Proc ACM Conf Health Inference Learn.*

Oakden-Rayner L, Gale W, Bonham TA, Lungren MP, Carneiro G, Bradley AP, Palmer L. (2022). Validation and Algorithmic audit of a deep learning system for the detection of proximal femoral fractures in patients in the emergency department: A diagnostic accuracy study, *Lancet Digital Health 4*, e351–58.

Poon, AIF, Sung, JJY. (2021). Opening the black box of AI-medicine. *Journal of Gastroenterology and Hepatology*, *36*(3), 581–584. https://doi.org/10.1111/jgh.15384.

Raji ID, Smart A, White RN, et al. (2020). Closing the AI accountability gap: Defining an end-to-end framework for internal algorithmic auditing. In: *Proceedings of the 2020 Conference on Fairness, Accountability, and Transparency*. New York, NY: Association for Computing Machinery.

Smith NT, Boonrod A, Boonrod A, Chindaprasirt J, Sirithhanaphol W, Chindaprasirt P, Twinprai P. (2022). Artificial Intelligence (AI) vs. Human in hip fracture detection. *Helion 2022*:e11366.

Wang S, et al. (2019). Deep Learning for image-based detection of femoral fracture. *International Journal of Computer Assisted Radiology and Surgery 14*, 9.

Yu, JS, Yu, SM, Erdal, BS, Demirer, M, Gupta, V, Bigelow, M, Salvador, A, Rink, T, Lenobel, SS, Prevedello, LM, & White, RD. (2020). Detection and localisation of hip fractures on anteroposterior radiographs with artificial intelligence: Proof of concept. *Clinical Radiology*, *75*(3), 237.e1–237.e9. https://doi.org/10.1016/j.crad.2019.10.022

17 Exploring Non-Fungible Tokens (NFTs)

Concepts, Applications, and Implications

Manisha Deep Andola and Deep Chandra Andola

INTRODUCTION

In recent years, Non-Fungible Tokens (NFTs) have emerged as a disruptive force in the digital landscape, captivating the attention of creators, collectors, investors, and technologists alike. Unlike cryptocurrencies such as Bitcoin or Ethereum, which are fungible and interchangeable, NFTs represent unique digital assets that cannot be replicated or substituted. Built on Blockchain technology, NFTs leverage smart contracts to certify ownership, authenticity, and provenance, ushering in a new paradigm of digital ownership and commerce. In the ever-evolving landscape of digital technology, NFTs have emerged as a revolutionary innovation with profound implications across various sectors. These unique cryptographic tokens, built on Blockchain technology, have redefined notions of ownership, authenticity, and value in the digital age.

The concept of digital ownership has evolved significantly over the past few decades. Initially, digital assets were easily replicable and lacked a concrete method of establishing true ownership. This was particularly problematic in industries such as digital art and music, where creators struggled to maintain control and monetize their works. The advent of Blockchain technology provided a solution to this issue through the use of decentralized ledgers and smart contracts, which ensure transparency, security, and immutability of transactions.

This chapter aims to provide a comprehensive exploration of NFTs, spanning their underlying concepts, diverse applications, economic implications, legal considerations, environmental impact, and societal ramifications. By examining the technical foundations of NFTs, elucidating their practical applications across industries, and critically assessing the opportunities and challenges they entail, this paper seeks to illuminate the multifaceted landscape of NFTs and its implications for technology, economics, and society. The advent of NFTs has democratized creative expression and ownership, empowering artists, musicians, and content creators to tokenize their work and engage directly with global audiences without relying on intermediaries.

This direct relationship between creators and consumers has reshaped industries like art, gaming, entertainment, and beyond, fostering new economic models and revenue streams.

The introduction of NFTs can be traced back to the development of the Ethereum Blockchain and the creation of the ERC-721 standard in 2017. This standard allowed developers to create tokens that are distinct from one another, each with unique properties and metadata. The popularization of NFTs began with projects like Crypto Kitties, which showcased the potential for unique digital collectibles. Since then, the NFT market has expanded exponentially, encompassing a wide range of applications from digital art and music to virtual real estate and beyond.

The NFT market has experienced rapid growth, attracting attention from artists, celebrities, investors, and major corporations. High-profile sales, such as Beeple's "Every days: The First 5000 Days" auctioned by Christie's for $69 million, have highlighted the economic potential of NFTs. Additionally, major platforms like OpenSea, Rarible, and Foundation have facilitated the creation and exchange of NFTs, further driving their adoption.

BRIEF HISTORY AND EVOLUTION OF NFTs

NFTs have revolutionized the digital landscape, reshaping how we perceive ownership, value, and the nature of digital assets. The journey of NFTs is intertwined with the broader evolution of Blockchain technology, highlighting significant milestones that have paved the way for their current prominence. This narrative explores the history, development, and multifaceted applications of NFTs, along with their societal and economic implications.

EARLY DAYS OF DIGITAL OWNERSHIP AND BLOCK CHAIN FOUNDATIONS

The concept of digital ownership precedes the advent of Blockchain technology. In the early days of the internet, digital assets were easily replicable, posing challenges for establishing verifiable ownership. The emergence of Blockchain technology, particularly Bit coin in 2009, introduced the concept of decentralized, immutable ledgers. This breakthrough laid the foundation for creating unique digital assets that could be securely owned and transferred.

The introduction of Ethereum in 2015 marked a pivotal moment in Blockchain evolution. Ethereum's smart contracts enabled programmable, self-executing agreements, expanding the possibilities for Blockchain applications. It was within this environment that NFTs began to take shape, offering a solution to the long-standing issue of digital asset uniqueness.

BIRTH AND EARLY DEVELOPMENT OF NFTs

The concept of NFTs was formally introduced with the launch of the ERC-721 token standard on the Ethereum Blockchain in 2017. ERC-721 enabled the creation of unique, indivisible tokens that could represent ownership of specific digital or physical assets. The pioneering project Crypto Kitties, launched in late 2017, showcased the potential of NFTs by allowing users to buy, sell, and breed unique digital cats. The game's popularity highlighted the novelty and value of digital scarcity, attracting widespread attention and demonstrating the viability of NFTs as a new asset class.

Following Crypto Kitties, the NFT ecosystem began to expand rapidly. Various platforms and projects emerged, exploring diverse applications ranging from digital art and collectibles to virtual real estate and gaming assets. Notable early projects included Decentraland, a virtual world where users could buy and develop land parcels, and Axie Infinity, a Blockchain-based game featuring unique creatures known as Axies.

MAINSTREAM ADOPTION AND MARKET EXPANSION

The year 2020 marked a significant turning point for NFTs, as mainstream interest and adoption surged. High-profile artists, musicians, and celebrities began exploring NFTs as a new medium for creative expression and monetization. The sale of digital art pieces by artists like Beeple, whose artwork "Every days: The First 5000 Days" sold for $69.3 million at Christie's auction, brought NFTs into the spotlight and showcased their potential to revolutionize the art world.

NFT marketplaces like OpenSea, Rarible, and Foundation gained traction, providing platforms for creators and collectors to trade digital assets. These marketplaces facilitated the growth of a vibrant NFT ecosystem, attracting a diverse range of creators, including visual artists, musicians, writers, and game developers. The unique attributes of NFTs, such as provenance tracking, verifiable ownership, and royalties for creators, offered new opportunities for artists to monetize their work and connect with their audiences.

TECHNOLOGICAL ADVANCEMENTS AND INNOVATION

As the NFT space evolved, technological advancements and innovations continued to shape its trajectory. Layer 2 scaling solutions, such as Polygon (formerly Matic), emerged to address the scalability and high transaction costs associated with Ethereum. These solutions enabled faster and cheaper transactions, making NFTs more accessible to a broader audience.

Interoperability between different Blockchain networks also became a focal point. Projects like Flow, developed by Dapper Labs, aimed to create specialized Blockchains optimized for NFTs and gaming applications. Flow's success with NBA (National Basketball Association) Top Shot, a platform for trading officially licensed NBA collectible highlights, demonstrated the potential for NFTs to engage mainstream audiences through familiar and popular content.

The development of NFT standards beyond ERC-721, such as ERC-1155, introduced the concept of semi-fungible tokens, allowing for the creation of both unique and fungible assets within a single contract. This flexibility opened up new possibilities for gaming, virtual goods, and other applications that require a mix of asset types.

SOCIETAL AND ECONOMIC IMPLICATIONS

The rise of NFTs has sparked significant discussions about their societal and economic implications. On one hand, NFTs have democratized access to creative markets, enabling artists and creators from diverse backgrounds to reach global audiences without traditional gatekeepers. This shift has the potential to redefine the economics of art and entertainment, empowering creators to retain greater control over their work and earnings.

However, the rapid growth of the NFT market has also raised concerns about environmental sustainability. The energy consumption associated with Blockchain transactions, particularly on proof-of-work (PoW) networks like Ethereum, has drawn criticism for its environmental impact. Efforts to address these concerns include the transition to Ethereum 2.0, which aims to implement a more energy-efficient proof-of-stake (PoS) consensus mechanism, and the adoption of eco-friendly Blockchains like Tezos.

LEGAL AND REGULATORY CHALLENGES

The rise of NFTs has also brought about a range of legal and regulatory challenges. Issues related to intellectual property (IP) rights, copyright infringement, and fraud have emerged as the market has grown. Cases of unauthorized minting and selling of digital assets have raised questions about the enforceability of digital ownership and the need for robust legal frameworks to protect creators and consumers.

Regulatory bodies around the world are grappling with how to classify and regulate NFTs. The intersection of NFTs with securities, taxation, and anti-money laundering (AML) laws presents complex challenges that require nuanced approaches. As the legal landscape evolves, stakeholders in the NFT space must navigate these challenges to ensure the sustainable and responsible growth of the market.

FUTURE PROSPECTS

Looking ahead, the future of NFTs holds immense potential for innovation and transformation. The convergence of NFTs with emerging technologies like virtual reality (VR), augmented reality (AR), and artificial intelligence (AI) promises to unlock new dimensions of digital experiences and interactions (Joshi & Tiwari, 2023). Virtual worlds and metaverses, where NFTs serve as the building blocks of digital economies, are poised to become integral parts of our digital lives.

The continued evolution of NFTs will likely see increased integration with traditional industries, such as fashion, real estate, and entertainment. Brands and businesses are exploring how NFTs can enhance customer engagement, loyalty, and brand experiences. As NFTs become more mainstream, their applications will extend beyond collectibles and art, encompassing a wide array of use cases that leverage their unique properties.

- **Importance and Relevance in the Digital Age**: NFTs have quickly become a significant innovation in the digital age, transforming how we perceive ownership, value, and authenticity in the digital realm. Their importance and relevance are underscored by several key factors that highlight their potential to reshape various industries and societal norms.

- **Redefining Digital Ownership**: In the digital age, the concept of ownership has been inherently challenging due to the ease of copying and distributing digital content. NFTs address this issue by providing a verifiable and immutable proof of ownership for digital assets. Each NFT is unique and cannot be replicated, ensuring that the owner possesses a distinct, original item. This shift in how ownership is defined and verified is particularly important for artists, creators, and collectors who seek to establish and maintain the provenance of their work.

- **Empowering Creators and Artists**: NFTs offer a new paradigm for creators and artists to monetize their work. By tokenizing their creations, artists can sell digital art, music, videos, and other content directly to consumers without the need for intermediaries. This direct-to-consumer model allows creators to retain a larger share of the revenue and maintain control over their IP. Additionally, smart contracts can be programmed to include royalties, ensuring that artists receive a percentage of sales whenever their NFTs are resold in the secondary market, providing ongoing revenue streams.

- **Expanding Digital Collectibles and Virtual Goods**: The popularity of NFTs has given rise to a burgeoning market for digital collectibles and virtual goods. From digital trading cards and virtual real estate to in-game items and fashion, NFTs enable the creation and exchange of unique digital assets that hold value for collectors and enthusiasts. This trend is particularly relevant in the context of virtual worlds and the metaverse, where digital identity and ownership of virtual assets are becoming increasingly important.

- **Enhancing Transparency and Security**: NFTs leverage Blockchain technology, which ensures transparency and security in transactions. Each NFT transaction is recorded on a decentralized ledger, providing a tamper-proof history of ownership and transfers. This transparency is crucial for establishing trust in digital marketplaces, reducing the risk of fraud, and ensuring the authenticity of digital assets. As a result, NFTs have the potential to enhance security and trust in various industries, from art and entertainment to real estate and finance.

- **Creating New Economic Opportunities**: The rise of NFTs has created new economic opportunities for individuals and businesses. NFT marketplaces, platforms, and related services have emerged, generating new revenue streams and employment opportunities. Additionally, NFTs have attracted significant investment and speculation, with high-profile sales and auctions driving interest and engagement. This economic impact extends to various sectors, including gaming, entertainment, sports, and even education, where NFTs can be used to represent achievements and credentials.

- **Promoting Digital Inclusion and Accessibility**: NFTs have the potential to promote digital inclusion by providing a platform for underrepresented and emerging artists to showcase and sell their work on a global stage. The decentralized nature of Blockchain technology ensures that anyone with internet access can participate in the NFT market, regardless of geographic location or socioeconomic status. This democratization of access can help bridge the digital divide and provide opportunities for diverse voices to be heard and valued.

- **Addressing Intellectual Property and Licensing**: NFTs offer a novel approach to managing IP and licensing in the digital age. By tokenizing IP assets, creators and rights holders can more effectively control and monetize their work. NFTs can also facilitate the licensing process, enabling automated and transparent enforcement of usage rights through smart contracts. This capability is particularly relevant for industries such as music, film, and publishing, where IP management is critical.
- **Contributing to the Development of the Metaverse**: The concept of the metaverse, a collective virtual shared space, is gaining traction, and NFTs play a crucial role in its development. In the metaverse, NFTs represent ownership of virtual land, assets, and experiences, enabling users to build, trade, and interact in immersive digital environments. The integration of NFTs in the metaverse enhances the sense of ownership and investment, driving engagement and innovation in virtual worlds.

The importance and relevance of NFTs in the digital age cannot be overstated. They represent a transformative innovation that redefines ownership, empowers creators, enhances transparency, and creates new economic opportunities. As the digital landscape continues to evolve, NFTs are poised to play a central role in shaping the future of digital content, commerce, and community. While challenges and controversies remain, the potential benefits of NFTs make them a critical area of focus for researchers, businesses, and policymakers alike.

TECHNICAL UNDERPINNINGS OF NFTs

NFTs are a revolutionary innovation built upon the robust and intricate framework of Blockchain technology. The technical underpinnings of NFTs involve various components, including Blockchain protocols, smart contracts, token standards, and cryptographic principles. Understanding these foundational elements is crucial for appreciating the mechanisms that enable NFTs to function as unique, verifiable digital assets. This narrative delves into the technical aspects of NFTs, elucidating the technologies and protocols that underpin their creation, management, and utility.

BLOCK CHAIN TECHNOLOGY: THE FOUNDATION OF NFTs

At the core of NFTs lies Blockchain technology, a decentralized and immutable ledger system. Unlike traditional databases, Blockchains are distributed across numerous nodes, ensuring transparency, security, and resistance to tampering. Each transaction on a Blockchain is recorded in a block, which is then linked to the previous block, forming a chain of blocks—hence the name "Blockchain." This structure ensures that once data is added, it cannot be altered or deleted, providing a reliable history of ownership and transactions.

The Ethereum Blockchain is the most widely used platform for NFTs, primarily due to its support for smart contracts. However, other Blockchains such as Binance Smart Chain, Flow, and Tezos are also gaining traction for NFT applications. Each Blockchain has its unique features, consensus mechanisms, and ecosystem, influencing the efficiency, scalability, and cost of NFT transactions.

SMART CONTRACTS: SELF-EXECUTING AGREEMENTS

Smart contracts are self-executing agreements with the terms directly written into code. They run on Blockchain networks and automatically enforce the rules and conditions set by the contract without the need for intermediaries. Smart contracts are pivotal to NFTs as they define the uniqueness, ownership, and transferability of the tokens.

The Ethereum Blockchain introduced the concept of smart contracts, enabling the development of decentralized applications (dApps) and complex automated systems. In the context of NFTs, smart contracts manage the creation (minting), ownership, and transfer of tokens. They ensure that each NFT is unique and cannot be replicated, embodying the concept of digital scarcity.

TOKEN STANDARDS: ERC-721 AND BEYOND

Token standards are predefined rules and protocols that govern how tokens behave on a Blockchain. The most notable standard for NFTs is ERC-721, introduced on the Ethereum Blockchain in 2017. ERC-721 tokens are unique and indivisible, meaning each token has distinct properties and cannot be exchanged on a one-to-one basis with another token.

The ERC-721 standard specifies a set of functions that allow for the creation, transfer, and tracking of NFTs. These functions include mint (to create a new NFT), transfer from (to transfer ownership), and token URI (Uniform Resource Identifier) (to store metadata associated with the NFT). The metadata typically includes information such as the token's name, description, and a link to the digital asset it represents.

While ERC-721 is the most widely used standard, other standards have emerged to address specific needs and improve functionality. ERC-1155, for example, allows for the creation of both fungible and NFTs within a single contract, enabling more efficient batch transfers and reduced transaction costs. This standard is particularly useful for gaming applications where different types of assets (e.g., in-game currency and unique items) need to coexist.

CRYPTOGRAPHIC PRINCIPLES: ENSURING SECURITY AND AUTHENTICITY

Cryptographic principles are fundamental to the security and authenticity of NFTs. Public-key cryptography, in particular, plays a crucial role in ensuring that only the rightful owner of an NFT can transfer or sell it. Each participant in the Blockchain network has a pair of cryptographic keys: a public key (which acts as an address) and a private key (which is used to sign transactions).

When an NFT is minted, a unique identifier is created and associated with the owner's public key. To transfer the NFT, the owner must use their private key to sign the transaction, which is then broadcast to the network and validated by nodes. This process ensures that ownership and transactions are secure, verifiable, and resistant to fraud.

Additionally, cryptographic hashing algorithms are used to link the metadata and digital assets associated with NFTs to the Blockchain (Joshi & Goyal, 2019). A hash function takes an input (e.g., a file or piece of data) and produces a fixed-size string of characters, which serves as a unique digital fingerprint. This hash is included in the token's metadata, ensuring that any changes to the associated digital asset can be easily detected.

DECENTRALIZED STORAGE SOLUTIONS

One of the challenges with NFTs is the storage of the digital assets they represent. Storing large files directly on the Blockchain is impractical due to limitations in storage capacity and cost. Instead, decentralized storage solutions like the InterPlanetary File System (IPFS) are used.

IPFS is a peer-to-peer network that enables the storage and sharing of files in a distributed manner. When a file is uploaded to IPFS, it is divided into smaller chunks, each of which is cryptographically hashed and stored across multiple nodes. The resulting hash (known as a content identifier (CID)) is unique to that file and can be used to retrieve it. By including the CID in the NFT's metadata, it ensures that the digital asset is accessible and tamper-proof, even if it is not stored directly on the Blockchain.

INTEROPERABILITY AND CROSS-CHAIN SOLUTIONS

As the NFT ecosystem expands, interoperability between different Blockchains has become increasingly important. Cross-chain solutions enable NFTs to be transferred and utilized across multiple Blockchain networks, enhancing their utility and accessibility.

Projects like Polkadot, Cosmos, and Wanchain are working on interoperability protocols that facilitate seamless communication and asset transfers between different Blockchains. Additionally, initiatives like Wrapped NFTs (WNFTs) allow NFTs from one Blockchain to be represented and traded on another, broadening the scope of NFT applications and markets.

SCALABILITY SOLUTIONS

Scalability is a significant challenge for Blockchain networks, especially those handling a high volume of NFT transactions. High gas fees and slow transaction times on the Ethereum network, for instance, have prompted the development of layer 2 scaling solutions and alternative Blockchains.

Layer 2 solutions like Polygon (formerly Matic) and Optimistic Rollups aim to alleviate congestion by processing transactions off the main Ethereum chain and then settling them in batches. These solutions significantly reduce transaction costs and improve throughput, making NFTs more accessible to a broader audience.

Alternative Blockchains such as Binance Smart Chain, Flow, and Tezos offer different consensus mechanisms and architectures designed to handle higher transaction volumes more efficiently. These Blockchains provide additional options for developers and users seeking scalable and cost-effective platforms for NFT projects.

FUTURE PROSPECTS

The technical underpinnings of NFTs are complex and multifaceted, involving a blend of Blockchain technology, smart contracts, token standards, cryptographic principles, decentralized storage, interoperability solutions, and scalability strategies. Together, these components create a robust framework that enables the creation, management, and utilization of unique digital assets.

As the NFT ecosystem continues to evolve, ongoing advancements in technology and infrastructure will likely address current limitations and unlock new possibilities. The integration of NFTs with emerging technologies such as VR, AR, and AI promises to enhance digital experiences and interactions further.

Thus, the technical foundation of NFTs is a testament to the ingenuity and innovation within the Blockchain space. By understanding the mechanisms that underpin NFTs, we can better appreciate their potential to transform various industries and redefine the concept of digital ownership and value. As the technology matures, NFTs are poised to play an increasingly integral role in the digital economy, offering new opportunities for creators, consumers, and businesses alike.

CHARACTERISTICS OF NFTs

NFTs possess unique characteristics that distinguish them from other digital assets and cryptocurrencies. These characteristics are the foundation of their functionality and utility in various applications.

Uniqueness: Each NFT is unique, meaning that no two NFTs are identical. This uniqueness is ensured through metadata that distinguishes one NFT from another. This characteristic is crucial for digital art, collectibles, and other assets where individuality and distinctiveness are valuable.

Indivisibility: Unlike cryptocurrencies such as Bitcoin or Ethereum, which can be divided into smaller units (satoshis or wei), NFTs are indivisible. They exist as whole items, and their value cannot be split into smaller parts. This indivisibility reinforces the concept of owning a complete, unique item.

Provenance and Ownership: NFTs provide a verifiable record of ownership and provenance. Each transaction involving an NFT is recorded on the Blockchain, creating a transparent and tamper-proof history of the asset. This feature is particularly important for art and collectibles, as it ensures the authenticity and origin of the item.

Interoperability: NFTs can be designed to be interoperable across different platforms and ecosystems. For instance, an NFT created on one Blockchain platform can be used or traded on another, provided there is compatibility. This interoperability enhances the flexibility and utility of NFTs, allowing them to be integrated into various applications and virtual environments.

Programmability: NFTs can incorporate programmable features through smart contracts. These smart contracts automate actions such as royalty payments to creators, transfer of ownership, and other conditions specified at the time of creation. This programmability adds a layer of functionality and innovation, enabling complex interactions and transactions.

Scarcity: Scarcity is a key characteristic that adds value to NFTs. Creators can set a limited supply of a particular NFT, ensuring its rarity. This scarcity drives demand and can increase the perceived and market value of the asset. Limited edition NFTs or one-of-a-kind digital art pieces leverage this characteristic to attract collectors.

Transferability: NFTs are easily transferable between parties. Ownership can be transferred through Blockchain transactions, making it straightforward to buy, sell, or trade NFTs. This transferability is facilitated by decentralized marketplaces and platforms that support NFT transactions.

Digital Representation of Physical Assets: NFTs can represent both digital and physical assets. While most commonly associated with digital art and collectibles, NFTs can also be used to tokenize physical items such as real estate, luxury goods, and event tickets. This digital representation can simplify the buying, selling, and tracking of physical assets.

Composability: NFTs exhibit composability, meaning they can be combined or integrated with other NFTs and digital assets. This characteristic allows for the creation of more complex and interactive digital experiences. For example, in gaming, multiple NFTs can be combined to create new in-game items or experiences.

Decentralization: NFTs operate on decentralized Blockchain networks, eliminating the need for intermediaries. This decentralization ensures that transactions are secure, transparent, and resistant to censorship or manipulation. It also enables global access and participation, broadening the market for NFTs.

The unique characteristics of NFTs—uniqueness, indivisibility, provenance, interoperability, programmability, scarcity, transferability, digital representation, composability, and decentralization—form the foundation of their utility and appeal. These features not only distinguish NFTs from traditional digital assets but also open up a wide range of possibilities for their application across various industries, from art and entertainment to real estate and beyond. Understanding these characteristics is essential for appreciating the transformative potential of NFTs in the digital age.

APPLICATIONS OF NFTs

NFTs have diverse applications across various industries and sectors, leveraging their unique properties and Blockchain technology. Here's an exploration of some key applications of NFTs:

- **Digital Art**: NFTs have revolutionized the art world by providing a way for digital artists to monetize their work. Artists can create, sell, and trade digital art pieces as NFTs, ensuring that each piece is unique and verifiable on the Blockchain. This has opened up new revenue streams and global exposure for artists.
- **Collectibles**: NFTs are widely used for digital collectibles, such as trading cards, virtual pets, and other unique items. Platforms like CryptoKitties and NBA Top Shot have popularized this use case, allowing users to buy, sell, and trade limited-edition collectibles.
- **In-Game Items**: NFTs can represent unique in-game items, such as weapons, skins, or virtual land. These items can be traded or sold within the game or on external marketplaces, providing players with real-world value for their digital assets.
- **Virtual Real Estate**: In virtual worlds and metaverses, NFTs are used to represent ownership of virtual land and properties. Platforms like Decentraland and The Sandbox allow users to buy, develop, and trade virtual real estate using NFTs.
- **Intellectual Property and Licensing**: NFTs can represent ownership and licensing rights for IP, such as music, videos, and written content. By tokenizing these assets, creators can maintain control over their work, automate royalty payments, and simplify the licensing process.
- **Real Estate**: NFTs can be used to tokenize physical real estate, representing ownership or shares in a property. This can simplify transactions, reduce fraud, and enable fractional ownership, making real estate investment more accessible.
- **Tokenized Assets**: Beyond real estate, NFTs can represent ownership of other physical assets, such as luxury goods, cars, and art. Tokenization allows for easier transfer and trade of these assets while ensuring authenticity and provenance.
- **Music**: Musicians can use NFTs to sell their music directly to fans, offering exclusive content, album releases, and concert tickets. NFTs can also automate royalty payments, ensuring that artists receive fair compensation for their work.
- **Entertainment**: NFTs are being used in the entertainment industry to create unique fan experiences, such as VIP (Very Important Person) access, behind-the-scenes content, and collectible memorabilia. This allows fans to engage with their favourite artists and creators in new and meaningful ways.
- **Digital Identity**: NFTs can represent digital identities, providing a secure and verifiable way to manage personal information. This can be used for authentication, access control, and identity verification in various online services.
- **Certification and Credentials**: NFTs can be used to issue and verify digital certificates and credentials, such as diplomas, professional licenses, and achievements. This ensures that certifications are tamper-proof and easily verifiable.

- **Virtual Fashion**: NFTs are being used to create and sell virtual fashion items, such as clothing and accessories for avatars in virtual worlds. This allows designers to explore new creative possibilities and reach a global audience.
- **Physical Fashion**: Fashion brands are using NFTs to represent ownership of physical items, offering unique digital counterparts to physical products. This can enhance the customer experience and provide added value through exclusive digital content.
- **Sports Memorabilia**: Sports teams and athletes are using NFTs to create and sell digital memorabilia, such as trading cards, highlights, and collectibles. This provides fans with a new way to engage with their favourite teams and players.
- **Fan Tokens**: Fan tokens, often issued as NFTs, give fans a stake in their favourite teams or events. These tokens can provide access to exclusive content, voting rights, and other perks, fostering a closer connection between fans and their favourite sports organizations.
- **Philanthropy and Social Impact**: NFTs are being used to raise funds for charitable causes and social impact initiatives. By auctioning unique digital assets, organizations can attract donations and support for various projects, ensuring transparency and accountability through Blockchain technology.

The applications of NFTs are vast and continually evolving, driven by their unique properties and the innovative potential they offer across different sectors. From digital art and gaming to real estate and identity verification, NFTs are reshaping how we interact with and value digital and physical assets. As the technology and market mature, we can expect even more creative and impactful uses of NFTs in the future.

ECONOMIC CONSIDERATIONS OF NFT

The rise of NFTs has significant economic implications, impacting various aspects of digital and physical markets. This section explores the key economic considerations associated with NFTs, including their market dynamics, valuation, investment potential, and broader economic impact.

- **Market Growth**: The NFT market has experienced explosive growth, driven by high-profile sales, increased adoption by creators and collectors, and the expansion of NFT platforms. This growth has led to substantial market capitalization, with billions of dollars traded in NFT marketplaces.
- **Volatility**: The NFT market is characterized by high volatility, with significant fluctuations in the prices of NFTs. Factors such as market sentiment, media coverage, and technological advancements can influence NFT values, leading to rapid changes in market conditions.
- **Liquidity**: Liquidity in the NFT market varies widely. While some NFTs, especially those from well-known artists or popular collections, can be highly liquid and easily tradable, others may have limited liquidity, making it challenging for owners to sell their assets quickly.

- **Determinants of Value**: The value of an NFT is influenced by several factors, including rarity, demand, historical significance, and the reputation of the creator. Unlike fungible assets, the value of an NFT is often subjective and can vary significantly based on buyer preferences and market trends.
- **Speculation and Bubbles**: The rapid appreciation of certain NFTs has led to speculative behaviour, with investors buying NFTs in the hope of reselling them at higher prices. This speculation can create market bubbles, where prices are driven to unsustainable levels, followed by sharp corrections.
- **Diversification**: NFTs offer a new asset class for investors, providing opportunities for portfolio diversification. Investing in NFTs allows exposure to the digital art, collectibles, gaming, and virtual real estate markets, among others.
- **Risk and Return**: Investing in NFTs carries both potential rewards and significant risks. While some investors have realized substantial returns, others have faced losses due to market volatility, illiquidity, and changes in demand. Thorough research and careful consideration are essential for NFT investment.
- **Institutional Interest**: Institutional investors and major corporations are increasingly exploring the NFT space. Their involvement can provide additional credibility and stability to the market, potentially leading to greater adoption and investment.
- **Revenue Streams**: NFTs create new revenue streams for creators, enabling them to monetize digital content directly. Artists, musicians, and other creators can sell their work as NFTs, bypassing traditional intermediaries and retaining a larger share of the proceeds.
- **Royalties and Residuals**: Smart contracts embedded in NFTs can automate royalty payments, ensuring that creators receive a percentage of sales whenever their NFTs are resold. This feature provides ongoing revenue for creators, incentivizing them to continue producing high-quality work.
- **Intellectual Property Rights**: NFTs raise important questions regarding IP rights. Ensuring that the creation, sale, and resale of NFTs respect copyright laws and the rights of creators is crucial to maintaining a fair and legally compliant market.
- **Taxation**: The taxation of NFT transactions is a complex and evolving area. Governments and tax authorities are beginning to establish guidelines for how NFTs should be taxed, including considerations for capital gains, income, and sales taxes.
- **Regulatory Frameworks**: Regulatory bodies are scrutinizing the NFT market to develop frameworks that protect consumers and ensure market integrity. Compliance with AML and know-your-customer (KYC) regulations is becoming increasingly important for NFT platforms.
- **Energy Consumption**: The environmental impact of NFTs, particularly those minted on energy-intensive Blockchains like Ethereum, has raised concerns. The process of minting and transacting NFTs can consume significant amounts of energy, contributing to carbon emissions.

- **Sustainable Solutions**: Efforts are underway to address the environmental impact of NFTs. These include transitioning to more energy-efficient Blockchain protocols, such as Ethereum 2.0 and other PoS networks, as well as developing carbon offset initiatives.
- **Democratization of Access**: NFTs can democratize access to art and collectibles, allowing creators from diverse backgrounds to reach global audiences. This inclusivity can foster cultural exchange and support underrepresented artists.
- **Economic Inequality**: The high prices of some NFTs have raised concerns about economic inequality in the digital art market. Ensuring that the benefits of the NFT market are accessible to a broad range of creators and collectors is essential for fostering an inclusive ecosystem.

The economic considerations of NFTs encompass a wide range of factors, from market dynamics and valuation to investment potential and regulatory challenges. While NFTs offer significant opportunities for creators, investors, and businesses, they also pose risks and challenges that must be carefully managed. Understanding these economic aspects is crucial for navigating the evolving NFT landscape and maximizing its potential benefits.

CHALLENGES IN NFTs

While NFTs offer numerous opportunities and innovations, they also present several challenges that need to be addressed for sustainable growth and broader adoption. These challenges span legal, technical, economic, and environmental domains.

1. Legal and Regulatory Challenges
   Intellectual Property Rights: Ensuring that NFTs respect IP rights is complex. There have been instances of NFTs being created and sold without the consent of the original creators, leading to legal disputes. Protecting creators' rights and preventing unauthorized use of content are ongoing challenges.
   Regulatory Uncertainty: The regulatory landscape for NFTs is still developing. Different jurisdictions are at varying stages of implementing regulations, leading to uncertainty for creators, investors, and platforms. Clear and consistent regulatory frameworks are needed to provide legal certainty and protect participants in the NFT market.
   Taxation Issues: Taxation of NFT transactions is complex and varies by country. Determining how to tax income from NFT sales, capital gains, and royalties can be challenging. Market participants need clear guidance on how to comply with tax laws to avoid legal issues and financial penalties.
2. Technical Challenges
   Scalability: The scalability of Blockchain networks is a significant concern. Popular Blockchains like Ethereum have faced congestion and high transaction fees, making it expensive and slow to mint, buy, and

sell NFTs. Solutions like layer 2 scaling and the transition to Ethereum 2.0 are being explored to address these issues.

Interoperability: Interoperability between different Blockchain platforms is limited. NFTs created on one platform may not be easily transferred or used on another, restricting their utility. Developing standards and protocols for cross-chain interoperability is essential for a more seamless NFT ecosystem.

Security: Security vulnerabilities in smart contracts and NFT platforms pose risks of hacks and fraud. Ensuring the security of NFT transactions and protecting users from potential losses requires robust security measures and ongoing audits of smart contract code.

3. Economic Challenges

Market Speculation and Bubbles: The NFT market has seen significant speculation, with prices of some NFTs reaching unsustainable levels. Market bubbles can result in volatility and lead to substantial financial losses for investors when the bubble bursts. Managing speculation and promoting long-term value creation are critical for market stability.

Liquidity Issues: Liquidity varies widely across different types of NFTs. While some NFTs, particularly those from high-profile creators or popular collections, are highly liquid, others may struggle to find buyers. Improving liquidity across the NFT market is important for supporting a healthy trading environment.

Valuation: Valuing NFTs is inherently challenging due to their unique and subjective nature. The absence of standardized valuation methods can lead to inconsistencies and market inefficiencies. Developing more transparent and reliable valuation frameworks can help address this issue.

4. Environmental Challenges

Energy Consumption: The energy consumption associated with Blockchain networks, particularly those using PoW consensus mechanisms like Ethereum, has raised environmental concerns. The process of minting and transacting NFTs can be energy-intensive, contributing to carbon emissions and environmental degradation.

Sustainable Practices: Addressing the environmental impact of NFTs requires the adoption of more energy-efficient Blockchain technologies, such as PoS consensus mechanisms. Additionally, initiatives to offset carbon emissions and promote sustainable practices within the NFT ecosystem are essential.

5. Social and Ethical Challenges

Accessibility and Inclusivity: While NFTs have the potential to democratize access to digital assets, there are concerns about accessibility and inclusivity. High transaction fees and technical barriers can exclude some creators and collectors from participating in the NFT market. Ensuring that the benefits of NFTs are broadly accessible is critical for fostering an inclusive ecosystem.

Digital Divide: The digital divide, characterized by unequal access to technology and the internet, can limit participation in the NFT market. Efforts to bridge this divide and provide resources and education to underrepresented communities are necessary to promote equitable access.

Ethical Considerations: Ethical issues, such as the use of NFTs for money laundering or illicit activities, pose challenges for the market. Implementing robust AML and KYC measures is essential to mitigate these risks and ensure the integrity of the NFT ecosystem (Kumar et al., 2024).

The challenges facing NFTs are multifaceted and require coordinated efforts from creators, investors, platforms, regulators, and the broader community to address. Legal and regulatory clarity, technical advancements, sustainable practices, economic stability, and ethical considerations are all critical for the long-term success and adoption of NFTs. By addressing these challenges, the NFT ecosystem can continue to innovate and thrive while minimizing risks and promoting positive social and economic impacts.

OPPORTUNITIES IN NFTs

The unique characteristics and innovative potential of NFTs offer a wide array of opportunities across various industries. These opportunities span from enhancing digital art and entertainment to transforming business models and creating new economic paradigms.

- **Monetization for Artists**: NFTs provide a new revenue stream for digital artists by enabling them to sell their work directly to collectors. This direct-to-consumer model allows artists to retain a larger share of the profits and eliminates the need for intermediaries such as galleries and agents.
- **Royalties and Residual Income**: Smart contracts embedded in NFTs can automate royalty payments, ensuring that artists receive a percentage of sales whenever their NFTs are resold. This feature provides ongoing income for creators and incentivizes the production of high-quality digital art.
- **Provenance and Authenticity**: NFTs establish a verifiable record of ownership and provenance for digital art. This transparency ensures the authenticity of the work and can increase its value by providing buyers with confidence in the asset's originality and history.
- **In-Game Assets**: NFTs can represent unique in-game items, such as weapons, skins, and virtual land, allowing players to own, trade, and sell these assets. This ownership model can enhance player engagement and create new revenue streams for game developers.
- **Cross-Platform Interoperability**: NFTs enable the creation of interoperable assets that can be used across multiple games and virtual worlds. This interoperability can create a cohesive digital ecosystem where players can transfer and use their assets in different environments.

- **Play-to-Earn Models**: NFTs support play-to-earn models, where players can earn valuable in-game assets through gameplay. These assets can be sold or traded for real-world value, creating new economic opportunities for gamers.
- **Fractional Ownership**: NFTs can represent fractional ownership of real estate and other physical assets, making it easier for individuals to invest in high-value properties. This fractionalization can democratize access to real estate investment and provide liquidity in traditionally illiquid markets.
- **Simplified Transactions**: Tokenizing real estate with NFTs can streamline the buying, selling, and transferring process by reducing paperwork and intermediaries. Blockchain-based transactions are transparent, secure, and can be executed quickly, enhancing efficiency in the real estate market.
- **Increased Market Access**: NFTs can enable global market access for real estate and other tokenized assets, allowing investors from anywhere in the world to participate. This increased accessibility can expand the investor base and drive market growth.
- **Digital Rights Management**: NFTs can revolutionize digital rights management by providing a transparent and automated system for licensing and royalty payments. Creators can maintain control over their IP and ensure fair compensation for its use.
- **Tokenized Licensing**: Licensing agreements can be tokenized using NFTs, allowing for more efficient and secure transactions. Smart contracts can automate compliance with licensing terms and conditions, reducing administrative overhead.
- **Protecting Copyrights**: NFTs can help protect copyrights by providing a verifiable record of ownership and usage rights. This can reduce instances of unauthorized use and piracy, ensuring that creators are properly credited and compensated.
- **Direct Fan Engagement**: NFTs enable artists and entertainers to engage directly with their fans by offering exclusive content, experiences, and merchandise. This direct engagement can strengthen fan loyalty and create new revenue streams.
- **Exclusive Content and Access**: Musicians and entertainers can use NFTs to offer exclusive content, such as unreleased tracks, behind-the-scenes footage, and VIP concert tickets. Fans can purchase and trade these NFTs, creating a new market for exclusive experiences.
- **Automated Royalties**: Smart contracts in NFTs can automate royalty payments for music and entertainment content, ensuring that creators receive fair compensation for their work. This automation reduces the need for intermediaries and increases transparency in royalty distribution.
- **Secure Digital Identities**: NFTs can be used to create secure digital identities that are verifiable on the Blockchain. This can enhance privacy and security in online transactions and interactions, reducing the risk of identity theft (Singh & Joshi, 2024).
- **Verifiable Credentials**: Educational institutions and professional organizations can issue verifiable credentials as NFTs, ensuring that diplomas,

certifications, and licenses are tamper-proof and easily verifiable. This can streamline verification processes for employers and other stakeholders.

- **Decentralized Identity Management**: NFTs enable decentralized identity management, allowing individuals to control their personal information and share it selectively. This decentralized approach can enhance privacy and give individuals greater control over their digital identities.
- **Fundraising and Charity**: NFTs can be used to raise funds for charitable causes by auctioning unique digital assets. This can attract donations and support for various initiatives, ensuring transparency and accountability through Blockchain technology.
- **Awareness Campaigns**: NFTs can be leveraged to create awareness campaigns for social and environmental issues. Artists and activists can use NFTs to generate attention and funding for important causes, fostering positive social impact.
- **Community Engagement**: NFTs can facilitate community engagement by offering unique rewards and incentives for participation in social and environmental projects. This can strengthen community bonds and encourage collective action.

The opportunities presented by NFTs are vast and varied, with the potential to transform numerous industries and create new economic paradigms. From enhancing digital art and gaming to revolutionizing real estate and IP management, NFTs offer innovative solutions to longstanding challenges. By leveraging the unique characteristics of NFTs, individuals, businesses, and organizations can unlock new value, drive engagement, and promote positive social impact.

FUTURE TRENDS

The rapid evolution of NFTs suggests several emerging trends that could shape the future of this technology. These trends span various sectors, including technology, finance, art, entertainment, and more. Understanding these trends can provide insights into the potential directions NFTs may take in the coming years.

- **Virtual Reality (VR) and Metaverses**: The integration of NFTs with VR is poised to transform digital experiences. NFTs can represent ownership of virtual assets within immersive VR environments, enabling users to own, trade, and interact with unique digital items in the metaverse. Platforms like Decentraland and The Sandbox are early examples of this trend.
- **Augmented Reality (AR)**: NFTs can be integrated with AR applications, allowing users to display and interact with their digital assets in the real world through AR interfaces. This can enhance the utility and engagement of NFTs, bridging the gap between digital and physical experiences.
- **Functional NFTs**: Beyond digital art and collectibles, NFTs with functional utility are gaining traction. These NFTs can provide access to services, software, exclusive content, and virtual events. For instance, NFTs can serve as digital keys or memberships, granting holders specific privileges and benefits.

- **Gaming and Play-to-Earn Models**: The gaming industry will continue to be a significant driver of NFT adoption. Play-to-earn models, where players earn NFTs and cryptocurrencies through gameplay, are becoming more popular. These models can create new revenue streams for both developers and players, enhancing the value proposition of games.
- **Increased Participation by Major Brands**: Mainstream brands and corporations are increasingly exploring NFTs to engage with consumers and create new business opportunities. Companies in fashion, sports, entertainment, and other sectors are launching NFT collections and integrating them into their marketing strategies.
- **Institutional Investment**: Institutional investors are beginning to recognize the potential of NFTs as an asset class. As financial products and services around NFTs mature, institutional participation is likely to increase, bringing more stability and credibility to the market.
- **Cross-Chain Interoperability**: The development of cross-chain interoperability solutions will enable NFTs to move seamlessly between different Blockchain networks. This will enhance the flexibility and utility of NFTs, allowing users to leverage their assets across multiple platforms and ecosystems.
- **Standardization**: The establishment of industry standards for NFTs will facilitate interoperability and ensure consistency in how NFTs are created, managed, and traded. Standards such as ERC-721 and ERC-1155 are early examples, but ongoing efforts will continue to refine and expand these frameworks.
- **Transition to Eco-Friendly Blockchains**: The environmental impact of NFTs has spurred efforts to transition to more energy-efficient Blockchain technologies. PoS networks and other low-energy consensus mechanisms are being adopted to reduce the carbon footprint of NFT transactions.
- **Carbon Offset Initiatives**: Projects and platforms are developing initiatives to offset the carbon emissions associated with NFTs. These efforts include investing in renewable energy projects and supporting environmental conservation programs, aiming to make the NFT ecosystem more sustainable.
- **Regulatory Clarity**: As the NFT market grows, regulatory bodies will continue to develop frameworks to govern NFT transactions. Clear regulations will help protect consumers, ensure market integrity, and provide legal certainty for creators, investors, and platforms.
- **Intellectual Property Protections**: Enhanced legal frameworks will address IP rights and ensure that NFTs respect the rights of creators. This will include measures to prevent unauthorized use and ensure that creators are fairly compensated for their work.
- **Decentralized Marketplaces**: The rise of decentralized marketplaces will provide greater transparency, security, and control for users. These platforms eliminate intermediaries, allowing for direct peer-to-peer transactions and reducing fees.
- **Enhanced User Experience**: Future NFT marketplaces will focus on improving the user experience, making it easier for creators and collectors to navigate, trade, and manage their assets. This includes user-friendly interfaces, better discovery tools, and comprehensive support services.

- **Democratization of Access**: NFTs have the potential to democratize access to art, entertainment, and investment opportunities. By lowering barriers to entry and providing new ways to engage with digital content, NFTs can foster greater inclusivity and diversity in the digital economy.
- **Community-Driven Projects**: Community-driven NFT projects will continue to grow, enabling collective ownership and governance. These projects can empower communities to create, manage, and benefit from their digital assets, fostering a sense of shared purpose and collaboration.

The future of NFTs is filled with exciting possibilities and transformative potential. As technology advances and the market matures, NFTs are likely to become an integral part of various industries, from art and entertainment to finance and real estate. By understanding and embracing these trends, stakeholders can navigate the evolving landscape and harness the opportunities that NFTs offer.

CONCLUSION

In conclusion, NFTs have emerged as a transformative force in the digital art market, offering artists, collectors, and stakeholder's unprecedented opportunities for creativity, collaboration, and economic empowerment. By tokenizing digital artworks on Blockchain networks, NFTs enable artists to establish provenance, ownership, and authenticity for their creations, while providing collectors with a secure and transparent way to buy, sell, and trade digital art assets.

Throughout this exploration, we've identified several key drivers and trends shaping the future of NFTs in digital art, including the integration with virtual and AR, the development of the metaverse, environmental sustainability initiatives, the rise of decentralized autonomous organizations, gamification and interactive experiences, regulatory developments, advancements in marketplaces and infrastructure, and the crossover with traditional art markets. While NFTs hold immense promise, they also come with challenges and considerations that need to be addressed, including regulatory uncertainties, environmental concerns, market fragmentation, scalability issues, and the protection of IP rights. By proactively addressing these challenges and leveraging emerging opportunities, stakeholders in the NFT ecosystem can work towards building a more inclusive, sustainable, and vibrant marketplace for digital art.

As the NFT market continues to evolve and mature, collaboration, innovation, and community engagement will be essential for driving positive change and realizing the full potential of NFTs in the creative industries. By embracing new technologies, exploring novel business models, and fostering a culture of creativity and experimentation, we can unlock new possibilities for artistic expression, economic empowerment, and cultural enrichment in the digital age.

In summary, the future of NFTs in digital art is bright and full of promise. By embracing innovation, addressing challenges, and embracing opportunities, we can create a more inclusive, diverse, and dynamic ecosystem for artists, collectors, and enthusiasts alike.

BIBLIOGRAPHY

Charney, N., & Schachter, K., *The NFT Book – Everything You Need to Know about the Art and Collecting of Non-Fungible Tokens*. Rowman & Littlefield Publisher (e-book), ISBN 9781538174760.

Fortnow, M., & Tery, Q., *The NFT Handbook How to Create, Sell and Buy Non-Fungible Tokens*. Wiley Publication, ISBN 9781119838395.

Johnston, A. *NFT for Beginners – The Ultimate Guide to Non-Fungible Tokens (Digital Art, Crypto and Collectibles)*. Independently Publisher, ISBN 9798747413016.

Joshi, A., & Goyal, S. B. "Comparison of Various Round Robin Scheduling Algorithms," *2019 8th International Conference System Modeling and Advancement in Research Trends (SMART)*, Moradabad, India, 2019, pp. 18–21, doi: 10.1109/SMART46866. 2019.9117345

Joshi, A., & Tiwari, H. (2023). An overview of Python libraries for data science. *Journal of Engineering Technology and Applied Physics*, 5(2), 85–90. https://doi.org/10.33093/jetap.2023.5.2.10

Kumar, R., Joshi, A., Sharan, H. O., Peng, S. L., & Dudhagara, C. R. (Eds.). (2024). *The Ethical Frontier of AI and Data Analysis*. IGI Global.

Nft Trending, *NFT (Non Fungible Tokens), Guide; Buying, Selling, Trading, Investing in Crypto Collectibles Art. Create Wealth and Build Assets*. Nft Cryptocurrency Investment Guides, ISBN 9781838365844.

Rich, O. J., *NFTs for Beginners Making Money with Non-Fungible Tokens*. Amazon Digital Services, ISBN 9798494272799.

Singh, B. P., & Joshi, A. (2024). Ethical Considerations in AI Development. In *The Ethical Frontier of AI and Data Analysis* (pp. 156–179). IGI Global.

The Financial Edits, *NFTs - Non-Fungible Tokens - A Precise Book to Learn All about NFTs*. Mocktime Publication (e-book).

18 Advancing Patient-Centric Care in Smart Hospitals via 6G-Enabled Healthcare Innovations
A Technical Framework

Prabh Deep Singh, Kiran Deep Singh,
Riya Sharma, and Roohi Naaz

INTRODUCTION

In recent years, "smart hospitals" (SHs) have emerged as an example of the Intelligent Medical Services (IMS) paradigm, which uses digital technologies to upgrade the operational efficiency, healthcare quality, and personalization of hospital services (Kanase & Gopal, 2016). Medical institutions are looking to use big data and other technologies to build electronic health records based on transparent and shared data, as well as intelligent diagnosis and treatment support systems, intelligent management and control systems, and other means to establish the SH platform. These efforts are driven by the demand for scientific and technological advancement in the healthcare industry and in medical facilities (Della Vecchia et al., 2012). SHs have significant value in the development of new services, based on IoT and other digital technologies, and can extend the principle of "patient-centric care" to improvements in medical and healthcare services. This paper explains the concept of sixth-generation (6G) and the patient-centric intelligent healthcare system and architecture requirements in "Introduction".

BACKGROUND AND RATIONALE

In the fourth industrial revolution, healthcare is undergoing a significant shift toward patient-centered, preventive, and other innovative care strategies. SHs, enabled by the Internet of Things (IoT), big data, and artificial intelligence (AI), play a substantial role in the advancement of healthcare (Hassan et al., 2019; Kanase & Gopal, 2016). The fifth-generation (5G) of wireless communication technology represents an important milestone in SH advancements, yet there remain substantial opportunities for the integration of advanced wireless technologies to revolutionize patient-centric care in

DOI: 10.1201/9781003516590-18

SHs. Toward the rapid growth of 5G and future 6G healthcare, outline the advances in SHs, particularly with respect to how advanced mobile technologies contribute to revolutionizing patient-centered care in an increasingly digital world (Holzinger et al., 2015). The evolution of healthcare embraces an emerging trend, moving from hospital-centered services toward patient-centered services. Combining with growing demands on an aging society, healthcare also begins to focus on preventive care instead of traditional disease treatment. To improve healthcare quality, the World Health Organization (WHO) recommends better coverage, increased access to services, and reduced healthcare costs. Additionally, the novel coronavirus pneumonia (COVID-19) has highlighted many other challenges in traditional hospitals, such as human infection transmission, shortage of medical resources, and overloaded healthcare systems (Moro Visconti & Martiniello, 2019). To address various healthcare demands and make rapid changes in the proposals, many of the options rely on digital technologies. As proposed in the fourth industrial revolution, healthcare is shifting towards patient-centered, innovative, and preventive care in an increasingly digital world. One of the key components enabling the concept of patient-centered, innovative, and preventive care is SHs.

SCOPE AND OBJECTIVES

In this paper, we lay out an early vision for pushing the innovation envelope of what SHs might ultimately be able to deliver to revolutionize patient-centric care using the next-generation wireless technology, 6G. Our initial work aims to provide an understanding of what is possible to enable as we embark on the roadmap for realizing future 6G mobile health facilities, i.e. Wi-Fi-free SHs, providing virtually untethered, high data rates in-wall/in-body environments, ultra-reliable and secure connectivity, and on-demand secure access to data. Although our paper focuses specifically on SHs as a use case for 6G (Estrela et al., 2023), our vision can be easily extrapolated to other mobile health facilities, such as a smart healthcare wearables ecosystem involving 6G repeaters and user health zones. Our overarching goal is to truly empower patients to reach their maximum potential in a way that was – for the most part of human history – never imaginable, let alone attainable.

SMART HOSPITALS: A CONCEPTUAL FRAMEWORK

With the passage of time, flexibility enables healthcare facilities to be more sustainable, resulting in building systems that remain versatile and lead to lower costs. Bio-hospitals and net buildings are examples of this development. These newly designed structures consider the environment in design and operation, in addition to the increasing patient-centric focus (in & 2024, 2024). There is also a focus on designing hospitals with a holistic approach. Technology advancements combined with digital technologies have enabled one to further fine-tune the concept of patient-centric care. Care processes and information exchange between patient and healthcare, by integrating patients with family and friends, are further improved by incorporating patient and patient-associated device data management (Srinivasu et al., 2022). These developments set the stage for a completely new service proposition in which the role of digital product-service is integrated into healthcare services. The digital initiative in healthcare started with the implementation of the healthcare system, and tremendous progress has been made with the implementation of e-health and tele-health on an ongoing basis. The commencement of the COVID-19 pandemic brought hospitals to an extremely challenging state. The digital revolution has highlighted the importance of increased demand and harnessing e-health real-time smart communication and data technology for rapid disease surveillance, early detection, and rapid response. SHs are a constituency of intelligent buildings, which are equipped with a combination of medical devices, ICT (Information and Communication Technology), and other technologies to ensure the efficient operation of healthcare at various levels. As an intelligent building, a SH facility effectively utilizes technology and space to enhance building design and building system efficiency to ensure that quality patient care and patient satisfaction needs are met in a cost-effective manner (Khattak et al., 2022). Patients receive treatment from hospital professionals, and they can expect to be integrated into the treatment program with more information and contact with healthcare service providers. This paper aims to set the stage for refining the vision and supporting the strategy of patient-centric care by setting up a conceptual discovery framework that highlights the key role of smart buildings and IoT, and 6G networks in SHs (Estrela et al., 2023). The study pursued structured mapping of previous literature that was analyzed and interpreted across multiple conceptual lenses, with the final paper ending in a strategy for supporting its vision as depicted in Figure 18.1.

DEFINITION AND EVOLUTION

The main objective is to develop the new 6GPPS (General Purpose Polystyrene) concept for the developing phase of SH with several key factors to leverage from these technologies to evolve 6G. The proposed solutions and methodologies have the ability to be adopted with the current ongoing technologies, like 5G, 802.11 working progress, information technologies, and connected hospitals. Six-Users Power Save Mode will be reviewed under the current 802.11 standard to verify the possibility of implementing the proposed solution to 6G (Kaiser et al., 2021). Additionally, considering the wearables federated body network support in 6G, the FLB-COFDM (Filtered Linearly Blocked Coded Orthogonal Frequency Division Multiplexing) modulation scheme is reviewed in order to verify the coexistence with the FLBCOFDM of SH services with the actual Wi-Fi communication. In addition to being an enabler of the Tactile Internet, which leads communication into true real-time, the 6G will radically transform healthcare services and particularly SHs. The healthcare of the future will move away from the current healthcare services approach based on the relationship between patient and doctor and focus on the health management of a patient's life journey that is continuously monitored by the SH. The concept presented both CO-FBMC/OQAM and highlighted both PTS techniques in order to review the proposed solutions. Considering the IoT for connecting the SH for regulating all services and in anticipation of 6G, the developed mainly solution performed a work in exploring the energy efficiency of compact architectures operating under low power conditions yet maintaining a cognitive approach

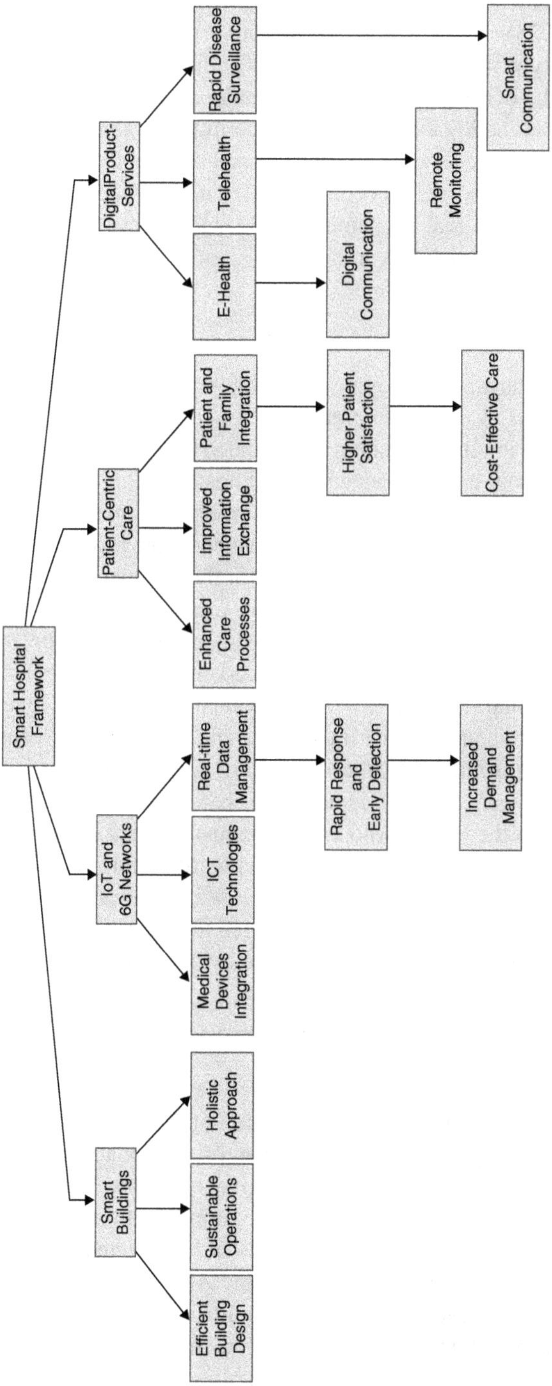

FIGURE 18.1 Conceptual framework for smart hospitals: integrating smart buildings, IoT, and 6G networks for enhanced patient-centric care.

allowing self-organization and self-reconfiguration capability under usual transmission scenarios in order to be ready to be integrated into the future 6GPPS concept (Nasralla et al., 2023). It has also provided both a theoretical and design approach to develop a prototype that can be part of the 6G chipset integrations and give a pioneer approach to the 6GPPS concept. Additionally, given the severization approach, the concept was that the logical entities must be implemented independently on the 6GPPS stages. At both the terminal equipment and in the middle anchor while opening new frontiers in healthcare, concepts presented in this chapter. In order to validate the principles and obtain real implementation results, these are provided as future work for the reader for further research.

Key Components

The idea of the SH starts by employing the technologies developed for the smart city within the hospital. It also aims to create patient-centric models of care to address patient needs through intelligent technologies. The SH coordinates technology together in a seamless and, from a patient viewpoint, almost invisible way to enable patient-centric models of care. The success of the SH is predicated on the use of vast numbers of sensors, connected to vast amounts of compute and storage, enabling significant AI to be done at the edge. This is how the benefits for the patient can be realized, through digital innovations which deliver better outcomes and experiences for patients. This can equally be employed to enable staff to meet care objectives. The architectures of SHs have developed through the IoT layers, placed on top of the operational and existing layers in the hospital (Deep, 2023). At the core, the SH remains an expert place of patient care. It does remain that, but it uses data and connectivity to enable networks across different areas, sometimes placed in situ or sometimes offsite using high-performance (Joshi & Tiwari, 2023). Despite these changes to the operation through data and connectivity, it is the patient who is at the center of what is delivered. Therefore, the principles of SHs are changing the focus and work performed within the hospital, but the confidence that is engendered in consultants and nurses within the hospital and their relationship with the patient can be leveraged to ensure future technology developments and the services they enable are trusted by the patient.

PATIENT-CENTRIC CARE IN SMART HOSPITALS

SHs make use of the IoT to enhance patient safety, ensuring patients are at the center of care. Widespread dissemination and integration of diverse health-related technologies into data about the people - patient, citizen, professional health, caregiver - can help make better diagnoses, faster disease treatment, and has been a general goal for personalized healthcare. Future next wireless communication networks, such as the 6G network, are helping to dynamize the vision of "connected patient". Adding virtual reality (VR) and augmented reality (AR) and AI technologies have the potential to change the state of the patient facing the current animation of clinical, therapeutic, and remote approach systems; audio, graphical, tactile, olfactory and taste-based 6G communications bear the objective of broadly offering XR in individual communications and possible collective environments (Ahad et al., 2024). A standard hospital room can be a source of stress and isolation, particularly for patients receiving treatment. To ensure patients receive the highest standard of treatment, it is important to provide a suitable hospital environment. There is a key need to transform the current hospital 4.0 (intelligent and smart) room into a 5G construction room linked to 6G VR and AR treatment. Indeed, intelligent room technologies can give our daily assistance a real safety, individualism, social requirement, and personal comfort. Individual attention changes medical practice and is also satisfaction from both patient and health workers (Zhang et al., 2018). This document describes an excellent hospital room structure and health and humanitarian services, as well as future VR and AR facilities, which are the foundation of 6G technologies, which aim to use various human omnidirectional sensations. Through the new software, it capitalizes on the patient's position and also with the outside and allows any type of remote and inclusive requirements to be met.

IMPORTANCE AND BENEFITS

Whilst SHs offer an advanced healthcare delivery paradigm, current hospitals do not meet the growing demands of futurized interconnected services, systems, and devices. In fact, in the post-COVID-19 pandemic era and beyond, the existing hospitals are expected to be excessively challenged. There are urgent and perhaps unmet needs to revolutionize hospital services to efficiently cater to growing and increasingly sophisticated healthcare needs in a connected, digital, technology-rich environment. Possible applications include remote patient care, mobility-assisted care, robotic-assisted and noncontact imaging diagnosis during chronic contagious disease pandemic, transparent end-to-end connected co-design, shared control and de-risking of ultra-recovery critical diseases, 100% accurate continual health status monitoring and health teasing, prescribing, treatment discussions, and self-administered online dynamic regulation in patient-centered hospital healthcare contacts. In previous years these solutions described were technically very immature and were still not accepted. There was widespread disbelief in the healthcare and hospital design communities that they could be realized, many others considered these to be futuristic work to be performed over decades. A fact that has been exacerbated since 2020 has shown, as we can witness, the COVID-19 pandemic has changed the whole world, and highlighted the unanticipated, unprecedented, and unimaginable hospital overload we are not equipped to manage, coupled with other many uncountable future challenges. Furthermore, without such patient-centric hospital healthcare innovation, innovations in other healthcare segments, such as digital or AI-assisted wearable for health teasing, health contactless or mobility-assisted care will come to nothing. With this, the containment of futuristic pandemics will also essentially fail. Therefore, an urgent comprehensive hospital care service innovation roadmap should be defined, and actively exploiting the potential of forthcoming 6G global wireless technology standardization could be particularly relevant.

CHALLENGES AND OPPORTUNITIES

5G has been introduced to address the challenges faced in SHs, and advancements in 6G will be a game-changer for the healthcare services sector, including SHs. Through a literature study, we have identified several issues faced by SHs that 6G innovations would overcome. The issues include the optimization of health data, increased security measures, faster networks, low latency, energy-efficient systems, and improved patient-centric services. The main takeaway from this study is to innovate, co-create, and collaborate in research to introduce SH methodologies to substantially improve healthcare services (Santhosh, 2019). These examples of the challenges indicate an advent of 6G to intensify patient-centric care in SHs. Consequently, our results provide a basis for future research to ascertain how beneficial 6G in SHs can be. 6G wireless communication is expected to be introduced to the public around 2030, and this most recent development of wireless technology has the potential to revolutionize every segment of human life. Of particular importance is the healthcare sector, which relies on its initiative to conduct innovative studies that can offer more effective, efficient, easily accessible, and patient-friendly healthcare services to the general public (Hassan et al., 2019). Many hospitals around the globe have piloted hospital administration system development to realize the growth of SHs; nevertheless, the explosion of medical data coming from a variety of directions, such as patient vital health-related data, patient clinical histories, and financial statistics, requires rapid and effective analyses. Consequently, the 5G wireless technology, termed 5G, has been designed and developed to address the diversity and enormity of wireless demand encountered.

6G TECHNOLOGY: ENABLING INNOVATIONS

SHs incorporate mobile health (m-health), IoT, electronic medical records (EMRs), and grid/acoustic technologies to provide high-quality, efficient, and intelligent care for patients with diverse healthcare needs. Even though many benefits and profound transformations have been derived from the revolutionary 5G technologies in many industries, 5G still has many shortcomings that impede the large-scale implementation of various innovative healthcare solutions. These problems include latency, bandwidth, energy consumption, peak data rate, device connectivity, reliability/availability, traffic density, deteriorating speed, spectral efficiency, positioning accuracy, short life cycle of up-to-date mobile communication technologies, high economic and environmental costs, and subversive technologies revolution (Della Vecchia et al., 2012). Very soon after the commencement of 5G structured design, global research, standardization, and 6G-technology-preparatory work began all over the world. As a result, 6G has received overwhelming participation and attention in academic research, industrial practice, and government strategies. The new 6G architecture, including generic connectivity like interconnection, collectively working, near-range access, medium-range access, large-range access, and deep space access, brings a range of outstanding innovations in hyperconnectivity, network architecture, IoT, high mobility, energy sustainability, and other groundbreaking high-order approaches (Hassan et al., 2019). These cutting-edge 6G technology innovations equip SHs with a more succinct and effective network infrastructure to serve the increasingly diverse healthcare needs of patients and contribute to three guaranteed resources. Additionally, with another tier of guaranteed resources granted by space resources, 6G extensively explores space science, application, development, and enhancement. Both business value and academic prospect are vivid and magnetic.

In this article, significant contributions are made that propose, discuss, develop, and evaluate 6G innovative applications and insights that have not previously been studied for healthcare. The main contributions are: to propose and deploy a 6G technology-based framework for realizing revolutionized patient-centric care in SHs. With 6G innovations, SHs can deliver better, faster, cheaper, and more secure services for remote patient monitoring, health-social collaboration, and clinical collaboration. These services not only help with early diagnosis, personalized intervention, easier access, price transparency, and efficient laying time saving, but they also enhance the healthcare process, set operation management, doctor-patient care interaction, medical resources distribution, and health supply chain information-sharing collaboration. Significant healthcare savings can be effectively achieved, which is particularly essential during the current crisis of the COVID-19 pandemic.

OVERVIEW AND KEY FEATURES

SHs are one of the critical application scenarios in the 6G era, where revolutionary innovations are required to achieve pandemic-proof patient-centric care effectively and efficiently. In this section, we first provide an overview of a SH and its technical requirements. Key features of a SH include high-quality 8K/4K multimedia sensory information acquisition, millions of devices per square kilometer ultra-reliable low-latency communication (URLLC), energy-efficient heterogeneous integration, and lightweight AI-based real-time decision-making assistance (Israni et al., 2023). We then present snapshots of the SH ecosystems by making 6G industry-specific scenarios in three stages of SH evolution. Furthermore, for the research community, we highlight a few essential technical issues and opportunities. In the 6G era, we envision that SHs would facilitate revolutionary advances in patient-centric care and ultimately realize the Sustainable Development Goal of good health and well-being for all. SHs provide full coverage for caregivers and patients to support various digital healthcare services with ultra-high-quality, real-time multimedia sensory information acquisition, AI-based analysis, and heterogeneous wireless connectivity. Their essential requirements are listed in this paragraph. SHs consist of several 5-dimensional access paradigms: caregiver dimension, patient dimension, multimedia dimension, AI dimension, and wireless connectivity dimension. SHs require holistic coverage for caregivers (e.g., medical staff, nurses, patient families, and support staff), patients, and a variety of their devices. The multimedia dimension covers not only high-quality video captured by high-resolution 8K/4K smart glasses/wearable cameras for remote diagnosis, monitoring, and surgery, but also other multimedia data, including medical images and reports, and other wireless sensor data like location, fall, elderly tracking, and environmental monitoring data (M. S. Kaiser et al., 2021). It should be noted that healthcare is reliant on integrated multimedia data to empower caregivers with the patient information necessary to make informed decisions. The AI dimension is defined to help caregivers better understand the acquired multimedia data and provide predictive care with the assistance of AI-based real-time data analytics. Finally, the wireless connectivity dimension is deemed essential to enable coverage for a myriad of medical and IoT devices. SHs with built-in communication technologies can support diverse low-latency control and remote surgical applications, enabling high-quality patient-centric care. Caregivers can also use real-time AI assistance, remote patient monitoring, and automated administrative processes to streamline workflows. Furthermore, patients can avail themselves of a wealth of digital healthcare services ranging from continuous in-hospital healthcare to pre-hospital and post-hospital care services, thus increasing patient experience while reducing outpatient visits to hospitals.

POTENTIAL APPLICATIONS IN HEALTHCARE

In general, super-broadband support will be provided across the entire hospital through 6G. Fixed wireless (Wi-Fi) to the end-user connection will provide continuous data access and a smooth experience of using multimedia services in different environments. Specifically, we will ensure that first-time decompression of full-quality 8K/12K transport video, including AR/VR, is delivered to hospital wards. Provide high-quality and low-latency video communication (fast and responsive tele-assistance/operation, virtual consultation, etc.) through robotic capabilities for diagnostic burns and remote communication with specialized workers (significant improvement in service quality and patient outcome). Specifically improve patient monitoring system capabilities based on high performance and support the next generation of the Internet of Medicine. High-value automated/assisted surgery and access to AI medical assistant services will be provided. Provide an Ambient Intelligence Environment with the supporting semantic and multimedia digital library. Patient-centric access to multimedia content/Ubiquitous communication-enabled wearables will allow patients and relatives to access and interact with their medical records and other services from their hospital rooms. Visually or manually control the stent platform of the hospital with user-in-hand services within a secure and reliable portable communication infrastructure. The ability to extend AI through the cloud way beyond the hospital level(Sun, 2023). The ability to transfer and concatenate personal data and biological data with high privacy standards to medical personnel, AI, and hospital services within the hospital. To elaborate, hospital infrastructure takes advantage of the global technician support by 6G/site reduction in hardware and batteries. The technician support agent, including tele-maintenance, is deployed in the cloud for less cost and the latest knowledge updates. Physical support and mobility-impaired individuals for individualized indoor navigation by 6G and robotic installation in the healthcare scenario domain. Improve the accuracy of indoor navigation and position localization to augment patient isolation and track patients in health operations. Support indoor map creation and update, and patient or robot localization and tracking without satellite signals to enable seamless autonomous operation in the health domain. In hospitals, 6G can be used to develop networks to support cloud computing and IT infrastructures with ultra-low latency and super-high broadband capability. The E-Health services are the primary usage scenario for 6G high data-rate communication systems, supporting dynamic off-site Magnetic Resonance Imaging (MRI)/CT scans (Computed Tomography Scan), emergency surgery assistance, remote appointments, live consultation, ambulance blue-light control, driver assistance, and similar real-time use cases. The performance of 6G sensors in these latency-sensitive applications will be closely scrutinized, and investment will be driven by patient experience improvements. There are numerous potential applications for innovative 6G technology in healthcare, both in terms of enhancing patient health and unlocking value from patient data through IoT (Ahmad et al., 2023). These can be broadly classified into low-latency, high-bandwidth real-time services; data-heavy and privacy-sensitive hospital systems; and patient-focused services. Over the next few years, 5G and 6G technologies are expected to help tackle some of the biggest challenges faced by healthcare systems across the world.

INTEGRATION OF 6G TECHNOLOGY IN SMART HOSPITALS

The integration of 6G in SHs, along with equally essential development aspects, to create a functional foundation, is discussed in this section. The envisioned key features of 6G technology in SHs pertain to hospital patients' diverse service requirements, ranging from area-specific and individualized needs to human-perceived services. The key feature is uniquely realized through economic data networking and several radio resource management-driven technologies that encompass implementations based on dynamic AI. At the epicenter of 6G technological integration into SHs is the integration of mobile phone devices using various system technologies, such as modular structure, new radio coverage, massive multiple input multiple output, and new radio-capable office situated radio installations. Development aspects, such as massive radio input, massive radio output design, R0 environment-associated design tools, and health AI technological integration, can be categorized as enabling and foundational technologies that further assist the hospital environment, guaranteeing in-hospital mobility. The integration of 6G technologies in SHs is perceived to be at the hospital environment-centric developmental stage and intended to trigger a combination of area 4, 5, 6, and 7 industry verticals. For effective economic data networking among patients, using these widely used devices can be undertaken through antidictionary communications, and the industrial revolution and scientific collaborations are extremely essential.

At the functional developmental stage, New Radio coverage and other design tools have evolved to be crucial, which is more important for smart in-hospital mobility compared to conventional smartphone devices. Also, technological integration of Health AI is critical for SHs, regardless of their occupancy rate and other hospital operation-specific practices. Approximately eighty percent of the industry work variable of patients are in different locations throughout the hospital. For the most obvious reason, healthcare is a human-centric service business whose focal point is the patient. Integer mobility in SHs is a key SH system design requirement, and economic networking for intelligent patient service must be realized before in-hospital mobility is realized. In this context, healthcare developments for in-hospital services are unique to intelligent patient services as depicted in Figure 18.2.

INFRASTRUCTURE REQUIREMENTS

The underlying infrastructure is primarily IoT, with increasing demands on data speed, security, and availability. 5G and its enhanced versions are being designed to address all these expectations. But emerging healthcare use cases are imposing

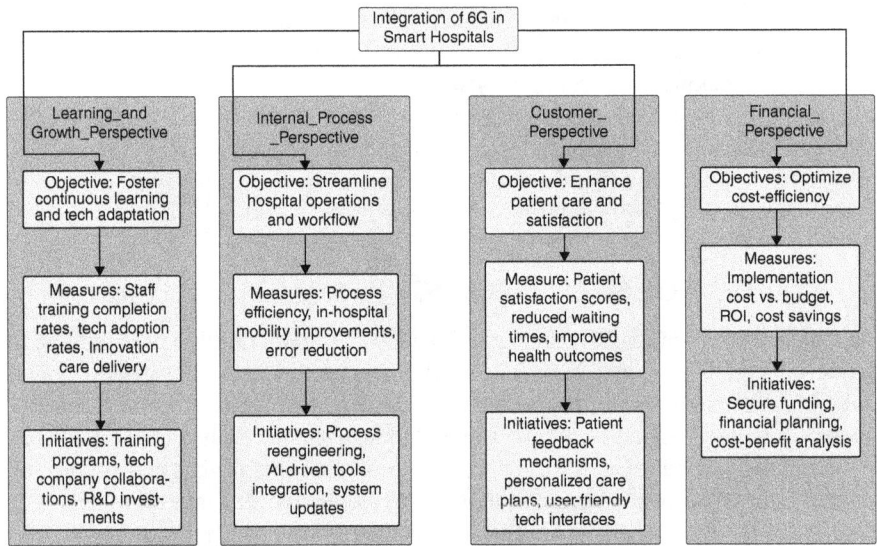

FIGURE 18.2 Integration of 6G in smart hospitals using the balanced scorecard framework.

new, stringent requirements on 5G, which are too challenging to be accommodated within the 5G evolution path. These include mission-critical machine-to-machine communication, extremely low-latency communication, ultra-reliable machine-type communication, and devices with no battery for a long time requirement. Beyond the mainstream technologies, emerging trends in networking solutions, and large-capacity decentralized storage devices are all expected to be in place for the 6G evolution. Prominent amongst these is the mixed reality platform. 6G needs to iterate and mature several existing and forthcoming technologies to enable future SHs.

To handle the above-discussed use cases, SHs draw inspiration from technologies that evolved in different vertical domains. Built on the legacy of IoT and 5G, SHs can realize a few of its applications, but without the string-edge requirements expected in the ensuing years; neither IoT nor 5G meets these expectations. Many of the envisaged capabilities are futuristic and necessitate a revolutionary technology vision. Now is the optimal time to contemplate and outline those requirements that are expected to frame the global 6G development trajectory. Among the emerging technologies, the healthcare sector is embracing mixed reality to address many of the pain points in healthcare delivery. In this next section, we re-imagine the SH experience with and without mixed reality and pinpoint the requirements thus derived.

DATA SECURITY AND PRIVACY CONSIDERATIONS

MRI is widely used in medical diagnosis, offering outstanding visualization of the human body, especially for soft tissues and organs, with no ionizing radiation. However, this medical imaging technology also has its own limitations, such as long imaging times, standard safety issues, such as the presence of metal implants for the patient, and the restricted availability of MRI services due to equipment complexity and power consumption, especially in remote areas and emerging economies. To address these challenges, there is increasing research interest in exploiting machine learning and deep learning (Mishra, 2024) to rebuild MRI. In SHs or regional tele-medicine health-care setups, 6G collaborations with applicable heterogeneous resources could securely support MRI data acquisition methods and image quality enhancements, while considering energy-efficient wireless communication of image reconstruction for constrained computation.

Pharmacogenomics is an important component of personalized medicine, aiming at identifying the genetic responders and adverse effects of drug treatments for each patient. However, current genetic data collection methods remain time-consuming and complex, and they lack scalability. Ideal genetic data collection would be non-invasive, reduce sample preparation time, and offer ultra-high throughput for quick data acquisition. Recent research has improved the detection and quantification of various biomolecules using terahertz technology. In particular, due to its better bio-logical molecule detection capabilities, the possibility for non-invasive genetic inter-rogation using terahertz spectroscopy has attracted significant attention. With 6G conditions that allow sensor fusion, on-site multi-dimensional high-throughput detection of genetic variants of pharmacogenomic interest could then be realized in these SHs with minimized sample preparation and reduced interference or concerns about data privacy.

Patient-centric data is extremely sensitive and critical. For all data acquisitions affecting any patients, sufficient data security and privacy protections must be implemented, such as data protection regulations (Kumar et al., 2024), encrypted transfer links, and access controls on a "must have" basis. Data privacy and security should be guaranteed from end to end. Data access, collection, processing, and transmission must all be logged and monitored, and appropriate rules must be embedded in all AI models that implement automatic audits. In general, only with the trust achieved by transparent and unbiased AI can patients confidently allow their data to be used by these models. In this case, a secure environment that is safe and guarantees high-quality medical decision-making for patient care purposes is non-negotiable.

CASE STUDIES AND BEST PRACTICES

Automated and autonomous technologies such as drones and robots can be utilized for various tasks in healthcare. Shifting the focus from COVID-19, a majority of the applications for robots are found in elderly care, but they are also used to help with a general set of care tasks for patients, or as social conversational partners. The imple-mentation of such technologies in healthcare is said to have the potential to increase the efficiency of healthcare services by reducing the need for human personnel. Such robots can also be utilized as communication tools and assist patients in communi-cating with healthcare professionals outside of physical meetings.

This section focuses on best practices in patient care with the goal of enhancing the SH through the lens of patient-centric care. The discussion underscores the opportunities that await with 6G as a new foundation for conceptualizing care deliv-ery and human health at the individual, community, and population levels.

SUCCESSFUL IMPLEMENTATIONS

IoT and 6G technologies will significantly boost the development of smart solutions for patient-centric care with personalized medicine at the focus. Several implementations of IoT and 6G innovations have been directly successful. In this regard, the authors in Cheng et al. improved the precision and the quality of diagnosis while streamlining the treatment process by solving the laboratory high-speed handover and examination problem in medical institutions. The work provides insights into 6G in the light of both laboratory and hospital requirements to build a smart, interconnected hospital ecosystem capable of smartly handling patient needs with diverse and rapid requests. The authors in Lenihan et al. dealt with the critical open issues experienced by healthcare institutes when looking after patients who benefit from IoT devices at home. The paper proposes VR can boost the reality aspect of the Health Smart Home devices in order to conduct a successful treatment of each patient. With the aim of decreasing the complexity of 5G in hospitals, Li et al. used channels of capacitive biosensors deployed onto the walls of hospital rooms and some state-of-the-art signal processing techniques to monitor the human presence forced by SH IoT devices. Nassar et al. had presented a future scenario with an implementation of IoT and LoRa wireless for SHs by offering a solution with a thermal camera for fever detection software that supports the multiple patient-centric capabilities currently demanded for hospital care. Santamaria et al. provided data-driven insights into building a COVID-19 recovery model for hospitals in a post-pandemic setting utilizing t-TSDFs (Treatment, Storage, and Disposal Facility). Their work is able to smartly plan hospital resources, especially bed occupation, to anticipate response and respond effectively to the cascade of follow-up health demands in the future.

It is already clear that technological advances in communication networks are capable of providing digital healthcare with huge benefits. Among the often-claimed advantages are network slicing, which increases the flexibility that can be built into network designs, the reduced latencies that can be achieved, and the ability to extend network reach. Notwithstanding well-chronicled and widely discussed challenges, network modernization can help with a number of these issues, providing connectivity and lower operational costs. Moreover, it is likely that healthcare will be a main driver of the deployment of 6G networks and associated technologies.

FUTURE TRENDS AND IMPLICATIONS

Life in SHs is still far from realization, and multiple challenges need to be properly addressed. First, the networking challenges are given, including energy efficiency, security, latency, and bandwidth. Energy efficiency is particularly challenging, as medical equipment typically consumes a non-negligible amount of energy. Therefore, large-scale wireless networking typically requires tremendous microcontrollers, sensors, and actuators during data sensing, processing, and feedback forwarding. The utmost security is mandatory (Singh & Joshi, 2024) for SHs. Note that intelligent healthcare devices are riddled with vulnerabilities, and the highly private and sensitive nature of medical data is continuously attracting criminal behaviors. Thus, flexible, secure, and trustworthy systems have to be designed and implemented. Third, models for analyzing large-scale Internet of

Medical Things (IoMT) and creating intelligence will be developed. Interoperability has to be satisfied, providing a means for different IoMT devices to connect to the network, and time efficiency has to be achieved, lessening the delay of processing information and creating intelligence-based healthcare models. With the maturity of the previously mentioned 6G characteristics in 2030, novel technologies that revolutionize patient-centric care in hospitals are given as follows. First, software will keep improving, with further cloudification, a large-scale interconnection and interplay between edge computing and edge AI, and even an increase in the potential operation of distributed future generation intelligent cells, massively becoming sustainable for managing a large-scale near real-time life-critical mission. Second, the deployment position of decentralized wireless networks is no longer just "axisymmetric". With the aid of high-frequency bands, wireless backscatter, and useful distributed intelligent cells, both the smaller homecare IoT network and the micro-scale intelligent cell network in the hospital are even more controllable, beneficial, and reliable. Third, such a visually intense 6G network would possess aggressive QoS (Quality of Service)guarantees for all patients in the hospital, being able to embrace a reliable, hyperconnected, and "no way out, anytime fast". In fact, the U versus k curve of the network could statistically achieve great progress, attracted by exabytes of data every minute flowing back and forth from countless patient-tailored intelligent devices and from "super manic" Immersive Via Drones (IVDs).

EMERGING TECHNOLOGIES

Several emerging technologies are being leveraged in SHs to cater to the ever-rising demand for patient-centric care. The next generation wireless networks – 6G, and other IoMT technologies such as blockchain, 5G, and edge/fog computing – enhance patient care by providing the required low-latency, high-throughput, efficient data storage, and secure and fast data access, among many other benefits. Contrary to existing works that focus extensively on harnessing the benefits of emerging technologies to improve the operations of SHs, no paper has systematically identified the potential of these methodologies to transform the SH industry, particularly in the next-generation 6G-enabled patient-centered care strategy. The development of 6G networks in general, and the 6G SH in particular, poses several challenges, including the design of the underlying marshaling information technologies. Although the industry is experiencing revolutionary breakthroughs in the development of advanced wireless technologies, the challenges are surmountable by leveraging emerging technologies such as micro/nano transmission and receiver devices, AI Integration, Software Lending Communication, Global Shrinkage, Full Duplication, Computing Phalanx, Terahertz, Enhanced Maternity, Quantum, Blockchain, and others. Such technologies have already been examined for performance improvement in the healthcare industry, focusing on physical conditions including cancer cells or skin infections.

POLICY AND REGULATORY FRAMEWORKS

The intersection of policy and regulation with spectrum – another key factor enabled through advanced use of AI in healthcare services, is compliance with policy and

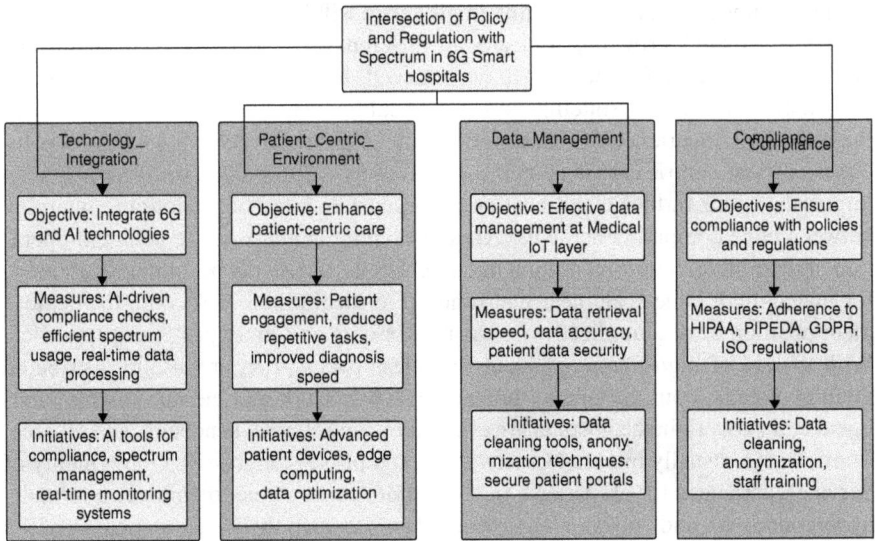

FIGURE 18.3   The intersection of policy and regulation with spectrum in the context of 6G integration in smart hospitals.

regulation by the hospital staff member. In an institutional environment such as a SH, especially one that relies heavily on data collection at the IoMT or Medical IoT layer, demands heightened data cleaning and anonymization to satisfy the regulatory bodies like HIPAA (Health Insurance Portability and Accountability Act), PIPEDA (Personal Information Protection and Electronic Documents Act), the General Data Protection Regulation, and/or ISO (International Organization for Standardization) regulations. Canadian Health Infoway reported that the retrieval of patient-initiated personal health information was primarily accomplished through the snap of technology enhancement of patient portals of patient engagement tools that some Canadian SH clients have already installed.

With 6G, it may be possible to extend the stored data on patients to be retrieved through advanced patient devices, which may aid with speedier and accurate diagnosis of a patient and may eliminate repetitive questions from hospital staff or painful blood typing and sampling tests for a patient. With the right regulatory frameworks in place, these 6G use case opportunities may be considered viable. They will require the use of edge computing and data optimization to work in a hospital environment. In the process, staff may inspect a nearby screen or tablet and identify a patient immediately, creating a more patient-centric environment in a SH as depicted in Figure 18.3.

CONCLUSION AND RECOMMENDATIONS

In conclusion, the increased pace of technological advances has allowed new opportunities for innovative ways in which patient-centric care is provided to patients in the modern hospital setting. SHs have benefited greatly from these systems, which have harnessed data about patient needs and used decision support to streamline and improve patient-centric care. 5G technology is at the forefront of driving advancements in the provision of these data, applications, and medical wearable devices. SHs have, for the most part, tended to use patient electronic health records or medical imaging IoT devices in providing the technology needed to drive patient-centric care. However, given that health services will be among the 6G non-technical enabling conservation, by harnessing 6G's photoacoustic sensing technology to drive "video speed imaging data transmission", SHs could further revolutionize their patient needs, providing normal or at-risk patient outcomes that will be vital in preventing disease or state and administering personalized medicine. Based on the findings of this paper, the following recommendations can be made. For healthcare professionals, with the anticipated advent of 6G technology, a future outlook should consider adapting to changing and evolving patient-centric care models that are driven by big patient data, medical wearable devices, and AI decision-making tools. The paper presents a forward-looking vision to inspire future initiatives and research applied in the emerging field. With their role in patient care and the increasing penetration of technology in healthcare, health systems and hospitals should become the seeds for new care models powered by digital health and driven by large medical data sources and applications. The increased focus of nursing professionals by the scientific community on care models enabled by digital health is an important area of development expected to enhance the potential value-based healthcare drivers for patient care.

REFERENCES

Ahad, A., Jiangbina, Z., Tahir, M., Shayea, I., & Mohammed, S. (2024). 6G and intelligent healthcare: Taxonomy, technologies, open issues and future research directions. *Internet of Things*, *25*, 101068. https://doi.org/10.1016/j.iot.2024.101068

Ahmad, H., Rafique, W., Rasool, R., Alhumam, A., Anwar, Z., & Qadir, J. (2023). Leveraging 6G, extended reality, and IoT big data analytics for healthcare: A review. *Computer Science Review*, *48*, 100558. https://doi.org/10.1016/j.cosrev.2023.100558

Deep, P. S. (2023). 5G+ smart healthcare. In S. Mumtaz, M. A. Jan, & J. Rodriguez (Eds.), *AI-enabled green communication for 5GtoB and 6G verticals* (pp. 199–214). Springer. https://doi.org/10.1007/978-981-99-4024-0_10

Della Vecchia, G., Gallo, L., Esposito, M., & Coronato, A. (2012). An infrastructure for smart hospitals. *Multimedia Tools and Applications*, *59*(1), 341–362. https://doi.org/10.1007/s11042-010-0695-8

Estrela, V. V., Deshpande, A., Stutz, D., de Assis, J. T., Laghari, A. A., Shi, F., & Lin, Y. D. (2023). 6G in healthcare – Anticipating needs and requirements. In A. L. Martins, J. M. R. S. Tavares, & R. N. Silva (Eds.), *Intelligent healthcare systems* (pp. 159–181). Taylor & Francis. https://doi.org/10.1201/9781003196822-9

Hassan, M. K., El Desouky, A. I., Elghamrawy, S. M., & Sarhan, A. M. (2019). Big data challenges and opportunities in healthcare informatics and smart hospitals. In A. E. Hassanien, K. Shaalan, & T. Gaber (Eds.), *The rise of big spatial data* (Lecture Notes in Intelligent Transportation and Infrastructure, Part F1404, pp. 3–26). Springer. https://doi.org/10.1007/978-3-030-01560-2_1

Holzinger, A., Röcker, C., & Ziefle, M. (2015). From smart health to smart hospitals. In A. Holzinger, C. Röcker, & M. Ziefle (Eds.), *Smart health: Open problems and future challenges* (pp. 1–20). Springer. https://doi.org/10.1007/978-3-319-16226-3_1

Israni, D. K., Chawla, N. S., & Israni, D. K. (2023). Human–machine interaction in leveraging the concept of telemedicine. In D. K. Israni (Ed.), *Human machine interface: Making healthcare digital* (pp. 211–245). Wiley. https://doi.org/10.1002/9781394200344.ch8

Joshi, A., & Tiwari, H. (2023). An Overview of Python Libraries for Data Science, *Journal of Engineering Technology and Applied Physics*, 5(2), 85–90. https://doi.org/10.33093/jetap.2023.5.2.10

Kaiser, M. S., Zenia, N., Tabassum, F., Mamun, S. A., Rahman, M. A., Islam, M. S., & Mahmud, M. (2021). 6G access network for intelligent Internet of Healthcare Things: Opportunity, challenges, and research directions. In K. Murugesan, M. Krishnamurthi, & A. Balasubramanian (Eds.), *Advances in intelligent systems and computing* (Vol. 1309, pp. 317–328). Springer. https://doi.org/10.1007/978-981-33-4673-4_25

Kanase, P., & Gopal, S. (2016). Smart hospitals using Internet of Things (IoT). *International Research Journal of Engineering and Technology (IRJET)*, 3(3), 2170–2174. https://www.academia.edu/download/54662780/IRJET-V3I3363.pdf

Khattak, S. B. A., Nasralla, M. M., & Rehman, I. U. (2022). The role of 6G networks in enabling future smart health services and applications. In *2022 IEEE International Smart Cities Conference (ISC2)* (pp. 1–7). IEEE. https://doi.org/10.1109/ISC255366.2022.9922093

Kumar, R., Joshi, A., Sharan, H. O., Peng, S., & Dudhagara, C. R. (Eds.). (2024). *The ethical frontier of AI and data analysis*. IGI Global Scientific Publishing. https://doi.org/10.4018/979-8-3693-2964-1

Mishra, G. (2024). A comprehensive review of smart healthcare systems: Architecture, applications, challenges, and future directions. *International Journal of Innovative Research in Technology & Science (IJIRTS)*, 12(210), 1–15. https://ijirts.org/index.php/ijirts/article/view/32

Moro Visconti, R., & Martiniello, L. (2019). Smart hospitals and patient-centered governance. *Corporate Ownership & Control*, 16(2). https://ssrn.com/abstract=3357473

Nasralla, M. M., Khattak, S. B. A., & Rehman, I. U. (2023). Exploring the role of 6G technology in enhancing quality of experience for m-health multimedia applications: A comprehensive survey. *Sensors*, 23(13), 5882. https://doi.org/10.3390/s23135882

Santhosh, M. P. (2019). *Smart hospitals: Challenges and opportunities* [Working paper]. Indian Institute of Management Kozhikode. https://iimk.ac.in/uploads/publications/3052smartHospitals_MPS2019.pdf

Singh, B. P., & Joshi, A. (2024). Ethical considerations in AI development. In R. Kumar, A. Joshi, H. Sharan, S. Peng, & C. Dudhagara (Eds.), *The ethical frontier of AI and data analysis* (pp. 156–179). IGI Global Scientific Publishing. https://doi.org/10.4018/979-8-3693-2964-1.ch010

Srinivasu, P. N., Ijaz, M. F., Shafi, J., Woźniak, M., & Sujatha, R. (2022). 6G driven fast computational networking framework for healthcare applications. *IEEE Access*, 10, 94235–94248. https://doi.org/10.1109/ACCESS.2022.3203061

Sun, P. (2023). 5G+ smart healthcare. In S. Mumtaz, M. A. Jan, & J. Rodriguez (Eds.), *Management for professionals* (Lecture Notes in Networks and Systems, Part F1199, pp. 217–246). Springer. https://doi.org/10.1007/978-981-99-4024-0_10

Zhang, H., Li, J., Wen, B., Xun, Y., & Liu, J. (2018). Connecting intelligent things in smart hospitals using NB-IoT. *IEEE Internet of Things Journal*, 5(3), 1550–1560. https://doi.org/10.1109/JIOT.2018.2792423

Index

Pages in *italics* refer to figures and pages in **bold** refer to tables.

For Product Safety Concerns and Information please contact our EU
representative GPSR@taylorandfrancis.com
Taylor & Francis Verlag GmbH, Kaufingerstraße 24, 80331 München, Germany

www.ingramcontent.com/pod-product-compliance
Lightning Source LLC
Chambersburg PA
CBHW060812220326
41598CB00022B/2601